Basic Clinical
Neuroanatomy

Basic Clinical Neuroanatomy

PAUL A. YOUNG, PH.D.

Professor & Chairman
Department of Anatomy & Neurobiology
St. Louis University School of Medicine
St. Louis, Missouri

PAUL H. YOUNG, M.D.

Associate Clinical Professor
Departments of Surgery (Neurosurgery) and
Anatomy & Neurobiology
St. Louis University School of Medicine
St. Louis, Missouri

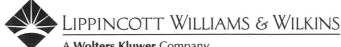

LIPPINCOTT WILLIAMS & WILKINS
A **Wolters Kluwer** Company

Philadelphia · Baltimore · New York · London
Buenos Aires · Hong Kong · Sydney · Tokyo

Editor: Jane Velker
Managing Editor: Crystal Taylor
Development Editor: Kathleen Scogna
Production Coordinator: Marette Magargle-Smith
Illustration Planner: Wayne Hubbel
Typesetter: Peirce Graphic Services, Inc.
Printer & Binder: Vicks Lithograph & Printing Corporation

351 West Camden Street
Baltimore, Maryland 21201-2436 USA

530 Walnut Street
Philadelphia, Pennsylvania 19106-3621 USA

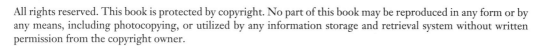

Accurate indications, adverse reactions and dosage schedules for drugs are provided in this book, but it is possible that they may change. The reader is urged to review the package information data of the manufacturers of the medications mentioned.

Printed in the United States of America

First Edition,

Library of Congress Cataloging-in-Publication Data

Young, Paul A., 1926–
    Basic clinical neuroanatomy / Paul A. Young, Paul H. Young. — 1st ed.
      p.   cm.
    Includes bibliographical references and index.
    ISBN 0-683-09351-7
    1. Neuroanatomy.   I. Young, Paul H. (Paul Henry), 1950– . II. Title.
    [DNLM: 1. Neuroanatomy. 2. Nervous System—anatomy & histology.
  WL 101 Y75b 1997]
  QM451.Y68   1997
  611.8—dc20
  DNLM/DLC
  for Library of Congress   96-17643
                                      CIP

The publishers have made every effort to trace the copyright holders for borrowed material. If they have inadvertently over-looked any, they will be pleased to make the necessary arrangements at the first opportunity.

To purchase additional copies of this book, call our customer service department at **(800) 638-3030** or fax orders to **(301) 824-7390.** For other book services, including chapter reprints and large quantity sales, ask for the Special Sales Department. International customers should call **(301) 714-2324.**

Visit Lippincott Williams & Wilkins on the Internet: **http://www.lww.com.** Lippincott Williams & Wilkins customer service representatives are available from 8:30 am to 6:00 pm, EST.

01
5 6 7 8 9 10

TO CATHERINE ANN, dear wife of Paul A. Young and mother of Paul H., Bob, Dave, Ann, Carol, Rick, Jim, Steve, Kevin, and Michael.

Preface

The main objective of this monograph is to provide the anatomical basis for neurologic abnormalities. Knowledge of basic clinical neuroanatomy will enable medical students to answer the first question asked when examining a patient with an injured or diseased nervous system: "Where is the lesion located?" Knowledge of basic clinical neuroanatomy will enable students in health-related fields such as nursing, physical therapy, occupational therapy, physician assistants, to understand the anatomical basis of the neurologic abnormalities in their patients. To accomplish these objectives, the anatomical relationships and functions of the clinically important structures are emphasized. Effort is exerted to simplify as much as possible the anatomical features of the brain and spinal cord.

This monograph is neither a reference book nor a textbook of neuroanatomy. Most neuroanatomy textbooks include much information about anatomical structures that aids in the understanding of a particular system or mechanism, but when these structures are damaged clinical signs or symptoms do not result. Such superfluous information is kept to a minimum in this book.

This basic clinical anatomy book is presented in three main sections: (1) the basic plan, (2) the functional systems, and (3) the associated structures. The basic plan includes the organization of the nervous system, its histologic features and supporting structures, distinguishing anatomical characteristics of the subdivisions of the brain and spinal cord, and an introduction to clinically important brain and spinal cord functional levels. Only those structures needed to identify the subdivisions and their levels are included in this part.

The second section deals with the functional systems and their clinically relevant features. This section is arranged so that the motor and somatosensory systems, of paramount importance because they include structures located in every subdivision of the brain and spinal cord, are described first. The remainder of this section includes the pathways associated with the special senses, higher mental functions, and the behavioral and visceral systems.

In the third section, the vascular supply and the ventricular cerebrospinal fluid system are presented.

The visualization of three-dimensional anatomical relationships plays a key role in localizing lesions and understanding the anatomical basis of neurologic disorders. Every effort has been made to include illustrations that enhance this visualization of three-dimensional images of the clinically important structures. In addition to the three-dimensional illustrations, schematic diagrams of the functional systems and drawings of myelin-stained sections from selected functional levels of the brain and spinal cord are used to provide the anatomical reltionships that enhance the understanding of the anatomical basis for neurologic disorders and their syndromes. Clinical relevance is emphasized throughout this book and illustrations of some neurologic abnormalities are included.

Review questions are found at the end of each chapter and an entire chapter is devoted to the principles of locating lesions and clinical illustrations. Answers to the chapter questions are found in the appendixes. Also in the appendixes are a section devoted to cranial nerve components and their clinical correlations, a glossary of terms, a list of suggested readings, and an atlas of the myelin-stained sections used throughout the book.

The authors are most grateful to Mr. Larry Clifford for his artistic skills in creating the illustrations, all of which are an invaluable part of this book. Our deep appreciation is expressed to Ms. Susan Quinn for her superb assistance in preparing the manuscript and to Ms. Susan McClain for her computer expertise in preparing the charts and tables. Finally, the authors are much indebted to the publisher, Williams & Wilkins, and its editorial and marketing staff for their interest, support, and patience throughout the project.

Contents

1 INTRODUCTION TO THE NERVOUS SYSTEM: ORGANIZATION, FUNCTIONAL UNITS, AND SUPPORTING STRUCTURES 1

2 SPINAL CORD TOPOGRAPHY AND FUNCTIONAL LEVELS 13

3 BRAINSTEM ANATOMY, TOPOGRAPHY, AND FUNCTIONAL LEVELS . . . 23

4 FOREBRAIN TOPOGRAPHY AND FUNCTIONAL LEVELS 35

5 LOWER MOTOR NEURONS: FLACCID PARALYSIS 45

6 THE PYRAMIDAL SYSTEM: SPASTIC PARALYSIS 61

7 BRAINSTEM MOTOR CENTERS: DECEREBRATE POSTURING AND POSTCAPSULAR LESION RECOVERY 73

8 THE BASAL GANGLIA: MOVEMENT DISORDERS 83

9 THE CEREBELLUM: ATAXIA 99

10 THE OCULAR MOTOR SYSTEM: VESTIBULO-OCULAR REFLEX AND CONJUGATE GAZE 117

11 THE SOMATOSENSORY SYSTEM: ANESTHESIA AND ANALGESIA 127

12 THE VISUAL SYSTEM: ANOPSIA 153

13 THE AUDITORY SYSTEM: DEAFNESS 167

14 THE GUSTATORY AND OLFACTORY SYSTEMS: AGEUSIA AND ANOSMIA 175

15 THE CEREBRAL CORTEX: APHASIA, AGNOSIA, AND APRAXIA 183

16 THE LIMBIC SYSTEM: ANTEROGRADE AMNESIA AND
INAPPROPRIATE BEHAVIOR 201

17 THE HYPOTHALAMUS: VEGETATIVE AND ENDOCRINE IMBALANCE . . . 209

18 THE AUTONOMIC SYSTEM: VISCERAL ABNORMALITIES 217

19 THE BLOOD SUPPLY OF THE CENTRAL NERVOUS SYSTEM:
STROKE 235

20 THE CEREBROSPINAL FLUID SYSTEM: HYDROCEPHALUS 251

21 PRINCIPLES FOR LOCATING LESIONS AND CLINICAL ILLUSTRATIONS 259

Appendixes

A CRANIAL NERVE COMPONENTS AND LESIONS 287

B ANSWERS TO CHAPTER QUESTIONS 298

C GLOSSARY 310

D SUGGESTED READINGS 323

E ATLAS OF MYELIN STAINED SECTIONS 324

Introduction to the Nervous System: Organization, Functional Units, and Supporting Structures

Two fundamental properties of animals, irritability and conductivity, reach their greatest development in the human nervous system. Irritability, the capability of responding to a stimulus, and conductivity, the capability of transporting signals, are specialized properties of the basic functional units of the nervous system: the nerve cells or neurons. Neurons respond to stimuli, transport signals, and process information that enable the awareness of self and surroundings; mental functions such as memory, learning, and speech; and the regulation of muscular contraction and glandular secretion.

Organization of the Nervous System

The basic functional unit of the nervous system is the neuron. Each neuron has a cell body that receives nerve impulses and an **axon** that transports the nerve impulse away from the cell body. The nervous system comprises neurons arranged in longitudinal series or spatial succession. The serial arrangement forms two types of circuits: reflex and relay. A reflex circuit transports the impulses that result in an involuntary response such as muscle contraction or gland secretion (Fig. 1–1A). A relay circuit transports impulses from one part of the nervous system to another. For example, relay circuits transport impulses from sensory organs in the skin, eyes, ears, etc. that become perceived by the brain as sensations (Fig.

1–1**B**). Relay circuits are categorized according to their functions and are called functional paths, e.g., pain path, visual path, or motor or voluntary movement path. A functional path may consist of a series of only two or three neurons, or as many as hundreds of neurons. Reflex circuits may overlap with parts of relay circuits (Fig. 1–1**C**).

A functional path may contain thousands or even millions of nerve cell bodies and axons. The nerve cell bodies may form pools or clumps, in which cases they are called nuclei or ganglia, or the nerve cell bodies may be arranged in the form of layers or laminae. The axons in a functional path usually form bundles called tracts, fasciculi, or nerves. Therefore, the entire nervous system is composed of functional paths whose neuronal cell bodies are located in nuclei, ganglia, or laminae and whose axons are located in tracts or nerves.

The human nervous system is divided into central and peripheral parts. The brain and spinal cord form the central nervous system (CNS), and the cranial, spinal, and autonomic nerves and their ganglia form the peripheral nervous system (PNS). The CNS integrates and controls the entire nervous system, receiving information (input) about changes in the internal and external environments, interpreting and integrating this information, and providing signals (output) for the execution of activities, such as movement or secretion. The PNS connects the CNS to the tissues and organs of the body. Hence, the PNS is responsible for conveying input and output signals to and from the

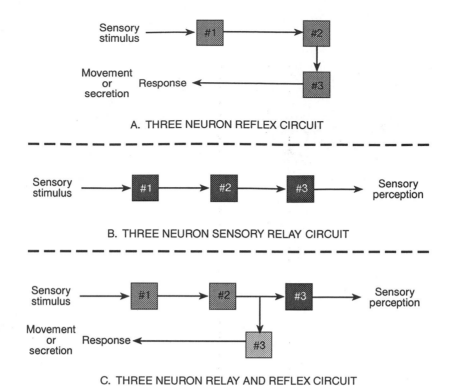

FIGURE 1–1. Simple reflex and relay circuits. **A.** Three neuron reflex circuit. **B.** Three neuron sensory relay circuit. **C.** Combined three neuron relay and reflex circuits.

CNS. Signals passing to the CNS are called **afferent,** whereas those passing away from the CNS are called **efferent.**

NEURONS

A neuron consists of a cell body or soma and of protoplasmic processes called **dendrites** and **axons** (Fig. 1–2).

The cell body is the metabolic center of a neuron and contains the nucleus and the cytoplasm. The nucleus contains nucleoplasm, chromatin, a prominent nucleolus, and in the female only, a nucleolar satellite. The cytoplasm contains the usual cellular organelles such as mitochondria, Golgi apparatus, and lysosomes. In addition, various-sized clumps of rough endoplasmic reticulum, called **Nissl bodies,** are prominent in the cytoplasm of neurons. However, the neuronal cytoplasm where the axon emerges is devoid of Nissl bodies; this area is called the axon hillock. Another cytoplasmic characteristic of neurons are neurofibrils, which are arranged longitudi-

nally in the cell body and the axons and dendrites.

Neurons are classified morphologically as unipolar, bipolar, or multipolar according to their number of protoplasmic processes (Fig. 1–3). The single process of a unipolar neuron is the axon. Unipolar neurons are located almost exclusively in the ganglia of spinal nerves and some cranial nerves. Bipolar neurons have an axon and one dendrite and are limited to the visual, auditory, and vestibular pathways. All the remaining nerve cells are multipolar neurons and have an axon and between 2 and 12 or more dendrites.

DENDRITES AND AXONS

Dendrites, cytologically similar to the neuronal cell body, are short and transport impulses toward the cell body (Table 1–1). Axons do not contain Nissl bodies, vary in length from microns to meters, and transport impulses away from the cell body.

The integrity of the axon, regardless of its

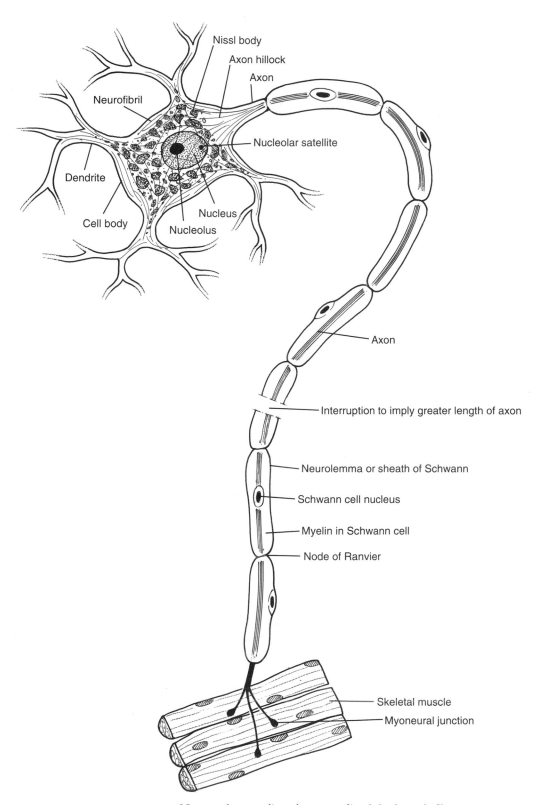

FIGURE 1-2. Neuron whose myelinated axon supplies skeletal muscle fibers.

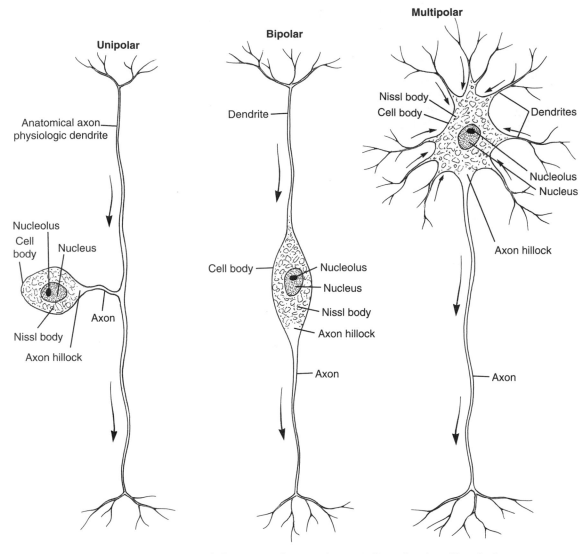

FIGURE 1-3.   Morphologic types of neurons (arrows indicate direction of impulses).

TABLE 1-1.   COMPARISON OF AXONS AND DENDRITES

	AXONS	DENDRITES
Function	Transport impulses from the cell body	Receive impulses and transports them toward the cell body
Length	Vary from microns to meters	Microns; seldom more than a millimeter
Branching Pattern	Limited to collaterals, preterminals, and terminals	Vary from simple to complex arborizations
Surface	Smooth	Vary from smooth to spiny
Coverings	Supporting cells and frequently myelin	Always naked

length, is maintained by the cell body via two types of axoplasmic flow or axonal transport. In **anterograde axonal transport,** the cell body nutrients are carried in a forward direction from the cell body to the distal end or termination of the axon. Anterograde axonal transport is vital for axonal growth during development, for maintenance of axonal structure, and for the synthesis and release of **neurotransmitters,** the chemicals that assist in the transfer of nerve impulses from one cell to another.

Besides anterograde transport, **retrograde axonal transport** occurs from the distal end of the axon back to the cell body. The function of retrograde axonal transport is the return of used or worn out materials to the cell body for restoration.

> Retrograde axonal transport is of clinical importance because it is the route by which toxins such as tetanus, and viruses such as herpes simplex, rabies, and polio are transported into the CNS from the periphery.

Axons may be myelinated or unmyelinated. Myelinated axons are insulated by a sheath of myelin that starts near the cell body and stops just before the axon terminates (Fig. 1–2). Myelin is a multilayered phospholipid located within axonal supporting cells. The myelin sheath increases the conduction velocity of the nerve impulse along the axon. The thicker the myelin sheath, the faster the conduction velocity.

SYNAPSES

Axonal endings or terminals occur in relation to other neurons, to muscle cells, or to gland cells. The junction between the axonal ending and the neuron, muscle cell, or gland cell is called the **synapse.** An important anatomical characteristic of the synapse is that the axonal ending is separated from the surface of the other nerve cell, muscle cell, or gland cell by a space, the synaptic cleft. An important physiologic characteristic of a synapse is polarization; that is, the impulse always travels from the axon to the next neuron in the circuit or to the muscle or gland cells supplied by the axon.

When a nerve impulse arrives at the synapse, chemicals called neurotransmitters are released into the synaptic cleft. Neurotransmitters, manufactured and released by the neurons, cross the synaptic cleft to affect the postsynaptic nerve, muscle, or gland cell. The transmitters at neuromuscular and neuroglandular synapses are excitatory; that is, they elicit muscle contraction or glandular secretion. However, the neurotransmitters at synapses between neurons may be excitatory, enhancing the production of an impulse in the postsynaptic neuron, or inhibitory, hindering impulse production in the postsynaptic neuron. All functions of the CNS, that is, awareness of sensations, control of movements or glandular secretions, and higher mental functions, occur as the result of the activity of excitatory and inhibitory synapses on neurons in various circuits.

DEGENERATION AND REGENERATION

All cells in the human body are able to reproduce, except nerve cells. As a result, the loss of neurons is irreparable; a neuron once destroyed can never be replaced. Conversely, axons can regenerate and regain their functions even after being completely transected or cut, as long as the cell body remains viable. This capacity to regenerate is limited, however, to axons in the PNS. Functional axonal regeneration has not occurred in the human CNS. Thus, the degeneration of neuronal cell bodies anywhere in the nervous system and the degeneration of CNS axons are irreparable.

NERVOUS SYSTEM SUPPORT AND PROTECTION

Nerve cells are extremely fragile and cannot survive without the protection of supporting cells. The brain and spinal cord, also very fragile, are protected from the surrounding bones of the cranial cavity and vertebral or spinal canal by three coverings or membranes, called the meninges.

SUPPORTING CELLS

Three basic types of supporting or glial cells exist: ependymal, microglial, and macroglial cells. The ependymal cells line the fluid-filled cavities or ventricles of the brain and the central canal of the spinal cord. The microglial cells are phagocytes that arise from macrophages and engulf the debris resulting from injury, infections, or diseases in the CNS. The macroglia consist of four cell types: **astrocytes** and **oligodendrocytes** in the CNS and **Schwann cells** and **capsular cells** in the PNS.

Astrocytes

Astrocytes are the most numerous cells in the CNS (Fig. 1–4). Each astrocyte has a star-shaped cell body and numerous irregularly shaped processes, some of which may be extremely long. Processes of some astrocytes have end-feet on the surface of the brain or spinal cord. These end-feet form a protective covering called the external limiting membrane or glial membrane. Many astrocytic processes have vascular endfeet, which surround capillaries. These processes form the **blood-brain barrier,** which selectively governs the passage of materials from the circulating blood into the CNS.

Astrocytes have other functions as well. They play a major role in the electrolyte balance of the CNS, produce neurotrophic factors necessary for neuronal survival, and remove certain neuro-

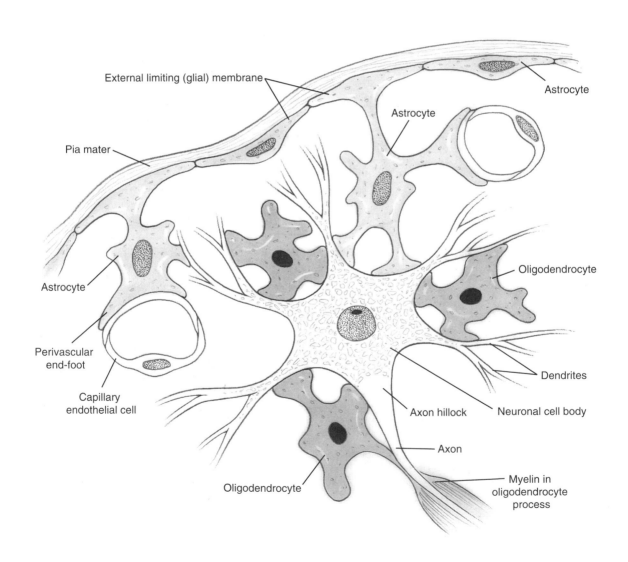

FIGURE 1–4.   Relation of neurons, glia, and capillaries.

transmitters from synaptic clefts. Astrocytes are the first cells to undergo alterations in response to CNS insults such as ischemia, trauma, or radiation. Also, astrocytes form scars resulting from CNS injury. Astrocytes are highly susceptible to the formation of neoplasms.

Oligodendrocytes

The formation and maintenance of CNS myelin are the primary functions of the oligodendrocytes, small glial cells with relatively few processes (Fig. 1–4). The myelin sheath is formed by oligodendrocyte processes, which wrap around the axon to form a tight spiral. The myelin itself is located within the processes. Each oligodendrocyte envelopes a variable number of axons depending on the thickness of the myelin sheaths. In the case of thin myelin sheaths, 1 oligodendrocyte may be related to 40 or 50 axons. Oligodendrocytes may also surround the cell bodies of neurons, but in this location they do not contain myelin. Recent research suggests that oligodendrocytes also produce neurotrophic factors, the most important of which is a nerve growth factor that may promote the growth of damaged CNS axons.

Schwann Cells

The PNS counterpart of the oligodendrocyte is the Schwann cell. Unlike the oligoden-

drocyte, which envelopes many myelinated axons, the Schwann cell envelopes only part of one myelinated axon. During development of the myelin sheath, the Schwann cell first encircles and then spirals around the axon many times, forming multiple layers or lamellae. The myelin is actually located within the Schwann cell lamellae (Fig. 1–5). The outermost layer of the Schwann cell lamellae is called the **neurolemma** or **sheath of Schwann.** Because each Schwann cell myelinates only a small extent of the axon, myelination of the entire axon requires a long string of Schwann cells. Between each Schwann cell, the myelin is interrupted. These areas of myelin sheath interruption are called **nodes of Ranvier** (Figs. 1–2, 1–5). Similar interruptions of myelin sheaths occur in the CNS. In unmyelinated fibers, one Schwann cell envelopes many axons.

Schwann cells not only form and maintain the myelin sheath but also are extremely important in the regeneration of damaged axons. When an axon is cut, the part of the axon separated from the cell body degenerates; however, the string of Schwann cells distal to the injury proliferates and forms a tube. Growth sprouts arising from the proximal end of the transected axon enter this tube and travel to the structures supplied by the axon before its injury. Such functional axonal regeneration is common in the PNS. Axonal regeneration has not occurred

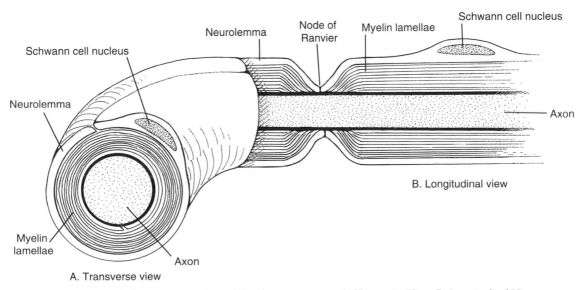

F I G U R E   1 – 5 .   Myelinated axon in the peripheral nervous system. **A.** Transverse View. **B.** Longitudinal View.

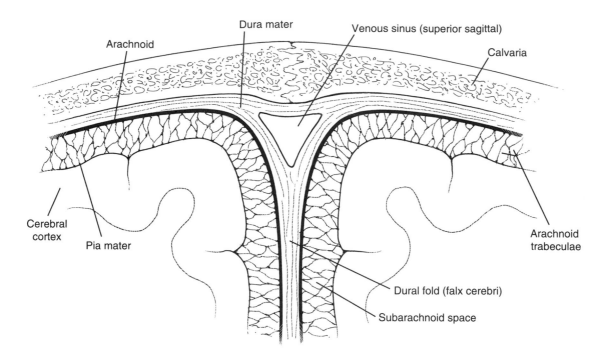

FIGURE 1-6. Coronal section of cranial meninges showing a venous sinus and dural fold.

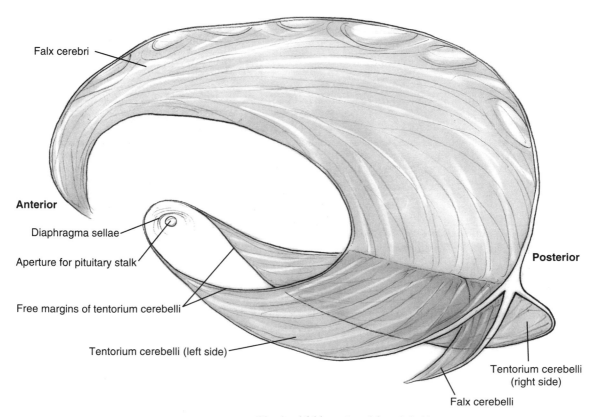

FIGURE 1-7. The dural folds as viewed from left side.

in the human CNS, and this lack of regeneration may be due, in part, to the absence of Schwann cells.

Capsular Cells

Capsular cells are the glial elements that surround the neuronal cell bodies in sensory and autonomic ganglia. The sensory ganglia of the spinal nerves and some cranial nerves contain large, round, unipolar neurons (Fig. 1–3). Each neuronal cell body is surrounded by a nearly complete layer of flattened capsular or satellite cells, thereby separating the ganglion cell from the non-neural connective tissue and vascular structures. The autonomic ganglion cells are multipolar neurons (Fig. 1–3). Although capsular cells are present, because of the irregular shape of the multipolar neurons, the capsules are less uniform and incomplete in autonomic ganglia.

SUPPORTING MEMBRANES

The CNS is supported and protected by the meninges, three connective tissue membranes located between the brain and the cranial bones and between the spinal cord and the vertebral column. The meninges are, from external to internal, the **dura mater,** the **arachnoid,** and the **pia mater.** The meninges around the brain and spinal cord are continuous at the foramen magnum, the large opening in the base of the skull where the brain and spinal cord are continuous.

Dura Mater

The dura mater is a strong, fibrous membrane that consists of two layers. In the cranial dura, which surrounds the brain, the two layers are fused and adhere to the inner surfaces of the cranial bones except in those regions where the layers split (Fig. 1–6) to form the venous sinuses that carry blood from the brain to the veins in the neck. The inner layer of the dura forms four folds that extend internally to partially partition various parts of the brain (Fig. 1–7). The sickle-shaped **falx cerebri** lies in the longitudinal groove between the upper parts of the brain, the cerebral hemispheres. The **falx cerebelli,** also oriented longitudinally, separates the upper parts of the hemispheres of the cerebellum,

or "little brain." The tentorium cerebelli is a flat dural fold that separates the posterior parts of the cerebral hemispheres above from the cerebellum below. The **diaphragma sellae** is a circular, horizontal fold beneath the brain that covers the sella turcica, in which the pituitary gland is located. The stalk of the pituitary gland pierces the diaphragma sellae and attaches to the undersurface of the brain.

The spinal dura consists of two layers: The outer layer forms the periosteal lining of the vertebral foramina that form the vertebral or spinal canal; the inner layer loosely invests the spinal cord and forms a cuff around the spinal nerves as they emerge from the vertebral canal.

Arachnoid

The arachnoid is a thin, delicate membrane that loosely surrounds the brain and spinal cord. The outer part of the arachnoid adheres to the dura (Fig. 1–8). Extending internally from this outer part are numerous cobweb-like projections or trabeculae that attach to the pia mater.

Pia Mater

The pia mater is the thin membrane that closely invests the brain and spinal cord. The pia is highly vascular and contains the small blood vessels that supply the brain and spinal cord.

Meningeal Spaces

Several clinically important spaces are associated with the meninges (Fig. 1–8). The **epidural space** is located between the bone and the dura mater, and the **subdural space** is located between the dura and arachnoid. Normally, both the epidural and subdural spaces are potential spaces in the cranial cavity. Both may become actual spaces if blood accumulates because of epidural or subdural hemorrhages caused by traumatic tearing of blood vessels that pass through the spaces. In the spinal cord, the subdural space is also potential, but the epidural space is actual and contains semifluid fat and thin-walled veins.

The **subarachnoid space** is located in the area between the arachnoid and pia mater and contains **cerebrospinal fluid.** The subarach-

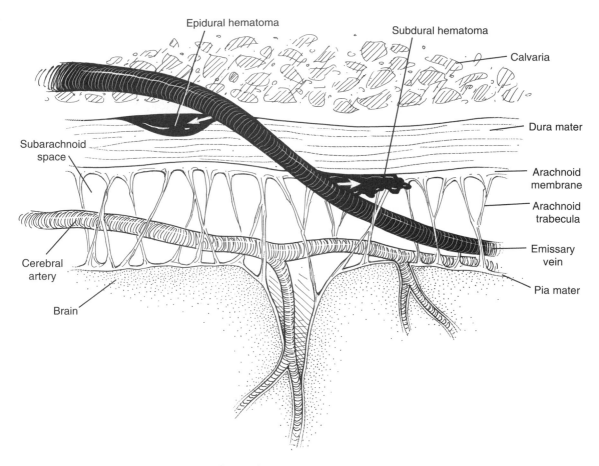

FIGURE 1-8.   Relation of meningeal spaces to blood vessels and hemorrhages.

noid space communicates with the cavities or ventricles of the brain where cerebrospinal fluid is formed. Also located within the subarachnoid space are the initial parts of the cranial and spinal nerves and numerous blood vessels on the surfaces of the brain and spinal cord. Vascular accidents involving the vessels here result in subarachnoid hemorrhage.

CHAPTER REVIEW QUESTIONS

1–1. What are the two main classes of cells in the CNS?

1–2. What is a synapse and what are the chief characteristics of synapses in the CNS?

1–3. What is the significance of axoplasmic transport?

1–4. Does functional regeneration occur in the nervous system?

1–5. What are the chief differences between astrocytes and oligodendrocytes?

1–6. Between which cranial structures are the following located:

    a. Subdural hematoma
    b. Cerebrospinal fluid
    c. Epidural hematoma

SPINAL CORD TOPOGRAPHY
AND FUNCTIONAL LEVELS

■ **A 19-year-old driver of an automobile is involved in an accident and suffers a severe flexion injury to his neck with subluxation (slippage) of the fifth and sixth cervical vertebrae and acute compression of the spinal cord at this level. The patient develops immediate paralysis and loss of all sensation below the C5 segment. In addition, the patient experiences loss of all skeletal muscle tone, reflex activity, and vasomotor function as well as paralysis of the bowel and bladder. This acute quadriplegia is complete and irreversible at the time of injury due to a physiologic transection of the spinal cord at the C5–C6 level.**

The spinal cord connects with the spinal nerves and is the structure through which the brain communicates with all parts of the body below the head. Impulses for the general sensations such as touch and pain that arise in the limbs, neck, and trunk must pass through the spinal cord to reach the brain where they are perceived. Likewise, commands for voluntary movements in the limbs, trunk, and neck originate in the brain and must pass through the spinal cord to reach the spinal nerves that innervate the appropriate muscles. Thus, damage of the spinal cord may result in the loss of general sensations and the paralysis of voluntary movements in parts of the body supplied by spinal nerves.

SPINAL CORD GROSS ANATOMY

The spinal cord is located within the vertebral canal, which is formed by the foramina of the 7 cervical (CV), 12 thoracic (TV), 5 lumbar (LV), and 5 sacral (SV) vertebrae that form the vertebral column, commonly called the spine. The spinal cord extends from the foramen magnum, the large opening in the base of the skull, to the intervertebral disc between the first and second lumbar vertebrae (Fig. 2–1). Superiorly, the spinal cord is continuous with the

> According to the U.S. Department of Health and Human Services, approximately 10,000 new spinal cord injuries occur in the United States each year, of which at least 50% result in permanent disabilities. Some 200,000 Americans must use wheelchairs because of spinal cord injuries. Most of these injuries result from trauma such as occurs in automobile or sports accidents. An estimated two thirds of the victims are 30 years of age or younger; the majority are men.

> The spinal cord is ordinarily protected by the strong bony ring formed by the vertebral column. However, high velocity objects (e.g., bullets) or high velocity impacts against immovable objects (e.g., trees, pavements, or automobile dashboards) can fracture vertebrae or dislocate them at the intervertebral articulations and compress or lacerate the spinal cord. The cervical vertebrae are the smallest and most fragile and, hence, most fractures occur here. Dislocations are most apt to occur at the points of greatest mobility, which are (in descending order of occurrence) the articulations between CV5–CV6, TV12–LV1, and CV1–CV2 (Fig. 2–1).

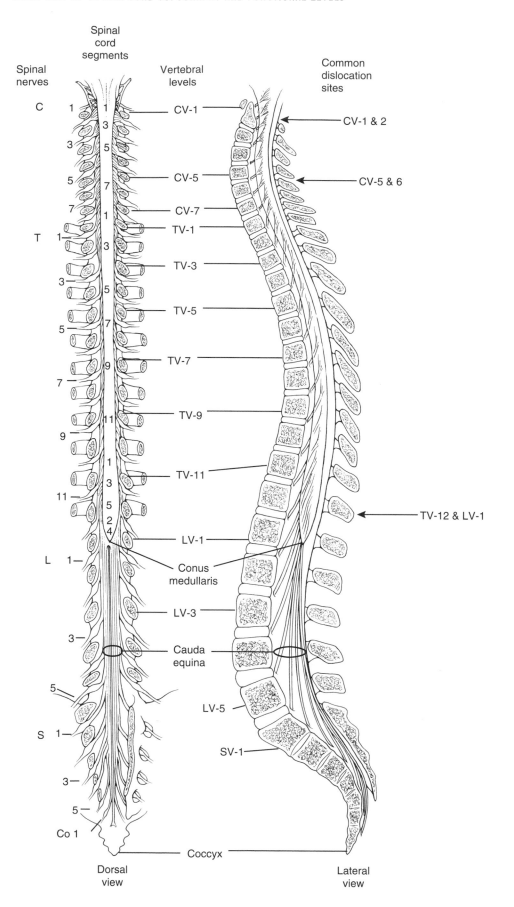

Spinal
cord
segments

Spinal
nerves

Vertebral
levels

Common
dislocation
sites

C 1 1

CV-1   CV-1 & 2

3

3

5

5   7   CV-5   CV-5 & 6

7   CV-7

T 1   1   TV-1

3

3   TV-3

5

5   TV-5

7

7   TV-7

9

9   TV-9

11

11   TV-11

1

3

5   TV-12 & LV-1

2
4   LV-1

L 1   Conus
medullaris

LV-3

3   Cauda
equina

5

LV-5

S 1   SV-1

3

5

Co 1

Coccyx

Dorsal
view

Lateral
view

brain, and, inferiorly, it ends by tapering abruptly into the conus medullaris (Fig. 2–1). In rare cases, its inferior end may be as high as the TV12 or as low as the LV3 vertebral level.

There are 31 spinal cord segments: 8 cervical (C), 12 thoracic (T), 5 lumbar (L), 5 sacral (S), and 1 coccygeal (Co)(Fig. 2–1). The segments are named and numbered according to the attachment of the spinal nerves. The spinal nerves are named and numbered according to their emergence from the vertebral canal. Spinal nerves C1–C7 emerge through the intervertebral foramina above their respective vertebrae. Because there are only seven cervical vertebrae, spinal nerve C8 emerges between CV7 and TV1. The remaining spinal nerves emerge below their respective vertebrae (Fig. 2–1).

Until the third month of fetal development, the position of each segment of the developing spinal cord corresponds to the position of each developing vertebra. After this time, the vertebral column elongates more rapidly than the spinal cord. At birth, the spinal cord ends at the disc between LV2 and LV3. Further growth of the vertebral column results in the inferior or

> The relation between spinal cord levels and vertebral levels is clinically important. The level of spinal cord lesions is always localized according to the spinal cord segment. Most spinal levels do not, however, correspond to vertebral levels. If neurosurgical procedures are to be performed, the spinal level must be correlated with the appropriate vertebral level.

caudal end of the spinal cord being located at the disc between LV1 and LV2 at adulthood. The approximate relation between spinal levels and vertebral levels is shown in Figure 2–1.

SPINAL MENINGES

The spinal cord is surrounded by three connective tissue membranes called the spinal meninges. From internal to external, the spinal meninges are called the pia mater, arachnoid, and dura mater (Fig. 2–2).

PIA MATER AND ARACHNOID

The pia mater completely surrounds and adheres to the spinal cord. The arachnoid loosely

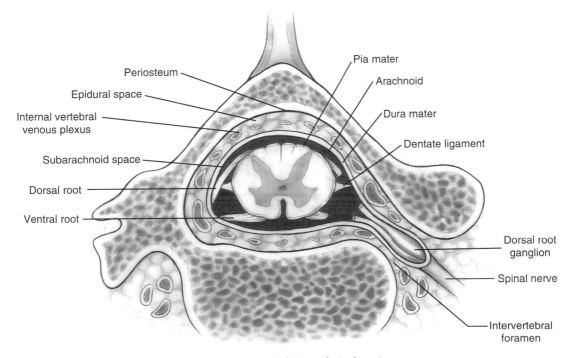

FIGURE 2–2. Relations of spinal meninges.

FIGURE 2–1. Relations of vertebral column, spinal cord, and spinal nerves.

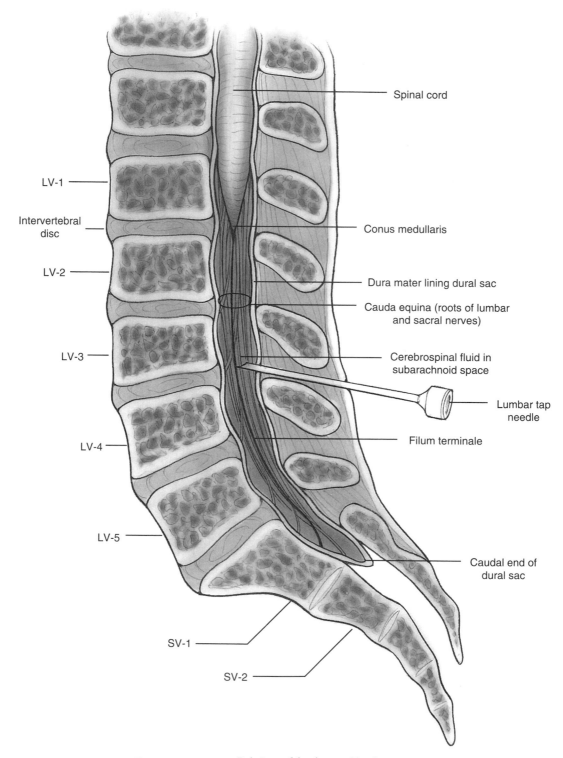

FIGURE 2-3.   Relations of dural sac and lumbar tap.

surrounds the spinal cord and is attached to the inner surface of the dura mater. The spinal cord is anchored to the dura by the **dentate ligaments** and by the spinal nerve roots. The dentate ligaments are 21 pairs of fibrous sheaths located at the sides of the spinal cord. Medially, the ligaments form a continuous longitudinal attachment to the pia mater. Laterally, they form triangular, tooth-like processes that attach to the dura. Due to their pial attachments midway between the posterior and anterior surfaces of the spinal cord, the dentate ligaments can be used as landmarks for surgical procedures. The spinal cord is also anchored by the roots of the spinal nerves, which are ensheathed by a cuff of dura where they perforate it near the intervertebral foramina.

DURA MATER

The spinal dura mater loosely surrounds the spinal cord. The area between the spinal dura and the periosteum lining the vertebral canal is the epidural space. Its contents include loose connective tissue, fat, and the internal vertebral venous plexus.

The internal vertebral venous plexus forms a valveless communication between the cranial **dural sinuses,** which collect blood from the veins of the brain, and the veins of the thoracic, abdominal, and pelvic cavities. It, therefore, provides a direct path for the spread of infections, emboli, or cancer cells from the viscera to the brain.

Inferior or caudal to the spinal cord, the dura mater forms the **dural sac** (Fig. 2–3), which extends inferiorly to the lower border of the second sacral vertebra. Caudal to this point, it surrounds the filum terminale, the thread-like extension of the pia mater, and descends to the back of the coccyx as the coccygeal ligament, which blends with the periosteum. The dural sac is located between the superior border of LV2, where the spinal cord ends as the conus medullaris, and the inferior border of SV2, where the dura ends. Because the arachnoid is attached to the inner surface of the dura lining the dural sac, the contents of the sac are in the

subarachnoid space. Therefore, the dural sac contains (*a*) the filum terminale; (*b*) the **cauda equina,** consisting of the lumbosacral nerve roots descending from the spinal cord to their points of emergence at the lumbar intervertebral and sacral foramina; and (*c*) cerebrospinal fluid.

The spinal cord ends just above LV2, whereas the subarachnoid space continues caudally to SV2. A hypodermic needle may be introduced into the subarachnoid space (Fig. 2–3) within the dural sac without danger of accidentally injuring the spinal cord, thereby causing irreparable damage, because regeneration or repair to neurons and axons in the spinal cord (or brain) does not occur.

This procedure, called **lumbar puncture,** may be used to withdraw cerebrospinal fluid for analysis, to measure cerebrospinal fluid pressure, and to introduce therapeutic agents, anesthetics, and contrast media. It is inadvisable to puncture above the LV2–LV3 interspace in adults and above the LV4–LV5 interspace in infants or small children.

SPINAL NERVES

Each spinal nerve (except the first and last) is attached to a spinal cord segment by posterior (dorsal) and anterior (ventral) roots (Fig. 2–4). Thus, each segment gives rise to four separate roots, one posterior and one anterior on each side. Each of these individual roots is attached to the spinal cord by a series of rootlets. The posterior and anterior roots take a lateral and descending course within the subarachnoid space (Fig. 2–1) and are encased in the dura mater as they approach the intervertebral foramina (Fig. 2–2). The posterior root or spinal ganglia, groups of neurons in the posterior root, are within the thoracic, lumbar, and sacral intervertebral foramina but slightly distal to the cervical foramina. The posterior and anterior roots unite immediately beyond the ganglia to form the spinal nerves, which then exit from the intervertebral foramina and immediately begin to branch.

SPINAL CORD TOPOGRAPHY

On the surface of the spinal cord are several longitudinal grooves (Fig. 2–4). The most prominent of these is the anterior median fis-

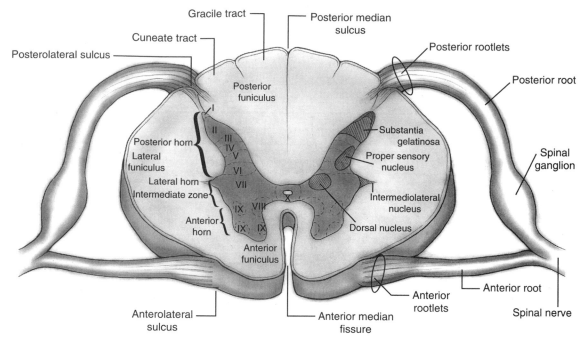

FIGURE 2–4. Transverse section showing a composite of the structures in various spinal cord segments and the formation of a spinal nerve.

sure, occupied by the anterior spinal artery and the proximal parts of its sulcal branches. On the opposite side is a far less conspicuous groove, the posterior median sulcus. The anterior and posterior rootlets of the spinal nerves arise somewhat lateral to these median grooves, at the anterolateral and posterolateral sulci, respectively. The small posterior spinal arteries are located in the latter sulci.

SPINAL CORD INTERNAL STRUCTURE

The spinal cord has external and internal parts that are similar throughout its extent. The external part is the white matter, which consists of millions of axons transmitting impulses superiorly or inferiorly. A large number of the fibers are myelinated, thus accounting for the white color in the fresh or unstained state.

The internal part is the gray matter, which consists of nerve cell bodies and the neuropil that includes the dendrites, preterminal and terminal axons, capillaries, and glia between the neurons. It contains some entering and exiting myelinated fibers but has a grayish color in the fresh or unstained state due to the virtual absence of myelin.

WHITE MATTER

The white matter is divided into three areas, called funiculi. Based on their positions, these are the posterior funiculus, the lateral funiculus, and the anterior funiculus (Fig. 2–4). Each funiculus is subdivided into groups of fibers called fasciculi or tracts. As an example, at cervical levels each posterior funiculus is divided into a medial part, the gracile tract, and a lateral part, the cuneate tract. A well-defined separation between these two tracts is not always evident. This is generally true of most of the tracts in the spinal cord; hence, the locations of the various tracts in the spinal white matter are based on postmortem studies of human subjects with known neurologic abnormalities.

GRAY MATTER

The gray matter is divided into four main parts:

1. The posterior or dorsal horns;

2. The anterior or ventral horns;

3. The intermediate zones;

4. The lateral horns.

For descriptive purposes, an imaginary horizontal line passing from side to side through the deepest part of each posterior funiculus and extending laterally through the gray matter, defines the anterior boundary of the posterior horns (Fig. 2–4). The posterior horns contain groups of neurons that are influenced mainly by impulses entering the spinal cord via the posterior roots. Hence, the posterior horns are primarily the "sensory" parts of the spinal gray matter, and many of their neurons give rise to axons that enter the white matter and ascend to the brain.

The anterior horns are located between the anterior and lateral funiculi. Most of their neurons play roles in voluntary movement and many of them give rise to axons that emerge in the anterior roots. Hence, the anterior horns are primarily the "motor" parts of the spinal gray matter.

The intermediate zones are located between the anterior and posterior horns and are continuous medially with the gray matter that crosses the midline at the central canal. The intermediate zones are composed mainly of association or interneurons for segmental and intersegmental integration of spinal cord functions. Hence, the intermediate zones are the "association" parts of the spinal gray matter, and most of the axons arising from their neurons remain in the spinal cord; some, however, do project to the brain.

The lateral horn is a small triangular extension of the intermediate zone into the lateral funiculus of the thoracic and the upper two lumbar segments. It contains cell bodies of preganglionic neurons of the **sympathetic** nervous system.

Nuclei or Cell Columns

The neurons of the spinal gray matter are arranged in longitudinal groups of functionally similar cells referred to as columns or nuclei (Fig. 2–4). Some of these nuclei extend through the entire length of the spinal cord, whereas others are found only at certain levels. For example, the substantia gelatinosa and the proper sensory nucleus, which are related to pain impulses from all spinal nerves, extend throughout the length of the spinal cord, but other nuclei such as the dorsal nucleus of Clarke and the intermediolateral nucleus, which are related to the cerebellar and autonomic systems, respectively, exist only in certain spinal cord segments.

Laminae

The spinal gray matter can also be divided into laminae or layers based on layerings of morphologically similar neurons (Fig. 2–4). Laminae provide a more precise identification of areas within the spinal gray and are very useful in describing the locations of the origins or terminations of the functional paths. Ten laminae make up the spinal gray matter, and, in general, they are numbered from posterior to anterior. The posterior horn includes laminae I–VI; the intermediate zone is mainly lamina VII; and the anterior horn contains part of lamina VII and all of laminae VIII and IX. Lamina X is in the commissural area surrounding the central canal.

REGIONAL DIFFERENCES

Myelin-stained transverse sections of the four major regions of the spinal cord can be distinguished from each other most readily by the size and shape of the respective gray matter (Figs. 2–5–2–8). Due to the large size of the lower limbs, the lumbar and sacral segments have massive posterior and anterior horns. In lumbar segments, the anterior horn has a distinct medial extension, whereas in sacral segments the anterior horn extends laterally. In addition, the rim of white matter surrounding the sacral gray matter is much thinner than that in the lumbar spinal cord.

The posterior horn in both thoracic and cervical segments is narrow compared to lumbar and sacral segments. However, due to the muscular volume of the upper limb, the cervical anterior horn is much larger than the thoracic, which mainly supplies the relatively small intercostal and subcostal muscles. The thoracic segments have the least amount of gray matter, both anteriorly and posteriorly.

Differences in the amount of white matter are subtle throughout the spinal cord. Nevertheless, because the white matter contains axons transmitting information between the spinal cord segments and the brain, the amount of white matter decreases in each segment proceeding from superior to inferior.

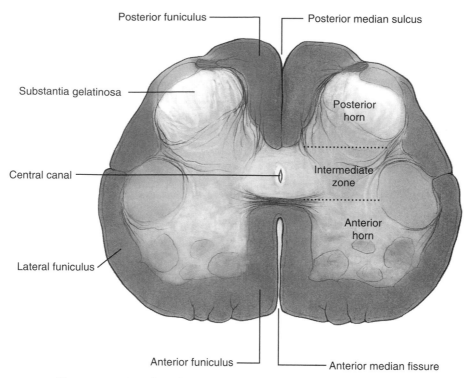

Posterior funiculus — Posterior median sulcus

Substantia gelatinosa — Posterior horn

Central canal — Intermediate zone

Anterior horn

Lateral funiculus

Anterior funiculus — Anterior median fissure

FIGURE 2–5. Transverse section of sacral spinal cord. Note the huge anterior and posterior horns surrounded by narrow white matter.

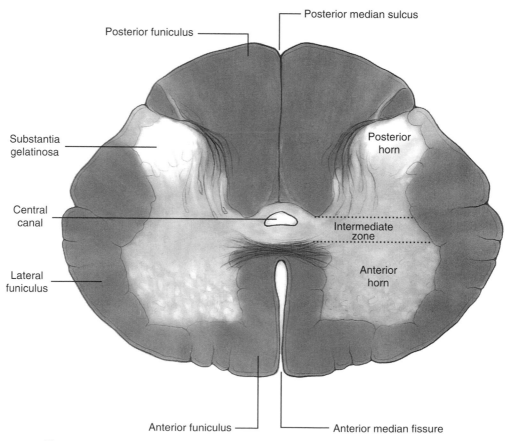

Posterior median sulcus

Posterior funiculus

Substantia gelatinosa — Posterior horn

Central canal — Intermediate zone

Lateral funiculus — Anterior horn

Anterior funiculus — Anterior median fissure

FIGURE 2–6. Transverse section of lumbar spinal cord. Note the large anterior and posterior horns and the large posterior funiculi.

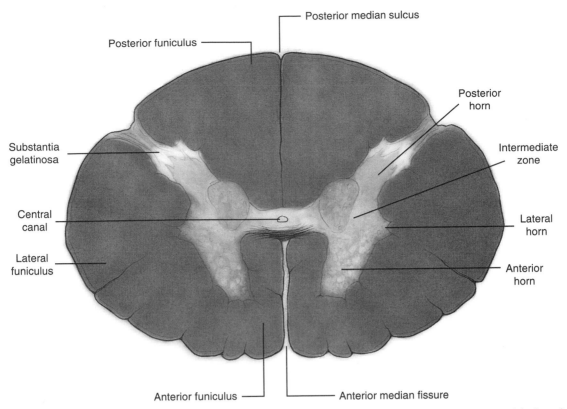

FIGURE 2-7. Transverse section of thoracic spinal cord. Note the slim anterior and posterior horns and the lateral horn indenting the lateral funiculus.

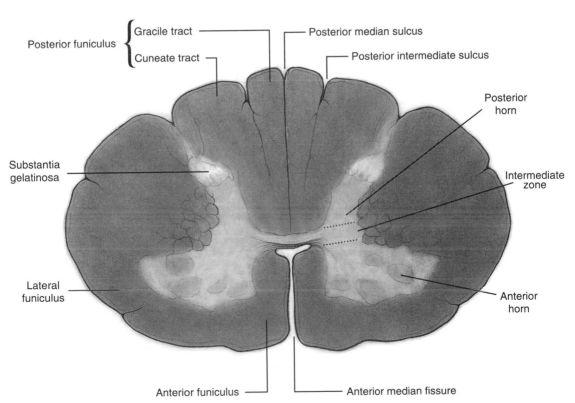

FIGURE 2-8. Transverse section of cervical enlargement. Note the slim posterior horn, large anterior horn, and the division of the huge posterior funiculus.

CHAPTER REVIEW QUESTIONS

2–1. What are the contents of the spinal epidural space?

2–2. What are the contents of the dural sac?

2–3. At what three intervertebral articulations are dislocations most likely to occur and what spinal cord segments are related to each?

2–4. Why are lumbar punctures done at the LV3–LV4 or LV4–LV5 levels in adults?

2–5. What are the distinguishing characteristics of transverse spinal cord sections at sacral, lumbar, thoracic, and cervical levels?

BRAINSTEM ANATOMY, TOPOGRAPHY, AND FUNCTIONAL LEVELS

The brainstem contains functional centers associated with all but 1 of the 12 cranial nerves. It also contains the long tracts that transmit somatosensory impulses from all parts of the body to the forebrain, as well as motor impulses for voluntary movements which originate in the forebrain. Damage to the brainstem is manifested by somatosensory or motor dysfunctions or both, accompanied by abnormalities in cranial nerve functions. The level of damage in a brainstem lesion can usually be determined by cranial nerve malfunction. Due to the vital nature of many functional centers located in the brainstem, especially at more caudal levels, brainstem lesions are frequently fatal.

The brainstem is the stalk-like part of the brain that is located in the posterior cranial fossa. It consists of the medulla oblongata, pons, and midbrain (Fig. 3–1). The medulla oblongata is continuous with the spinal cord at the foramen magnum and the midbrain is continuous with the forebrain at the tentorial notch, the opening at the free margins of the tentorium cerebelli.

The brainstem is covered posteriorly by the cerebellum to which it is connected by huge masses of nerve fibers that form the three pairs of **cerebellar peduncles.** Its anterior surface is

A life-threatening event involving the brainstem can occur when a lumbar puncture is performed in a patient with increased intracranial pressure. In this circumstance, the brainstem is thrust downward as the overlying mass of the cerebellum herniates through the foramen magnum against the medulla oblongata. Pressure on cardiovascular and respiratory centers in the medulla quickly results in death.

closely related to the clivus, the downward sloping basal surface of the posterior cranial fossa between the dorsum sellae and foramen magnum (Fig. 3–2).

BRAINSTEM ANATOMY

MEDULLA OBLONGATA

The medulla oblongata, more simply called the medulla, extends from the spinal cord to the pons (Figs. 3–1, 3–2). The posterior surface of its rostral part is anatomically related to the cerebellum to which it is connected by the inferior cerebellar peduncles.

The caudal half of the medulla contains a prolongation of the central canal of the spinal cord and is referred to as the closed part of the medulla. The posterior surface of the rostral half of the medulla forms the caudal or medullary part of the floor of the fourth ventricle, the cerebrospinal fluid-filled cavity between the cerebellum and the pons and open medulla (Fig. 3–2). The rostral half of the medulla is referred to as the open part. The medulla contains nuclei related to the vestibulocochlear (VIII), glossopharyngeal (IX), vagus (X), cranial part of the accessory (XI), and hypoglossal (XII) cranial nerves and also contains centers that are associated with equilibrium, audition, deglutition, coughing, vomiting, salivation, tongue movements, respiration, and circulation.

PONS

The pons extends from the medulla to the midbrain. Posteriorly, it forms the floor of the

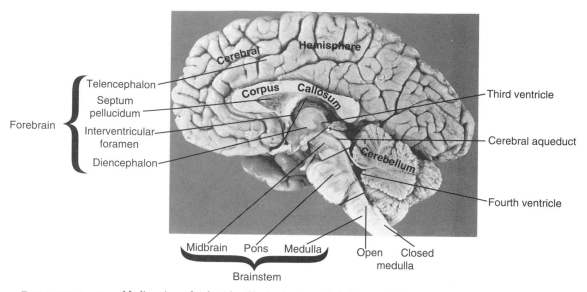

FIGURE 3-1. Median view of right side of brain showing subdivisions and their parts of the ventricular system.

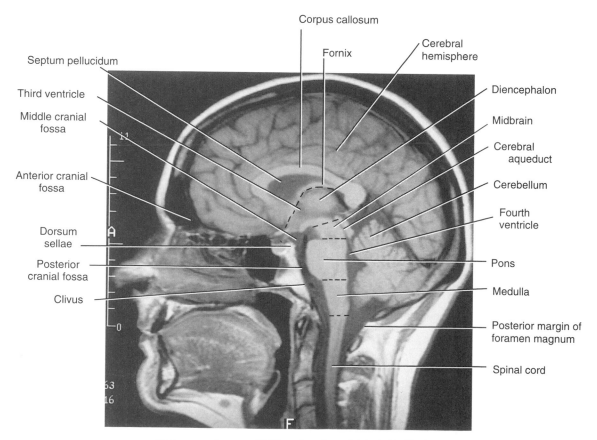

FIGURE 3-2. MRI median view of right half of brain.

rostral part of the fourth ventricle and it is covered by the cerebellum to which it is attached by the middle cerebellar peduncles or brachii pontis. The pons contains nuclei related to the trigeminal (V), abducent (VI), and facial (VII) cranial nerves and contains centers associated with mastication, eye movements, facial expression, blinking, salivation, equilibrium, and audition.

MIDBRAIN

The midbrain lies between the pons and the forebrain and is located in the tentorial notch. It is the shortest part of the brainstem and contains the nuclei of the oculomotor (III) and trochlear (IV) cranial nerves as well as centers associated with auditory, visual, and pupillary reflexes. It contains the **cerebral aqueduct** (Figs. 3–1, 3–2), the narrow channel that is the only route by which cerebrospinal fluid can exit from the ventricles of the forebrain to the fourth ventricle. An imaginary line passing from side to side through the cerebral aqueduct divides the midbrain into a posterior part or roof, the tectum, and an anterior part, the cerebral peduncle.

BRAINSTEM TOPOGRAPHY

As stated in the Preface, prior to covering the clinically important functional paths, it is imperative for the reader to become familiar with the distinguishing characteristics of the subdivisions of the brain and their functionally important levels. Because only the most conspicuous anatomical landmarks are necessary to distinguish the subdivisions and their functional levels, these alone are described here. Other structures of clinical importance are described with the functional paths.

ANTERIOR SURFACE

Medulla

On the anterior surface of the medulla (Fig. 3–3) are the pyramids, a pair of elongated elevations on either side of the anterior median fissure. Lateral to the rostral part of each pyramid is a prominent elevation, the olive. The shallow groove between the olive and pyramid is the preolivary sulcus where the hypoglossal (XII)

nerve rootlets emerge. The sulcus posterior to the olive is the postolivary sulcus and this sulcus is where the rootlets of the glossopharyngeal (IX) and vagus (X) nerves attach (from superior to inferior). The rootlets of the cranial accessory (XI) nerve emerge in line with those of the vagus but inferior to the postolivary sulcus.

Pons

The anterior portion of the pons is the basilar part. Its surface consists of transverse bands formed by bundles of fibers that become continuous laterally with the middle cerebellar peduncles. The shallow basilar sulcus near the midline is normally occupied by the basilar artery.

The abducent (VI) nerve emerges at the pontomedullary junction near the lateral border of the pyramid. Attaching more laterally at the pontomedullary junction are the facial (VII) and vestibulocochlear (VIII) nerves. On the anterolateral surface of the pons about midway between the medulla and midbrain is the attachment of the trigeminal (V) nerve. This nerve consists of a larger inferolateral sensory root (portio major) and a small superomedial motor root (portio minor).

Midbrain

The anterior surface of the midbrain is formed by the cerebral peduncles. These consist of the converging cerebral crura (the most anterior parts of the cerebral peduncles), which are separated from each other by the **interpeduncular fossa.** The oculomotor (III) nerves emerge from the walls of the interpeduncular fossa.

POSTERIOR SURFACE
Medulla

The posterior surface of the closed or caudal half of the medulla contains the gracile tubercles on either side of the posterior median sulcus (Fig. 3–4). Lateral to each gracile tubercle and extending slightly more rostral is the cuneate tubercle. The posterior surface of the open half of the medulla and the posterior surface of the pons form the floor of the fourth ventricle.

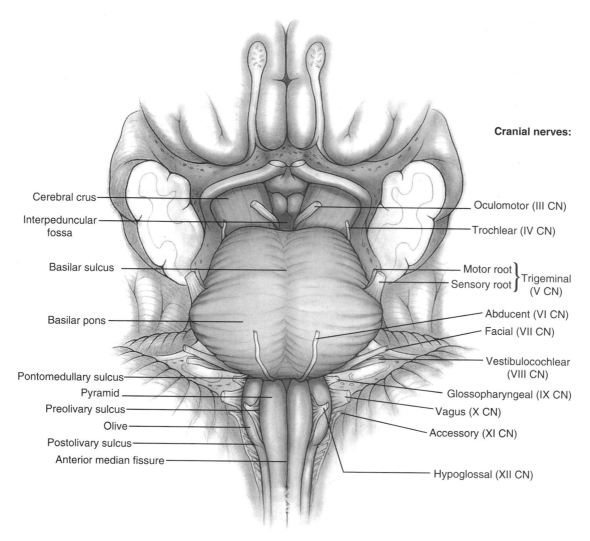

Cranial nerves:

Cerebral crus

Interpeduncular fossa

Basilar sulcus

Basilar pons

Pontomedullary sulcus
Pyramid
Preolivary sulcus
Olive
Postolivary sulcus
Anterior median fissure

Oculomotor (III CN)

Trochlear (IV CN)

Motor root ⎫
Sensory root ⎬ Trigeminal (V CN)

Abducent (VI CN)
Facial (VII CN)

Vestibulocochlear (VIII CN)

Glossopharyngeal (IX CN)
Vagus (X CN)
Accessory (XI CN)

Hypoglossal (XII CN)

FIGURE 3-3.   Anterior surface of brainstem.

Fourth Ventricle

The floor of the fourth ventricle can be divided into medullary and pontine parts by drawing an imaginary horizontal line between the lateral recesses, which are found at the widest point of the fourth ventricle. In most brains, the rostral part of the medullary floor contains a variable number of white strands called the striae medullares, which extend laterally from the median sulcus toward the lateral recess.

The median sulcus divides the floor of the fourth ventricle into symmetrical halves. Each half is further subdivided into medial and lateral parts by the superior and inferior foveae, small depressions at pontine and medullary levels, re-

spectively. These foveae indicate the boundary between motor structures, which are medial, and sensory structures, which are lateral. Hence, extending laterally from the two foveae to the lateral recess is the vestibular area and at the lateral recess is a small eminence, the acoustic tubercle. Both the vestibular area and acoustic tubercle are sensory structures. Between the inferior fovea and the median sulcus are two small triangular areas, the hypoglossal trigone positioned medially, and the vagal trigone positioned laterally, both of which are motor structures. Between the superior fovea and the median sulcus is the medial eminence. Its caudal part enlarges and is the facial colliculus, a motor structure. The caudal tip of the fourth ventricle

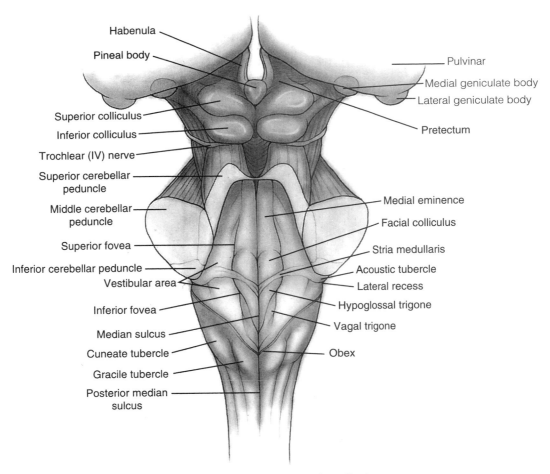

FIGURE 3–4.   Posterior surface of brainstem.

lies between the gracile tubercles and is called the obex.

Cerebellar Peduncles

The cut surfaces of the cerebellar peduncles are at the lateral aspects of the pons and in the roof of the fourth ventricle. The massive **middle cerebellar peduncle** or brachium pontis is continuous with the basilar part of the pons. At its inferomedial part is the **inferior cerebellar peduncle** or restiform body, which connects the medulla to the cerebellum. The **superior cerebellar peduncle** or brachium conjunctivum passes from the roof of the fourth ventricle into the tegmentum of the rostral pons.

Midbrain

The posterior surface of the midbrain is composed of the tectum. The tectum consists of two pairs of mounds, the corpora quadrigemina or inferior and superior colliculi. The trochlear (IV) nerves emerge caudal to the inferior colliculi. The small area rostral to the superior colliculi is the pretectum.

BRAINSTEM RETICULAR FORMATION

Extending through the central part of the medulla, pons, and midbrain is a complex intermingling of loosely defined nuclei and tracts that forms the brainstem reticular formation (Fig. 3–5). As its central location (Figs. 3–6 to 3–13) might suggest, it is intimately associated with ascending and descending paths and cranial nerve nuclei. As a result, it receives input from all parts of the nervous system and, in turn, exerts widespread influences on virtually every CNS function.

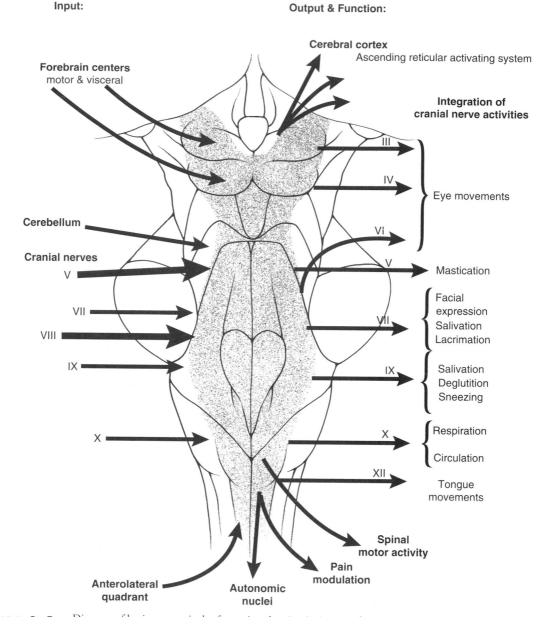

FIGURE 3–5.   Diagram of brainstem reticular formation showing its input and output. Reticular formation forming central core (*shaded area*).

BRAINSTEM FUNCTIONAL LEVELS

After the surface features of the brainstem are familiar, these same structures can be identified in transverse sections at the levels that are used in localizing lesions or injuries. By locating on the brainstem specimen the same surface landmarks in a transverse section, one is able to determine precisely from where the section was taken. For example, refer to the brainstem drawings in Figures 3–3 and 3–4 and compare them closely with the transverse sections in Figures 3–6 to 3–13. Because the brainstem sections are referred to repeatedly as the functional systems are studied, knowing precisely where they are located in the brain will enhance the development of a three-dimensional image of the functional paths. This is important because the clinician must project knowledge of the nervous system, no matter what the source, onto the gross brain and ultimately to the living brain in situ.

ROSTRAL PART OF CLOSED MEDULLA

The pyramids are anterior and separated by the anterior median fissure (Fig. 3–6). The gracile and cuneate tubercles are posterior and separated by the posterior intermediate sulcus. The posterior median sulcus is between the gracile tubercles.

CAUDAL PART OF OPEN MEDULLA

Positioned anteriorly are the pyramids and olives with the rootlets of the hypoglossal nerve between them (Fig. 3–7). The preolivary and

postolivary sulci are anterior and posterior to the olive, respectively. Posteriorly, the floor of the fourth ventricle contains from medial to lateral, the hypoglossal and vagal trigones, the inferior fovea, and the vestibular area.

ROSTRAL PART OF OPEN MEDULLA

Anteriorly, the surface of the medulla presents, from medial to lateral, the anterior median fissure, the pyramids, the preolivary sulci, the olives, and the postolivary sulci (Fig. 3–8). Posteriorly, the widest part of the floor of the fourth ventricle is relatively smooth except at the lateral recess where there is an eminence, the acoustic tubercle. Lateral to this tubercle is the lateral aperture, the opening into the subarachnoid space. Most of the ventricular floor consists of the vestibular area. The bundles of myelinated fibers in the floor are the striae medullares of the fourth ventricle.

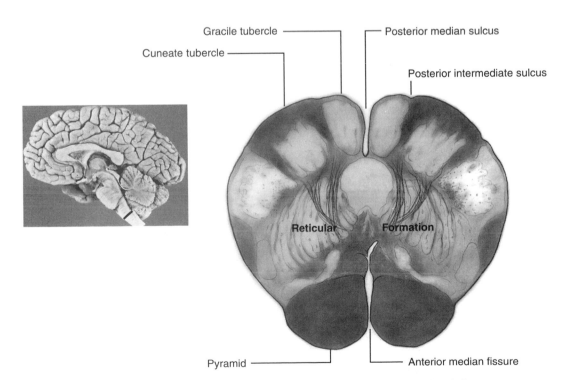

Gracile tubercle — Posterior median sulcus

Cuneate tubercle — Posterior intermediate sulcus

Reticular Formation

Pyramid — Anterior median fissure

FIGURE 3–6. Transverse section of the rostral part of the closed medulla.

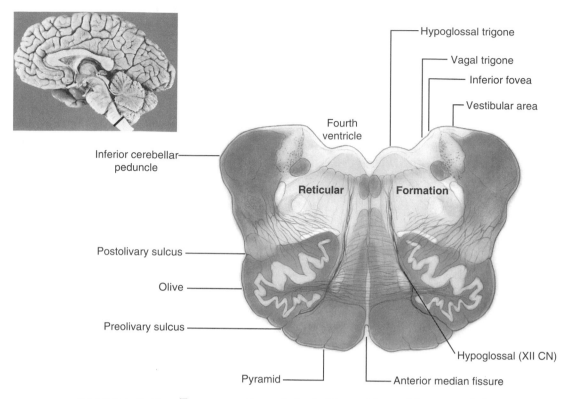

FIGURE 3–7.   Transverse section at the level of the caudal part of the open medulla.

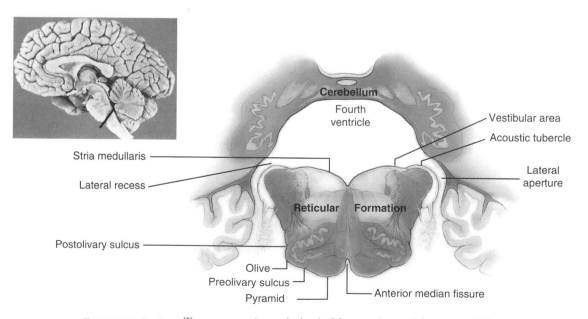

FIGURE 3–8.   Transverse section at the level of the rostral part of the open medulla.

CAUDAL PART OF PONS

The anterior or basilar part of the pons consists of gray matter, the pontine nuclei, and white matter, large circular bundles of descending fibers, and smaller bundles of transverse fibers, which laterally enter the middle cerebellar peduncle (Fig. 3–9). The most conspicuous structures in the posterior or tegmental part of the pons are the intramedullary parts of the abducent (VI) and facial (VII) nerves and the abducent nucleus, which is deep to the facial colliculus.

MIDDLE PART OF PONS

This section is at the midpontine level where the trigeminal nerve attaches (Fig. 3–10). Although its size and shape may vary, the basilar part of the pons appears similar at all pontine levels. The most conspicuous structures in the lateral part of the pontine tegmentum are the large, oval motor trigeminal nucleus and the smaller sensory trigeminal nucleus lateral to it. The superior cerebellar peduncles are in the roof of the fourth ventricle. The **superior medullary velum** is between them.

ROSTRAL PART OF PONS

At the posterior surface of the rostral pons is the decussation and emergence of the trochlear (IV) nerves, the only cranial nerves emerging from the posterior surface of the brainstem (Fig. 3–11). The fourth ventricle has narrowed to become the cerebral aqueduct. The massive superior cerebellar peduncles have entered the tegmentum and are beginning to decussate or cross. The basilar part contains larger bundles of fibers separated by the pontine nuclei.

CAUDAL PART OF THE MIDBRAIN

Posteriorly, the inferior colliculi are separated by the periaqueductal gray matter surrounding the cerebral aqueduct (Fig. 3–12). Anteriorly is located the cerebral peduncle which, from posterior to anterior, consists of the tegmentum, substantia nigra, and **cerebral**

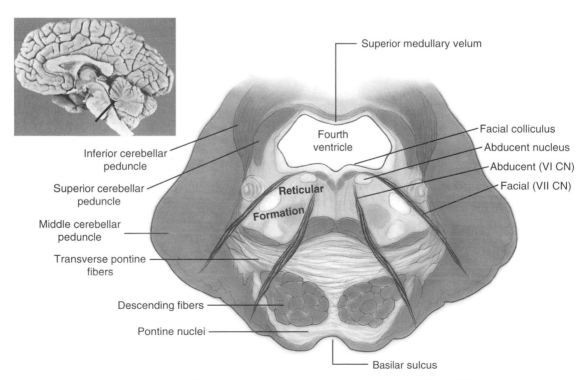

FIGURE 3–9.   Transverse section at the level of the caudal pons (VI and VII CN).

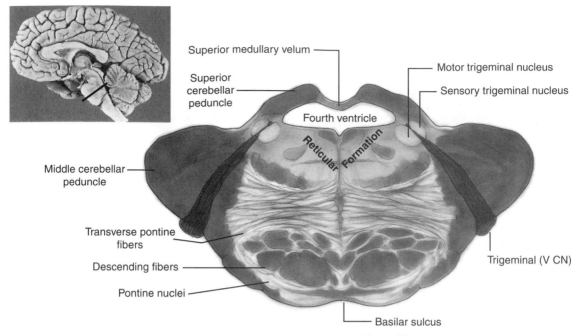

FIGURE 3–10. Transverse section at the level of the middle pons (V CN).

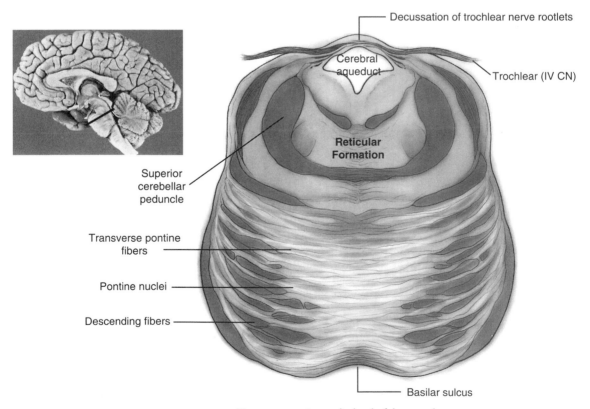

FIGURE 3–11. Transverse section at the level of the rostral pons.

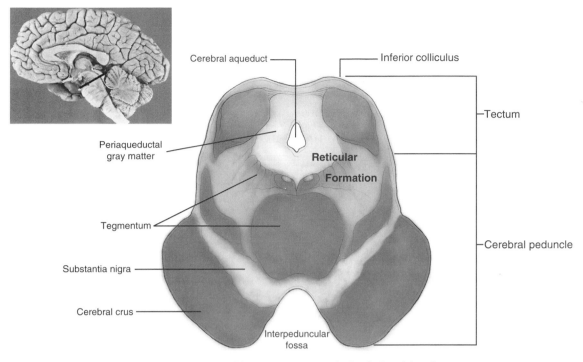

FIGURE 3-12. Transverse section at the level of caudal midbrain.

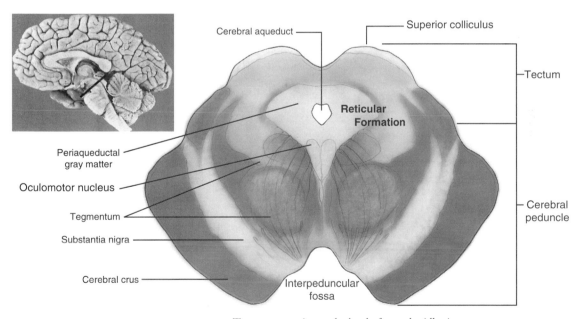

FIGURE 3-13. Transverse section at the level of rostral midbrain.

crus. The large interpeduncular fossa is between the cerebral crura.

ROSTRAL PART OF MIDBRAIN

Posteriorly, the superior colliculi are partially separated by the periaqueductal matter and cerebral aqueduct (Fig. 3–13). The oculomotor nuclei are in the V-shaped anterior part of the periaqueductal gray matter. Anteriorly, the cerebral peduncle is composed of the tegmentum, substantia nigra, and cerebral crus. The oculomotor (III) nerves emerge from the walls of the interpeduncular fossa.

CHAPTER REVIEW QUESTIONS

3–1. To which parts of the brainstem do cranial nerves III–XII attach?

3–2. What are the distinguishing characteristics of the ventral surface of the (*a*) medulla, (*b*) pons, and (*c*) midbrain?

3–3. What are the distinguishing characteristics of the dorsal surface of the (*a*) closed medulla, (*b*) open medulla, (*c*) pons, and (*d*) midbrain?

3–4. What and where is the brainstem reticular formation?

3–5. At which specific brainstem level is each of the following?

  a. Hypoglossal trigone
  b. Motor trigeminal nucleus
  c. Superior colliculus
  d. Decussation of trochlear nerve
  e. Acoustic tubercle
  f. Gracile tubercle
  g. Facial colliculus
  h. Inferior colliculus

FOREBRAIN TOPOGRAPHY AND FUNCTIONAL LEVELS

Damage to the forebrain may result in disturbances involving hormonal imbalance, temperature regulation, emotions, or behavior. Forebrain lesions may also affect sensory perception and voluntary movements as well as memory, judgment, and speech. The most common vascular lesions in the entire nervous system are "capsular strokes" that occur deep within the forebrain.

The forebrain consists of the diencephalon and the paired cerebral hemispheres. The diencephalon contains functional centers for the integration of all information passing from the brainstem and spinal cord to the cerebral hemispheres as well as the integration of motor and visceral activities. The two cerebral hemispheres integrate the highest mental functions such as the awareness of sensations and emotions, learning and memory, intelligence and creativity, and language.

The diencephalon (interbrain) receives the optic (II) nerves and is subdivided into four parts: thalamus, hypothalamus, subthalamus, and epithalamus. The cerebral hemispheres receive the olfactory (I) nerves. The diencephalon contains the third ventricle and the cerebral hemispheres contain the lateral ventricles, which are separated from each other in part by the septum pellucidum (Figs. 3–1 and 3–2).

DIRECTIONAL TERMINOLOGY

The forebrain is located in the anterior and middle cranial fossae and is supratentorial in position, that is, superior or above the tentorium cerebelli. It is oriented almost perpendic-

ular to the brain and spinal cord (Figs. 3–1, 3–2, 4–1). The change in direction occurs at the junction between the midbrain and forebrain, and at this junction there is a change in directional terms. In descriptions of the spinal cord and brainstem, the terms anterior or ventral indicate toward the front of the body, and the terms posterior or dorsal mean toward the back. Moreover, superior or rostral indicate higher or toward the top or above, and inferior or caudal mean lower or toward the bottom or below.

With the change in direction at the midbrain-forebrain junction, the directional terms used in anatomical descriptions of the forebrain are as follows:

Anterior—toward the *front* of the skull
Posterior—toward the *back* of the skull
Ventral or inferior—toward the *base* of the skull
Dorsal or superior—toward the *top* of the skull

DIENCEPHALON

The cerebrospinal fluid-filled cavity found in the middle of the diencephalon is the third ventricle (Figs. 3–1, 3–2, 4–2). Posteriorly, the third ventricle is continuous with the cerebral aqueduct. Anteriorly, it is continuous with the two lateral ventricles at the interventricular **foramina (of Monro).** The hypothalamic sulcus traverses the lateral wall of the third ventricle from the interventricular foramen to the cerebral aqueduct and separates the thalamus, above, from the hypothalamus, below.

The diencephalon includes the thalamus, a

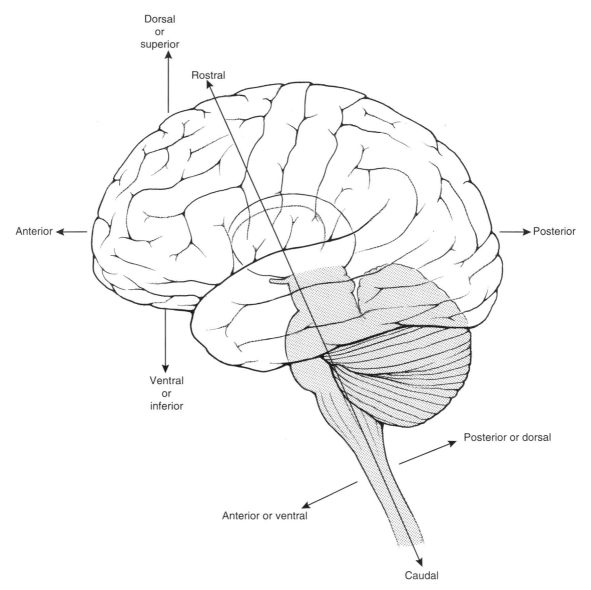

FIGURE 4–1. CNS directional terminology. The midbrain, hindbrain, and spinal cord (*stippled*) are oriented almost vertically, whereas the forebrain is oriented horizontally. Because of this change in orientation at the midbrain-forebrain junction, the terms dorsal and ventral have different connotations rostral and caudal to this junction.

large nuclear mass forming the dorsal part of the wall of the third ventricle; the hypothalamus, which lines the ventral part of the wall of the third ventricle and extends ventrally from the medial part of the thalamus to the base of the brain; the subthalamus, ventral to the lateral part of the thalamus and lateral to the hypothalamus, but not reaching the surface of the brain; and the epithalamus, a small area dorsal to the most posterior part of the third ventricle.

THALAMUS

The thalami are two egg-shaped masses bordering the third ventricle, dorsal to the hypothalamic sulcus (Fig. 4–2). In most brains, the right and left thalami are partially fused across the third ventricle by the interthalamic adhesion or massa intermedia. At the interventricular foramen is a swelling, the anterior tubercle, and on the dorsomedial surface of the thalamus is a bundle of fibers, the medullary stria. Poste-

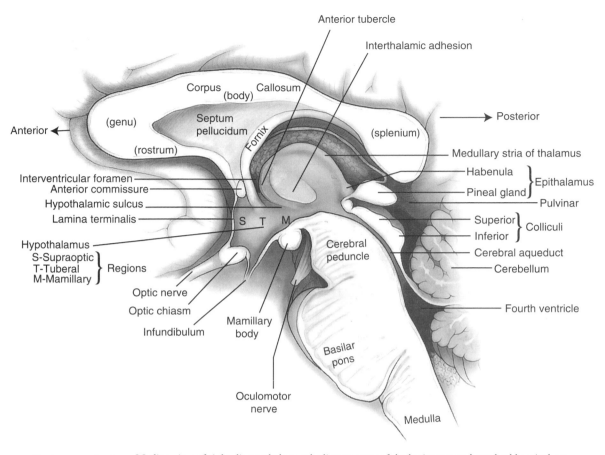

FIGURE 4–2. Median view of right diencephalon and adjacent parts of the brainstem and cerebral hemisphere.

riorly, the pulvinar overhangs the midbrain like a pillow.

Thalamic Nuclei

The thalamus consists of a large number of nuclei that form eight nuclear masses named according to their anatomical locations (Fig. 4–3). The internal medullary lamina, a thin sheet of bundles of myelinated fibers, separates the thalamus into three major subdivisions: anterior, medial, and lateral. The anterior subdivision is located at the anterior tubercle of the thalamus and consists of the anterior nuclei (A). The medial subdivision chiefly includes a large medial dorsal nucleus (MD) and a thin midline nucleus (M) along the wall of the third ventricle. The interthalamic adhesion is a bridge of midline nuclei.

The lateral subdivision is composed of two nuclear masses. The more ventral nuclear mass is subdivided into ventral anterior (VA), ventral lateral (VL), and ventral posterior (VP) nuclei. The ventral posterior nucleus is further divided into ventral posterolateral (VPL) and ventral posteromedial (VPM) nuclei. The more dorsal mass consists of lateral nuclei, the lateral dorsal (LD) and lateral posterior (LP) anteriorly and the pulvinar (P) posteriorly. On the undersurface of the pulvinar are the metathalamic nuclei, the lateral geniculate (LG), and medial geniculate (MG) nuclei.

Two other nuclear masses are anatomically related to the medullary laminae. Within the internal medullary lamina are several intralaminar nuclei, the most prominent of which is the centromedian (CM). Lateral to the external medullary lamina is the reticular (R) nucleus, a thin nucleus forming the most lateral part of the thalamus.

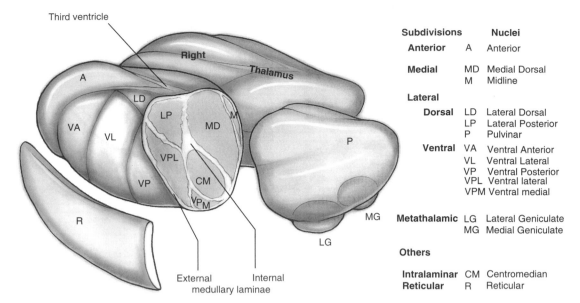

FIGURE 4-3. Lateral view of left thalamic nuclei, including a coronal section through the posterior part of the thalamus.

HYPOTHALAMUS

The only subdivision of the diencephalon on the ventral surface of the brain is the hypothalamus (Fig. 4–2). It is located in the median part of the middle cranial fossa (Fig. 3–2) above the diaphragma sellae. The hypothalamus is subdivided into three main areas in the anterior-posterior plane. Positioned posteriorly is the mamillary region which is related to the mamillary bodies, paired spherical masses about the size of small peas located in the rostral part of the interpeduncular fossa. Found anteriorly is the supraoptic region located dorsal to the optic chiasm. Between the mamillary and the supraoptic regions is the tuber cinereum after which the tuberal region is named. The anterior part of the tuberal region contains the **infundibulum** or stalk of the pituitary gland and is sometimes referred to as the infundibular region.

SUBTHALAMUS

The **subthalamus** consists of a wedge-shaped area ventral to the thalamus and lateral to the hypothalamus. It contains several nuclei, the most prominent of which is the subthalamic nucleus.

EPITHALAMUS

Posteriorly, the dorsal surface of the diencephalon is formed by the epithalamus. The epithalamus consists of the pineal gland and the **habenula** (Figs. 3–4, 4–2).

CEREBRAL HEMISPHERE

The right and left cerebral hemispheres consist of cortical, medullary, and nuclear parts. The cortical portion of each hemisphere is located externally and consists of gray matter that is folded or convoluted to form gyri, which are separated by sulci. Underlying the cortex are masses of nerve fibers that form the white matter or medullary region of the hemisphere, commonly called the centrum semiovale. Embedded deeply in the white matter are the telencephalic nuclei, the most prominent of which are the caudate and lentiform.

LATERAL SURFACE

The lateral surface (Fig. 4–4) is convex and conforms to the concavity of the cranial vault. The most prominent cleft on the lateral surface of the cortex is the lateral sulcus or **fissure of**

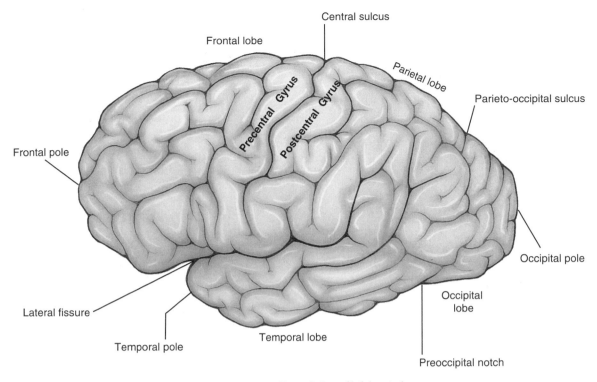

FIGURE 4–4. Lateral view of left hemisphere.

Sylvius, which begins at the base of the brain, extends to the lateral surface of the hemisphere, and proceeds posteriorly and slightly superiorly. It separates the frontal and parietal lobes (superiorly) from the temporal lobe (inferiorly). The next most prominent cleft is the central sulcus or fissure of Rolando, which is between the frontal and parietal lobes. This sulcus is oriented in the dorsoventral direction behind the most anterior gyrus that extends uninterruptedly from the lateral sulcus to the superior margin of the hemisphere. The anterior and posterior walls of the central sulcus are formed by the precentral and postcentral gyri, respectively.

The frontal lobe extends anteriorly from the central sulcus to the anterior tip of the hemisphere, called the frontal pole. The parietal lobe is superior to the lateral sulcus and behind the central sulcus. The temporal lobe is inferior to the lateral sulcus. It is shaped like the thumb of a boxing glove and its most anterior part is called the temporal pole. Posteriorly, the parietal and temporal lobes become continuous with the occipital lobe. The occipital lobe is de-

marcated from the parietal and temporal lobes by an imaginary line between the parieto-occipital sulcus and the preoccipital notch. The occipital pole is the most posterior part of the cerebral hemisphere.

MEDIAL SURFACE

The medial surfaces of the hemispheres (Fig. 4–5) are flat and vertical and form the walls of the longitudinal fissure between the two hemispheres. The most conspicuous clefts on the medial surface are two horizontally oriented sulci, the callosal and cingulate, and the vertically oriented parieto-occipital sulcus. The callosal sulcus is dorsal to the corpus callosum, the huge mass of nerve fibers connecting the two hemispheres. The cingulate sulcus encircles the cingulate gyrus, which is dorsal to the callosal sulcus. The parieto-occipital sulcus, located a short distance posterior to the corpus callosum, separates the parietal and occipital lobes. The central sulcus reaches the medial surface of the hemisphere in the posterior part of the paracentral

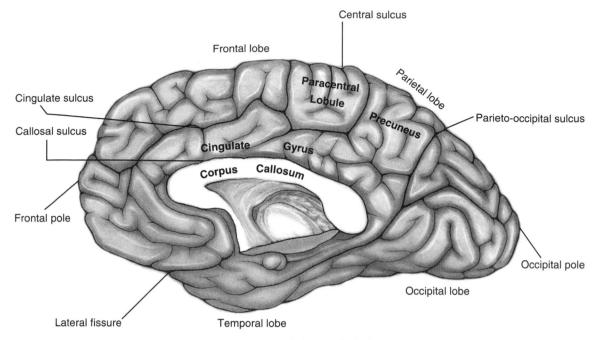

FIGURE 4–5. Medial view of right hemisphere.

lobule. Between the paracentral lobule and the parieto-occipital sulcus is the precuneus.

FOREBRAIN FUNCTIONAL LEVELS

POSTERIOR THALAMIC

This level is at the posterior part of the thalamus and the underlying rostral part of the cerebral peduncle (Fig. 4–6). The level also includes parts of the cerebral hemisphere: the corpus callosum, lateral ventricles, and the caudate and lentiform nuclei. The caudate and lentiform nuclei are telencephalic nuclei.

As found in the midbrain sections, the midbrain here also comprises, from anterior to posterior, the cerebral crus, substantia nigra, and tegmentum. Dorsal to the midbrain is the thalamus. The most prominent thalamic nuclei are the round, centrally located centromedian nucleus in the internal medullary lamina, and the ventral posteromedial nucleus located ventrolateral to it. The ventral posterolateral nucleus lies lateral and somewhat dorsal to the ventral posteromedial nucleus. Other thalamic nuclei at this level are the medial dorsal, lateral posterior, and reticular nucleus which is lateral to the external medullary lamina. In the walls of the third ventricle, medial to the dorsal parts of the thalamus, are the habenulae of the epithalamus and the medullary striae.

MAMILLARY

This level includes the diencephalon at the mamillary bodies and surrounding parts of the cerebral hemispheres (Fig. 4–7). In the midline, from ventral to dorsal, are the hypothalamic area between the mamillary bodies, the third ventricle, the interthalamic adhesion, and the corpus callosum. The walls of the third ventricle are formed by the hypothalamus ventrally and the thalamus dorsally. The thalamus extends laterally to the **internal capsule,** a huge mass of hemispheric white matter or nerve fibers. Many of these fibers are continuous with the cerebral crus. The area bounded by the hypothalamus medially, the thalamus dorsally, the internal capsule laterally, and the cerebral crus ventrally is the subthalamus. The biconvex structure dorsal to the cerebral crus is the subthalamic nucleus.

The lateral ventricle is beneath the lateral part of the corpus callosum. The caudate nucleus is found in the lateral wall of the lateral

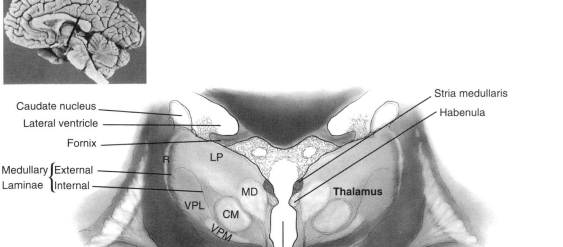

Caudate nucleus

Lateral ventricle

Fornix

Medullary {External
Laminae {Internal

R

LP

VPL

CM

VPM

MD

Stria medullaris

Habenula

Thalamus

Thalamic Nuclei :

CM- Centromedian
LP- Lateral Posterior
MD- Medial Dorsal
R- Reticular
VPL- Ventral Posterolateral
VPM- Ventral Posteromedial

Third ventricle

Cerebral crus
Substantia nigra
Midbrain tegmentum

} Cerebral peduncle

FIGURE 4–6. Coronal section at posterior thalamus. Note the overlap with the rostral cerebral peduncle.

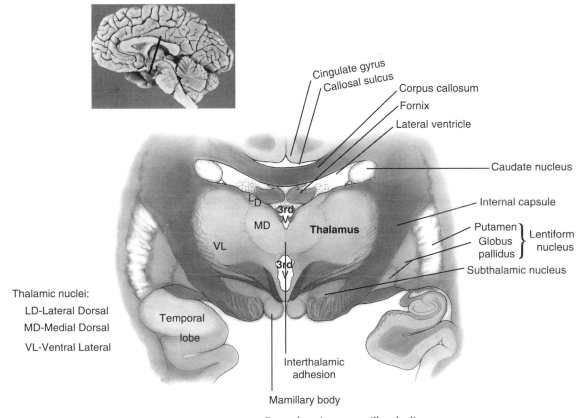

Cingulate gyrus
Callosal sulcus
Corpus callosum
Fornix
Lateral ventricle

Caudate nucleus

LD

3rd V

MD

VL

Thalamus

3rd V

Internal capsule

Putamen
Globus
pallidus

} Lentiform
nucleus

Subthalamic nucleus

Thalamic nuclei:

LD-Lateral Dorsal

MD-Medial Dorsal

VL-Ventral Lateral

Temporal
lobe

Interthalamic
adhesion

Mamillary body

FIGURE 4–7. Coronal section at mamillary bodies.

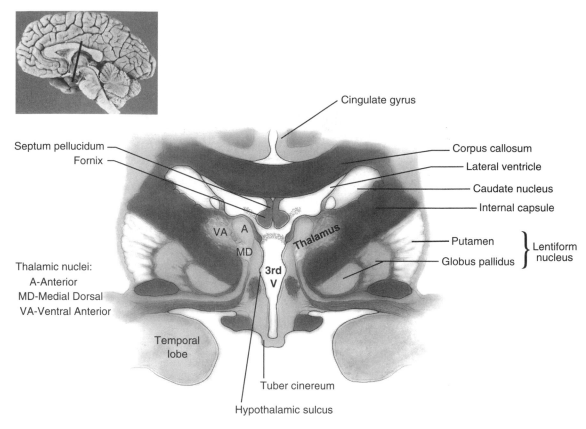

FIGURE 4–8. Coronal section at tuber cinereum.

ventricle. More ventrally, lateral to the internal capsule, is the lentiform nucleus, which comprises two medial segments, the globus pallidus, and a lateral segment—the putamen.

TUBERAL

The tuberal level is at the anterior part of the thalamus and the surrounding cerebral hemisphere (Fig. 4–8). In the midline, from ventral to dorsal, are the tuber cinereum of the hypothalamus, the third ventricle, and the corpus callosum. The **fornix,** a group of nerve fibers arching beneath the corpus callosum, is suspended from the corpus callosum by the septum pellucidum. The walls of the third ventricle are formed by the hypothalamus ventrally and the thalamus dorsally. Lateral to the thalamus is the internal capsule. In the angle between the internal capsule and corpus callosum is the caudate nucleus and lateral ventricle. Lateral to the internal capsule are the putamen and globus pallidus, the two nuclei that form the lentiform nucleus.

CHAPTER REVIEW QUESTIONS

4–1. How do cranial nerves differ from spinal nerves?

4–2. Which cranial nerves attach to the forebrain, which to the midbrain, and which to the hindbrain?

4–3. In which divisions of the brain are the various parts of the ventricular system located?

4–4. When are the terms "anterior or ventral" and "posterior or dorsal" synonymous in regard to the CNS?

LOWER MOTOR NEURONS:
FLACCID PARALYSIS

■ A 22-year-old medical student awakened one morning and found the left side of his face paralyzed. The left nasolabial groove was smoothed out and his lips were drawn toward the right side. He was unable to retract the left corner of his mouth or to pucker his lips as in whistling. Frowning and raising his eyebrow on the left were impossible, and he was unable to close the left eye tightly. No other motor abnormalities and no sensory abnormalities were present.

The motor system consists of neurons and pathways whose integrated activity allows normal movements to occur. For convenience of description, this complex system is traditionally divided into five groups of neurons: lower motor, pyramidal system, basal ganglia, cerebellar, and brainstem control (Fig. 5–1). All of these participate in the sequence of events that occurs when a voluntary movement is desired. The idea or desire to perform the movement occurs in association areas of the cerebral cortex. Impulses from these areas pass to the basal ganglia and cerebellum. The basal ganglia contain the programming for the initiation and necessary postural adjustments, whereas the cerebellum controls the programming for coordination of the movements. Both the basal ganglia and cerebellum exert their influences on the premotor and motor areas of the cerebral cortex. The pyramidal system, which arises from the premotor and motor areas, then carries the cortical commands to the lower motor neurons located in the brainstem and spinal cord. In turn, the

lower motor neurons carry the commands to the contractile units of the voluntary muscles, and the movement occurs. During the execution of the movement, muscle receptors that record stretch, send information back to the lower motor neurons and to the cerebellum in order to fine-tune the coordination of the movement as it continues. The fine-tuning occurs via connections of the cerebellum with the motor cortex and the brainstem motor control centers, both of which influence the lower motor neurons. It should be remembered that even though the five subdivisions are described separately, all participate in commanded movements and all must be intact for normal voluntary movements to occur.

THE MOTOR UNIT

Lower motor neurons are also called **α-motoneurons.** Whether in the spinal cord or brainstem, α-motoneurons and their axons are the only connections between the CNS and skeletal muscle contraction units, the **extrafusal muscle fibers.** These huge multipolar neurons are influenced by impulses from many sources. Because all CNS influences on the contraction of skeletal muscles must be mediated through these units, they are designated as the **"final common path."** Their large myelinated axons, which may be over 1 m in length in tall individuals, synapse as **motor end-plates** (myoneural junctions) on muscle fibers. Acetylcholine is the neurotransmitter at these junctions.

The α-motoneuron, its axon, and the extra-

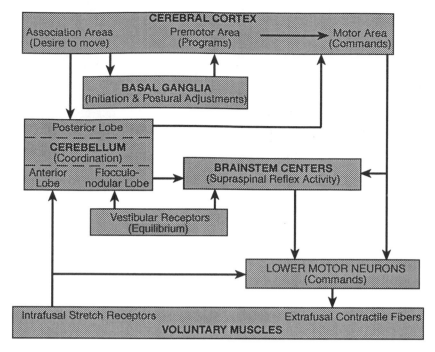

FIGURE 5–1.   Motor system interconnections.

fusal muscle fibers it innervates form the **motor unit** (Fig. 5–2). The number of muscle fibers within a motor unit varies considerably and depends on the delicacy or coarseness of the movement produced by the muscle. Thus, motor units in muscles involved in delicate movements such as the extraocular, lumbrical, or interosseus muscles include less than a dozen muscle fibers; motor units in muscles involved in coarse movements such as the biceps, gluteus maximus, or soleus muscles may contain a thousand or so muscle fibers.

In addition to α-motor neurons, skeletal muscles are also supplied by **γ-motor neurons.** The axons of the γ-motor neurons innervate the intrafusal fibers of the **muscle spindles,** which are sensory organs that are stimulated by lengthening or stretching the muscle. The intrafusal fibers are located at the poles of the muscle spindles. When activated by the γ-motor neurons, the intrafusal fibers increase the tension on the muscle spindle receptors, thereby decreasing the

thresholds of these receptors. The γ-motor neurons play an important role in muscle tone.

BRAINSTEM LOWER MOTOR NEURONS

All cranial nerves, except the olfactory, optic, and vestibulocochlear nerves, contain axons of lower motor neurons. The cell bodies of these lower motor neurons are clumped in paired nuclei located from the level of the superior colliculus to the caudal part of the medulla (Fig. 5–3).

OCULOMOTOR NUCLEUS AND CRANIAL NERVE III

The oculomotor nucleus is located in the V-shaped ventral part of the periaqueductal gray of the midbrain at the level of the superior colliculus (Fig. 5–4). The oculomotor (III CN)

FIGURE 5–2.   Schematic drawing of a motor unit. A lower or α-motor neuron and the extrafusal muscle fibers it innervates. The cell body is located in the spinal cord or brainstem and its myelinated axon courses in a spinal or cranial nerve to synapse on a variable number of extrafusal muscle fibers. Figure 1–2 contains cellular details.

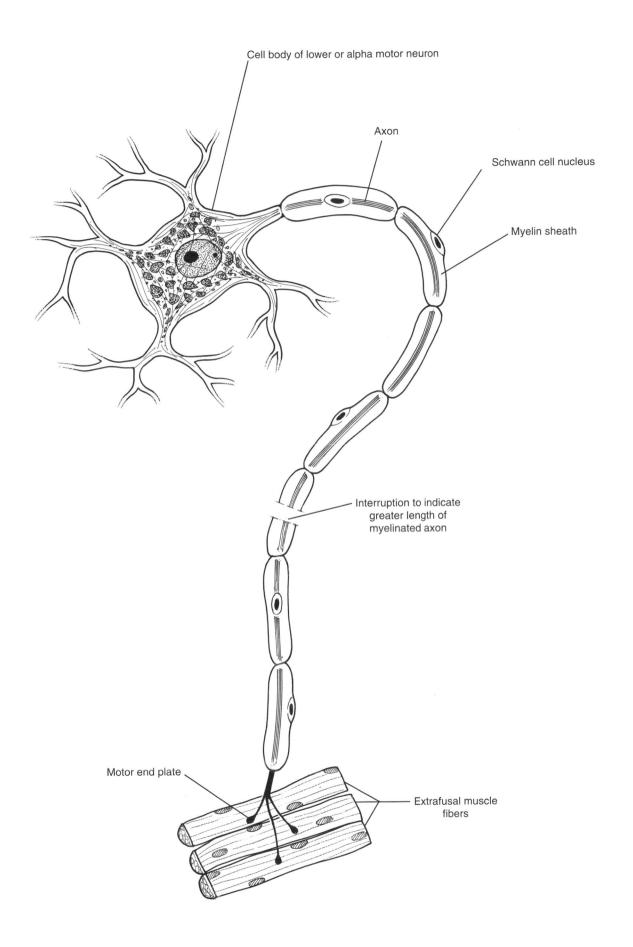

Cell body of lower or alpha motor neuron

Axon

Schwann cell nucleus

Myelin sheath

Interruption to indicate greater length of myelinated axon

Motor end plate

Extrafusal muscle fibers

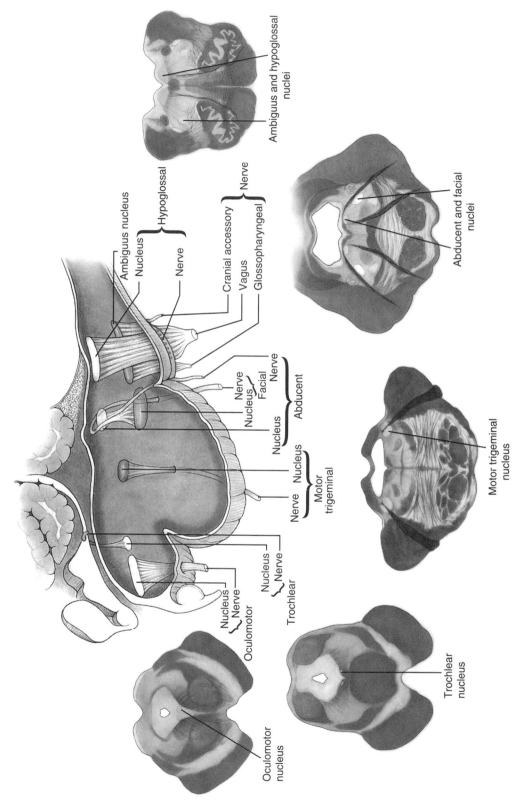

FIGURE 5-3. Distribution and relations of brainstem motor nuclei.

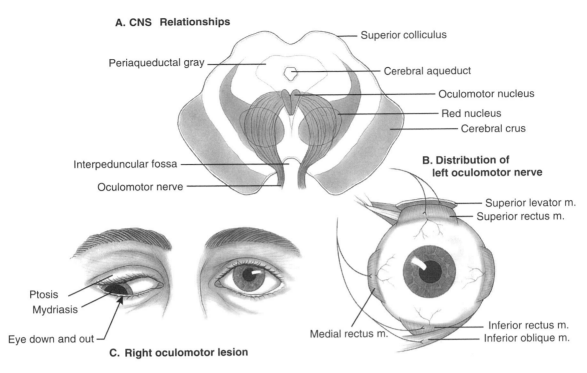

FIGURE 5–4. Oculomotor nucleus and nerve (III CN). **A.** CNS relations; **B.** Distribution; **C.** Lesion results.

rootlets pass ventrally and emerge in the wall of the interpeduncular fossa, just medial to the cerebral crus. The oculomotor nerve innervates five muscles: four external ocular muscles (superior, medial, and inferior rectus, and inferior oblique) and the levator of the superior eyelid.

> A lesion of the oculomotor nucleus or nerve results in ipsilateral ophthalmoplegia, in which the eye turns downward and outward, and **ptosis,** or sagging of the upper eyelid. In addition, because of the presence of the visceromotor components, an ipsilateral **mydriasis,** a dilated pupil, usually occurs, often as the initial sign of oculomotor **palsy.** Also, accommodation of the lens for near vision is lost. The affected eye is turned downward and outward because of the unopposed actions of the lateral rectus and superior oblique muscles, which are not supplied by the oculomotor nerve. The ptosis occurs because of paralysis of the levator muscle of the superior eyelid.

TROCHLEAR NUCLEUS AND CRANIAL NERVE IV

The trochlear nucleus is located at the ventral border of the periaqueductal gray of the mid-brain at the level of the inferior colliculus (Fig. 5–5). The trochlear (IV CN) rootlets arch dorsally and caudally in the outer part of the periaqueductal gray to reach the most rostral part of the pons. Here, they decussate in the superior medullary velum before emerging from the dorsal surface of the brainstem immediately caudal to the inferior colliculus. The trochlear nerve innervates the superior oblique muscle of the eye. The trochlear nerve differs from all other cranial nerves in two ways: It emerges at the dorsal surface of the brainstem and all of its fibers arise from the trochlear nucleus in the opposite side.

> Lesions of the trochlear nucleus are rare, but when they do happen, two abnormalities occur in the contralateral eye: a slight extorsion or outward rotation of the superior part of the globe, which is compensated for by a tilting of the head slightly downward and toward the contralateral shoulder, and a slight impairment of depression after the eye is adducted. The diplopia resulting from a trochlear palsy is most noticeable to the patient when walking down a stairway. When the trochlear nerve is damaged, these abnormalities are in the ipsilateral eye.

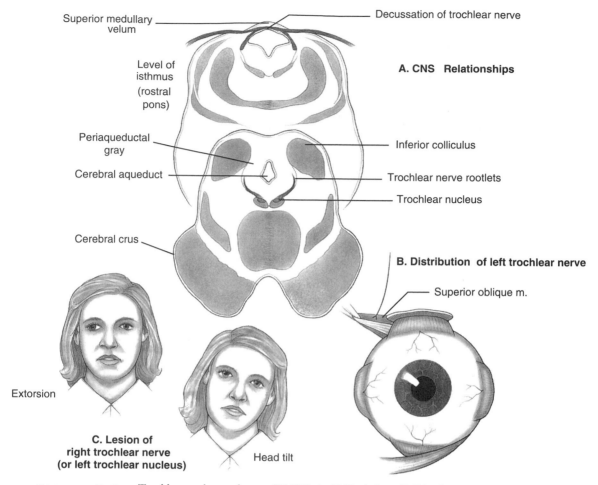

A. CNS Relationships

B. Distribution of left trochlear nerve

C. Lesion of right trochlear nerve (or left trochlear nucleus)

FIGURE 5–5. Trochlear nucleus and nerve (IV CN). **A.** CNS relations; **B.** Distribution; **C.** Lesion results.

MOTOR TRIGEMINAL NUCLEUS AND MOTOR ROOT OF CRANIAL NERVE V

The motor trigeminal nucleus lies in the dorsolateral part of the tegmentum at the mid-pontine level (Fig. 5–6). Its axons emerge in the motor root of the trigeminal nerve, and after entering the mandibular division they innervate mainly the muscles of mastication—the mas-seter, temporalis, and medial and lateral ptery-goid muscles.

ABDUCENT NUCLEUS AND CRANIAL NERVE VI

The abducent nucleus is located beneath the facial colliculus in the floor of the fourth ven-tricle in the caudal pons (Fig. 5–7). The abdu-cent (VI CN) rootlets pass ventrally near or through the lateral parts of the medial **lemnis-cus** and pyramidal tract and emerge in the pon-

> A lesion of the trigeminal motor nucleus, the motor root, or the mandibular nerve results in paralysis and wast-ing of the ipsilateral muscles of mastication. The opened jaw may also deviate to the ipsilateral side due to the unopposed action of the intact contralateral lateral pterygoid muscle.

> Lesions of the abducent nucleus or nerve result in medial deviation or **esotropia** and paralysis of abduction of the ipsilateral eye.

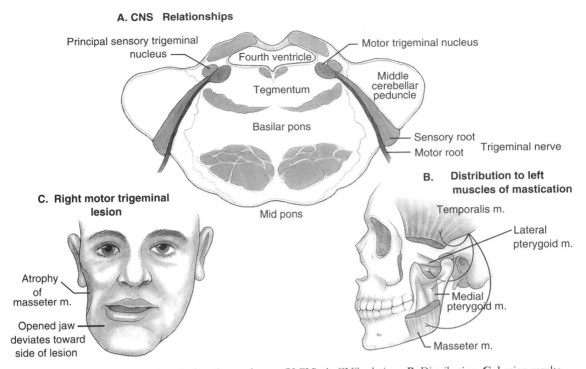

A. CNS Relationships

Principal sensory trigeminal nucleus

Fourth ventricle

Motor trigeminal nucleus

Tegmentum

Middle cerebellar peduncle

Basilar pons

Sensory root

Motor root

Trigeminal nerve

Mid pons

C. Right motor trigeminal lesion

Atrophy of masseter m.

Opened jaw deviates toward side of lesion

B. Distribution to left muscles of mastication

Temporalis m.

Lateral pterygoid m.

Medial pterygoid m.

Masseter m.

FIGURE 5–6. Motor trigeminal nucleus and nerve (V CN). **A.** CNS relations; **B.** Distribution; **C.** Lesion results.

A. CNS relationships

Facial colliculus

Fourth ventricle

Abducent nucleus

Medial lemniscus

Pyramidal tract

Abducent nerve

Caudal pons

B. Distribution of left abducent nerve

Lateral rectus muscle

Left eye

Esotropia

C. Right abducent lesion

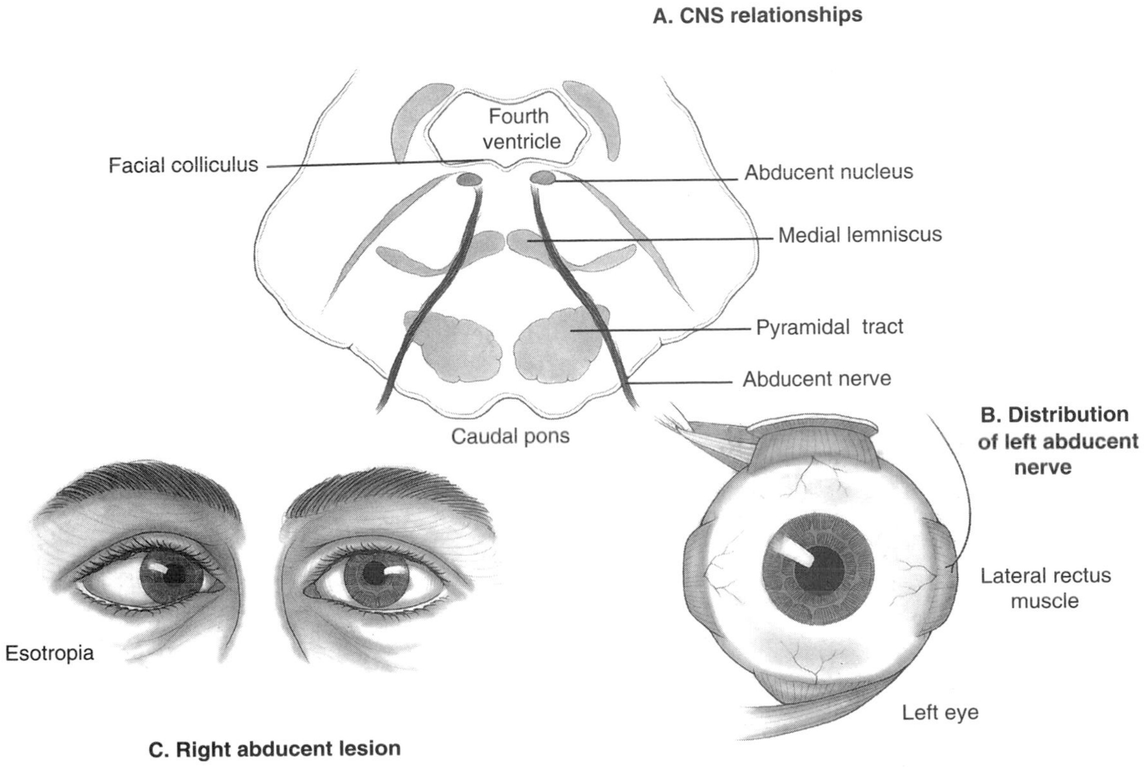

FIGURE 5–7. Abducent nucleus and nerve (VI CN). **A.** CNS relations, **B.** Distribution; **C.** Lesion results.

tomedullary junction, near the pyramid. The abducent nerve innervates the lateral rectus muscle of the eye.

FACIAL NUCLEUS AND MOTOR ROOT OF CRANIAL NERVE VII

The facial nucleus lies in the lateral part of the tegmentum of the caudal pons (Fig. 5–8). This motor nucleus is divided into two parts: a small part that innervates the upper facial muscles and a larger part that supplies the lower facial muscles.

The facial root fibers, on emerging from the nucleus, stream dorsomedially as individual fibers or in small groups (unobservable in myelin-stained sections) to the floor of the fourth ventricle where they form the ascending root of the facial nerve, a compact bundle directed rostrally for about 2 mm. The ascending root is located medial to the abducent nucleus, and at the rostral border of this nucleus the fibers of the ascending root arch over it as

the genu of the facial nerve. The fibers then course ventrolaterally, passing lateral to the facial nucleus before emerging in the lateral part of the pontomedullary junction in the **cerebellar angle.** The facial nucleus innervates the muscles of facial expression and several other muscles, including the stapedius.

Lesions of the facial nucleus or nerve result in paralysis of the ipsilateral facial muscles, both upper and lower. The most common lesion of the facial nerve occurs in **Bell palsy,** which produces weakness of both upper and lower facial muscles and inability to close the eye tightly (as given in the case at the beginning of this chapter). In addition, lacrimation, salivation, and taste may be impaired (due to involvement of secretory and gustatory fibers), accompanied by **hyperacusis** (abnormal loudness of hearing due to paralysis of the stapedius muscle). An inflammatory reaction of the nerve as it courses in the facial canal is the presumed cause of Bell palsy. The accompanying abnormalities depend on the location of the inflammation in the facial canal. Fortunately, most Bell palsy patients recover completely within a month or two.

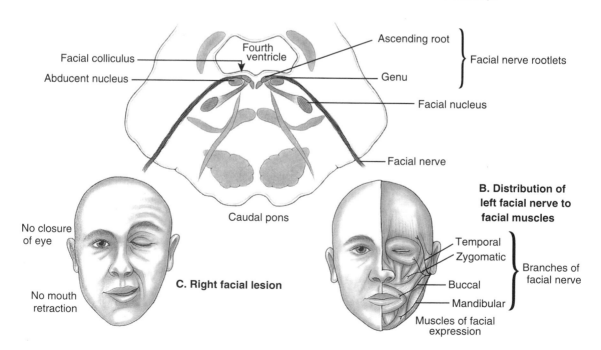

A. CNS Relationships

Facial colliculus — Fourth ventricle — Ascending root } Facial nerve rootlets
Abducent nucleus — Genu
Facial nucleus
Facial nerve

B. Distribution of left facial nerve to facial muscles

Temporal
Zygomatic } Branches of facial nerve
Buccal
Mandibular
Muscles of facial expression

Caudal pons

No closure of eye
No mouth retraction

C. Right facial lesion

FIGURE 5–8.   Facial nucleus and nerve (VII CN). **A.** CNS relations; **B.** Distribution; **C.** Lesion results.

NUCLEUS AMBIGUUS AND MOTOR ROOTS OF CRANIAL NERVES IX, X, AND XI

The nucleus ambiguus is an elongated column of α-motoneurons in the ventrolateral part of the reticular formation of the medulla (Fig. 5–9). Its axons emerge with the glossopharyngeal and vagus nerves and with the cranial part of the accessory nerve. The latter joins the vagus at the jugular foramen. The nucleus ambiguus supplies the skeletal muscles of the palate, pharynx, larynx, and upper esophagus; hence, it is involved in deglutition and phonation.

HYPOGLOSSAL NUCLEUS AND CRANIAL NERVE XII

This elongated motor nucleus is located in the floor of the medullary part of the fourth ventricle near the midline (Fig. 5–10). The rootlets pass ventrally through the medulla and emerge at the preolivary sulcus. Along their route they lie next to or in the lateral parts of the medial lemniscus and pyramidal tract. The hypoglossal nerve supplies the ipsilateral muscles of the tongue.

> A lesion of the rostral part of the nucleus, which gives axons to the glossopharyngeal nerve, results in **dysphagia** due to paralysis of the stylopharyngeus muscle. A lesion of the remainder of the nucleus, which supplies axons to the vagus and cranial accessory nerves, results in paralysis of the vocal muscles (causing hoarseness and vocal weakness). Paralysis of the palatal muscles results in sagging of the ipsilateral palatal arch and deviation of the uvula to the contralateral side. Bilateral lesions involving the vagal nerves or vagal components of the nucleus ambiguus may result in a closing of the airway severe enough to require tracheostomy.

> Lesions of the hypoglossal nucleus or nerve result in a paralysis and atrophy of the ipsilateral muscles of the tongue. Moreover, when protruded, the tongue deviates toward the side of the lesion due to the unopposed actions of the normal genioglossus and transverse muscles on the other side.

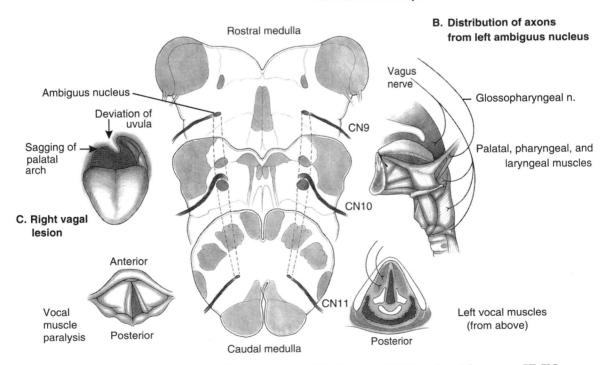

A. CNS Relationships

B. Distribution of axons from left ambiguus nucleus

Rostral medulla

Ambiguus nucleus

Deviation of uvula

Sagging of palatal arch

C. Right vagal lesion

Vocal muscle paralysis

Anterior

Posterior

Caudal medulla

Vagus nerve

Glossopharyngeal n.

CN9

CN10

Palatal, pharyngeal, and laryngeal muscles

CN11

Posterior

Left vocal muscles (from above)

FIGURE 5–9. Ambiguus nucleus and glossopharyngeal (IX CN); vagus (X CN); and cranial accessory (XI CN) nerves. **A.** CNS relations; **B.** Distribution; **C.** Lesion results.

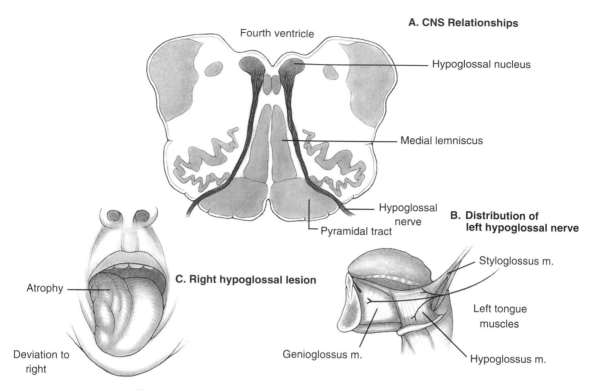

A. CNS Relationships

Fourth ventricle

Hypoglossal nucleus

Medial lemniscus

Hypoglossal nerve

Pyramidal tract

B. Distribution of left hypoglossal nerve

C. Right hypoglossal lesion

Atrophy

Deviation to right

Styloglossus m.

Left tongue muscles

Genioglossus m.

Hypoglossus m.

FIGURE 5–10.   Hypoglossal nucleus and nerve (XII CN). **A.** CNS relations; **B.** Distribution; **C.** Lesion results.

SPINAL CORD LOWER MOTOR NEURONS

In the spinal cord, the lower motor neurons make up two main cell columns forming lamina IX in the anterior horn. The medial column is uniform in size and, for the most part, extends through the length of the cord; it supplies the paravertebral or paraxial musculature. The lateral column varies segmentally; it is relatively small in the thoracic segments because its neurons here innervate only the intercostal and abdominal muscles. In contrast, the lateral column is extremely large in the cervical and lumbar enlargements, where it is subdivided into a number of nuclei. The more lateral nuclei of the lateral column supply the more distal muscles of the limbs, whereas the more medial nuclei supply muscles located more proximally (Figs. 5–11, 5–12).

The spinal α-motoneurons innervating any muscle (other than an intercostal muscle), are found in more than one spinal cord segment. Thus, in addition to a medial-lateral represen- tation of muscles in the spinal cord, a segmen- tal representation is present as well. The mus- cles innervated by a single spinal cord segment form a **myotome.** The segmental innervation of some important groups of muscles is given in Table 5–1.

Three groups of motor neurons, the spinal accessory nu- cleus and phrenic nucleus in the cervical region and Onuf nucleus in the sacral, are of special interest. The spinal accessory nucleus is located in the upper 5 or 6 cervical segments. It gives rise to the spinal part of the accessory nerve, which innervates the sternomastoid and trapezius muscles. Lesions of this component of the accessory nerve result in weakness in turning of the head to the opposite side and in shrugging the ipsilat- eral shoulder. The phrenic nucleus, whose axons inner- vate the diaphragm, is located in cervical segments 3, 4, and 5. Lesions of this nucleus, or of the descending fibers to it, result in paralysis of the ipsilateral hemidi- aphragm or, if bilateral, in respiratory failure. Onuf nu- cleus makes up a distinct group of α-motor neurons in sacral segments 2, 3, and 4. These neurons innervate the external urethral and anal sphincters and, hence, play a major role in continence mechanisms.

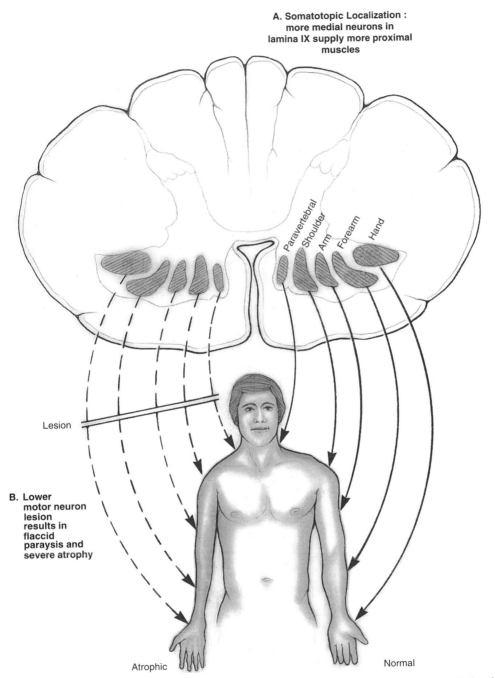

A. Somatotopic Localization :
more medial neurons in
lamina IX supply more proximal
muscles

Paravertebral
Shoulder
Arm
Forearm
Hand

Lesion

B. Lower
motor neuron
lesion
results in
flaccid
paraysis and
severe atrophy

Atrophic   Normal

FIGURE 5–11.   Lower motor neurons of cervical enlargement. **A.** Somatotopic localization; **B.** Results of lesions.

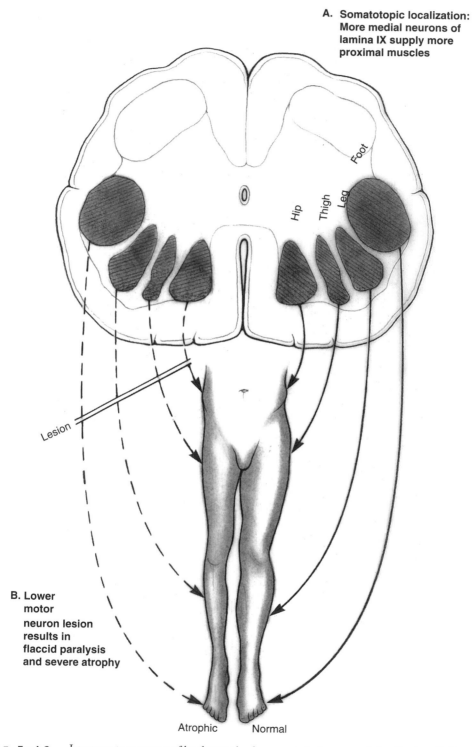

A. Somatotopic localization:
More medial neurons of
lamina IX supply more
proximal muscles

Foot

Leg

Thigh

Hip

Lesion

B. Lower
motor
neuron lesion
results in
flaccid paralysis
and severe atrophy

Atrophic   Normal

FIGURE 5–12.   Lower motor neurons of lumbosacral enlargement. **A.** Somatotopic localization; **B.** Results of lesions.

TABLE 5-1. SEGMENTAL INNERVATION OF SELECTED MUSCLES

MUSCLES	NERVES
Trapezius	C3, C4 and spinal part of XI CN
Deltoid	C5*, C6
Biceps	C5, C6*
Triceps	C6, C7*, C8
Flexor digitorum profundus	C7, C8*, T1
Thenar, hypothenar, interossei	C8, T1*
Abdominal	T6–L1
Quadriceps	L2, L3, L4*
Extensor hallucis	L4, L5*, S1
Gastrocnemius	L5, S1*, S2
Rectal sphincter	S3, S4

Provide major innervation.

TABLE 5-2. MORE COMMONLY TESTED MYOTATIC REFLEXES

MUSCLE OR TENDON	NERVE	CRUCIAL SPINAL CORD SEGMENT
Biceps	Musculocutaneous	C6
Triceps	Radial	C7
Patellar	Femoral	L4
Achilles	Tibial and sciatic	S1

REFLEX ACTIVITY OF SPINAL MOTONEURONS

The lower motor neurons in the spinal cord are involved in numerous reflex mechanisms, three of which are of clinical importance—the **myotatic**, the **inverse myotatic**, and the **γ-loop reflexes.**

MYOTATIC REFLEX

The myotatic reflex is the contraction of a muscle when it is stretched. The myotatic reflex, which is also called the tendon or stretch reflex, is monosynaptic (Fig. 5–13). To initiate the re-flex, the muscle is stretched by tapping either the muscle itself or its tendon with a reflex hammer. The afferent limb of the reflex consists of **Ia afferent fibers** and their **annulospiral stretch receptors** located at the center of muscle spindles. An Ia afferent fiber is the peripheral branch of the axon of a unipolar neuron in a dorsal root or spinal ganglion. The central branch of the unipolar neuron's axon has excitatory synapses on lower motor or α-motor neurons in lamina IX of the anterior horn. The axons of the lower motor neurons enter the appropriate spinal nerves via their ventral roots and synapse in the muscle that has been stretched, thereby causing it to contract. The more commonly tested myotatic reflexes and their central and peripheral components are given in Table 5–2.

INVERSE MYOTATIC REFLEX

The contraction of voluntary muscle is influenced by tendon receptors that respond to increases in tension. Such receptors are the **Golgi tendon organs,** which are the endings of nerve

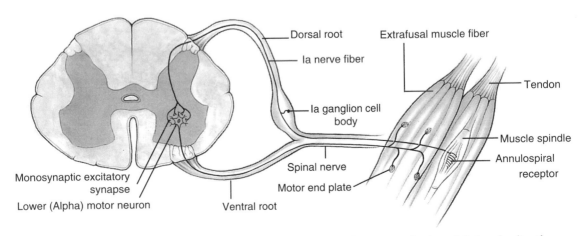

FIGURE 5-13. The myotatic reflex. Muscle stretch → annulospiral receptor activation → Ia impulse directly excites lower motor neuron → contraction of muscle stretched.

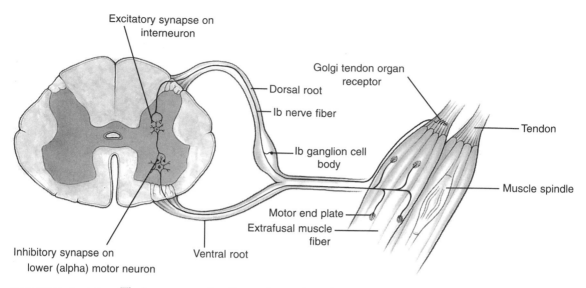

FIGURE 5–14.   The inverse myotatic reflex: tendon tension → Golgi tendon organ activation → Ib impulse excites interneuron which, in turn, inhibits lower motor neuron → relaxation of muscle whose tendon had increased tension. Prevents tendon tear.

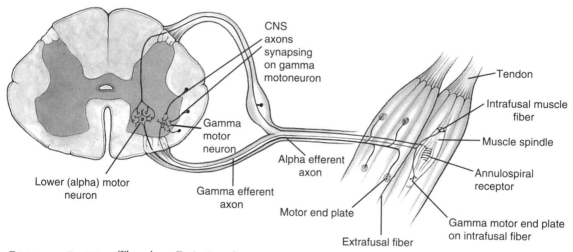

FIGURE 5–15.   The γ-loop. Excitation of γ-motor neuron → contraction of intrafusal muscle fibers at poles of muscle spindle → stretch of annulospiral receptor. Regulates muscle spindle excitability.

fibers belonging to the Ib afferent system. The **Ib afferent fibers** decrease the contraction of their own muscles by inactivation or inhibition of the α-motoneurons that supply these muscles. This α-motoneuron inactivation occurs through inhibitory interneurons on which the Ib afferent fibers synapse (Fig. 5–14). The inverse myotatic reflex, also called the lengthening or autogenic inhibition reflex, protects the tendon from an injury that would result from too much tension. It also plays an important

role in mechanisms related to fatigue and hyperextension or hyperflexion of a joint.

THE γ-LOOP

In addition to the populations of large lower or α-motoneurons in the anterior horn of the spinal cord, numerous small γ-motoneurons exist here. The axons of the γ-motoneurons, which are about one third of the total ventral root fibers, supply the **intrafusal muscle fibers** at the poles of muscle spindles. On contracting, the intrafusal muscle fibers stretch the central parts of the muscle spindles, where the annulospiral stretch receptors are located. By regulating the stretch or tautness in the central receptor part of the muscle spindle, the γ-motoneuron can maintain the sensitivity of the muscle spindles when an entire muscle is contracting or shortening during voluntary or reflex contractions.

The γ-system of motoneurons can participate in the activation and control of movements by producing enough muscle spindle tautness to stimulate the annulospiral stretch receptors, thereby eliciting myotatic reflexes. This mechanism, referred to as the γ-loop (Fig. 5–15), can be influenced by various centers in the brain.

LOWER MOTOR NEURON SYNDROME

Injury to lower motor neurons interrupts the flow of impulses along the final common path and results in **flaccid paralysis,** or paralysis accompanied by hypotonia (because lower motor neurons maintain normal tone). In addition, there occur decreased or absent superficial and deep reflexes (because lower motor neurons form the efferent limbs of all skeletal muscle reflexes). Spontaneous twitches or fasciculation may also take place. Finally, pronounced decrease in bulk (atrophy) occurs in the denervated muscles after weeks to months (Figs. 5–11, 5–12).

The **lower motor neuron syndrome** may occur from either CNS or PNS lesions. In the former, cell bodies or intramedullary rootlets are involved, whereas in the latter the axons within peripheral nerves are involved. Another feature of the lower motor neuron syndrome is that the paralysis and atrophy are segmental, i.e., these abnormalities are limited to the individual muscles denervated by the lesion; no other muscles are involved.

CHAPTER REVIEW QUESTIONS

5–1. Define the term "motor unit" and compare those involved in delicate and coarse movements.

5–2. What is the most clinically important feature of lower motor neurons?

5–3. What abnormalities result from the lesion, appearing as a cross-hatched area, in each section below?

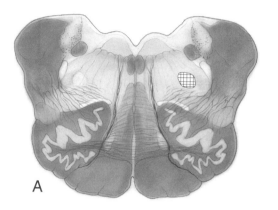

A

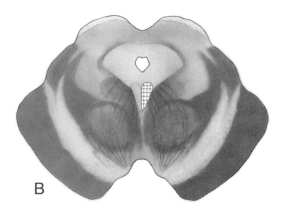

B

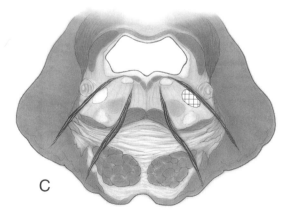

C

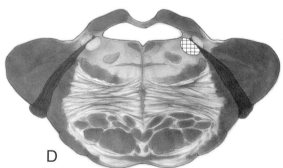

D

THE PYRAMIDAL SYSTEM: SPASTIC PARALYSIS

■ **A 60-year-old hypertensive man has sudden headache accompanied by spastic hemiplegia on the right side of the body. An extensor plantar response is present on the right side, tendon reflexes of the right limbs are exaggerated, and resistance to passive movements are increased. Also, the lower facial muscles on the right are weak.**

The pyramidal system is composed of the upper motor neurons in the cerebral cortex. Their axons pass without interruption to lower motoneurons or their interneuronal pools for the purpose of initiating and regulating voluntary movements (especially the more skilled movements). Most pyramidal system neuronal cell bodies are located in the precentral gyrus and anterior part of the paracentral lobule.

Axons of the pyramidal system destined for the spinal motor nuclei form the pyramidal or corticospinal tract, those destined for brainstem motor nuclei form the corticobulbar (or corticonuclear) tract.

THE PYRAMIDAL OR CORTICOSPINAL TRACT

The pyramidal tract arises from upper motor neurons mostly in the primary motor area (MI) located in the precentral gyrus and anterior part of the paracentral lobule (Figs. 6–1, 6–2). A large number of neurons in the premotor area, immediately anterior to MI, and the primary sensory area in the postcentral gyrus and posterior part of the paracentral lobule also contribute fibers. Whether the neurons in the primary sensory area

should be considered "upper motor neurons" is questionable because their function is to modulate secondary sensory neurons in the spinal cord.

Those corticospinal neurons influencing the upper limb are located in the more dorsal parts of the precentral gyrus, where contralateral upper limb movements are represented. The corticospinal neurons influencing the lower limb are located in the anterior part of the paracentral lobule, where contralateral lower limb movements are represented.

After leaving the cortex, the pyramidal tract axons descend through the **corona radiata** to reach the posterior limb of the internal capsule (Figs. 6–1, 6–2). After passing through the internal capsule, the pyramidal tract enters the cerebral crus, where it is located in the middle third (Fig. 6–3). The cerebral crus is said to contain about 20 million fibers; only a minority of these, 1 to 2 million, are corticospinal fibers. Most of the others are corticopontine fibers that are associated with the cerebellar system.

At the caudal end of the midbrain, the pyramidal tract separates into bundles, which enter the basilar part of the pons. These bundles are separated from one another by the pontine nuclei and the transversely directed pontine fibers. As the pyramidal bundles descend through the pons, they gradually move closer together, so that on entering the medulla, they again form one bundle, the medullary pyramid (after which the pyramidal tract was named).

The pyramid extends through the rostral two thirds of the medulla. In the caudal third of the medulla, its fibers cross in the pyramidal decussation. Here, the decussating fibers (ordinarily

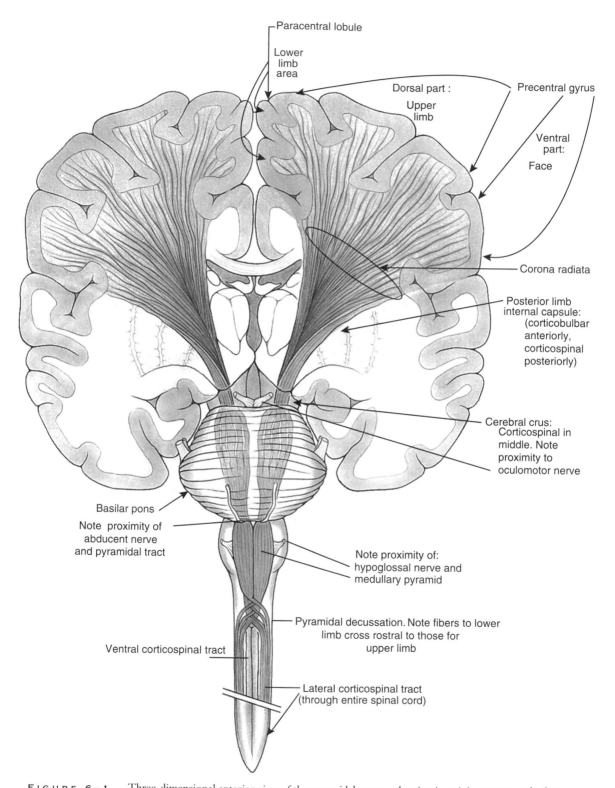

FIGURE 6-1.   Three-dimensional anterior view of the pyramidal system, showing its origin, course, and relations.

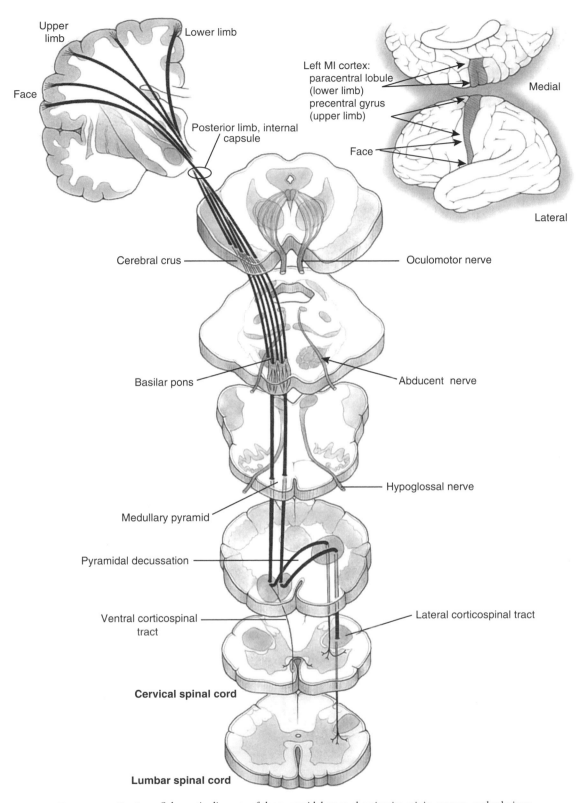

FIGURE 6-2. Schematic diagram of the pyramidal tract, showing its origin, course, and relations.

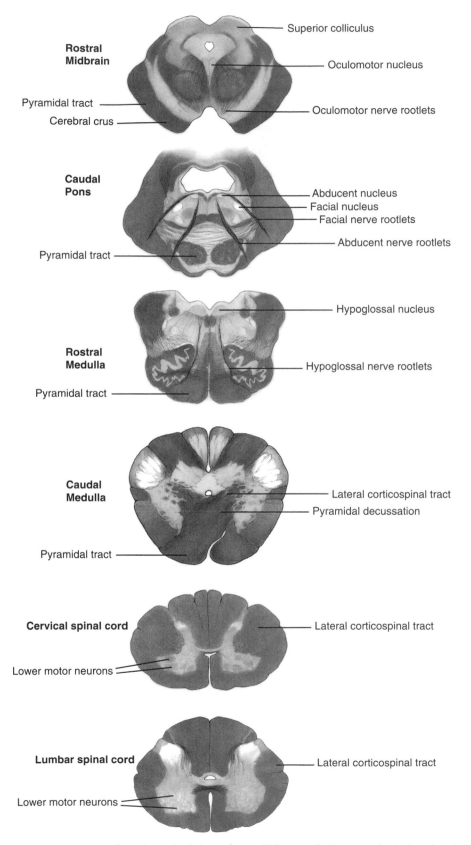

Rostral Midbrain

Superior colliculus

Oculomotor nucleus

Pyramidal tract

Oculomotor nerve rootlets

Cerebral crus

Caudal Pons

Abducent nucleus
Facial nucleus
Facial nerve rootlets

Abducent nerve rootlets

Pyramidal tract

Rostral Medulla

Hypoglossal nucleus

Hypoglossal nerve rootlets

Pyramidal tract

Caudal Medulla

Lateral corticospinal tract
Pyramidal decussation

Pyramidal tract

Cervical spinal cord

Lateral corticospinal tract

Lower motor neurons

Lumbar spinal cord

Lateral corticospinal tract

Lower motor neurons

FIGURE 6-3.   Location and relations of pyramidal tract in brainstem and spinal cord sections.

composing about 90% of the pyramidal tract), pass dorsolaterally and form the lateral corticospinal tract, which descends through all spinal cord levels in the dorsal half of the lateral funiculus. The uncrossed pyramidal fibers continue directly into the anterior funiculus of the spinal cord as the ventral corticospinal tract (usually limited to the cervical segments). Most fibers of the ventral corticospinal tract decussate in the ventral white commissure at the level at which they terminate. They bilaterally innervate the most medial motor nuclei, which supply paraxial muscles that act in unison with each other. As far as the limbs are concerned, the corticospinal tracts should be considered completely crossed.

THE CORTICOBULBAR OR CORTICONUCLEAR TRACT

The corticobulbar tract is formed from the upper motoneurons located primarily in the ven-

tral part of the precentral gyrus, the face region of the motor cortex. The corticobulbar tract accompanies the pyramidal tract through the corona radiata and the internal capsule (Figs. 6–1, 6–2).

For many years it was thought that within the internal capsule, the corticobulbar fibers are located at the **genu** whereas the corticospinal fibers are located in the adjacent part of the posterior limb. Recent evidence, based on electrical stimulation in humans and studies of autopsy specimens, suggests that both groups of fibers are located in the posterior half of the posterior limb. Actually, depending on the capsular level, both views are true. Careful dissections show that the tracts gradually shift from anterior to posterior as they descend through the capsule en route from the corona radiata to the cerebral crus. As a result, a lesion in the posterior half of the posterior limb in the dorsal part of the internal capsule does not damage the corticobulbar tract, whereas a similarly located lesion in the ventral part does damage this tract.

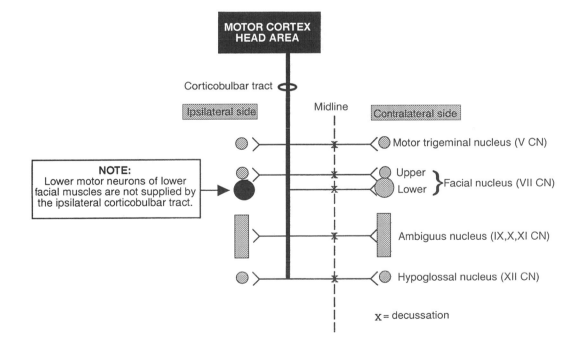

Below the internal capsule the corticobulbar fibers are difficult to identify. Some descend in relation to the corticospinal fibers, others descend within the tegmentum of the pons and medulla. As the corticobulbar tract passes caudally through the brainstem, it continuously gives off fibers to the various motor nuclei of the cranial nerves.

Limb movements are controlled by the contralateral cerebral cortex. However, muscles on both sides of the trunk or head that ordinarily act in unison are influenced by the motor cortex of both sides. Thus, the motor nuclei associated with mastication, deglutition, phonation, and lingual movements are influenced by corticobulbar fibers arising from both the contralateral and ipsilateral hemispheres (Fig. 6–4). As a result, unilateral lesions of the corticobulbar tract above the level of the facial nucleus are manifested by abnormalities that are most pronounced in the lower part of the face contralaterally. Because the cerebral cortex exerts a more powerful influence even on contralateral muscles that work in unison with their homologues on the opposite side, transient contralateral abnormalities may occur after acute unilateral cortical or capsular lesions. Such transient abnormalities occur especially in the case of the soft palate and tongue.

The nuclei innervating the external ocular muscles are not under the direct influence of the cerebral cortex. Voluntary eye movements are so intricate that they are controlled by cortical centers, which influence specialized gaze centers in the brainstem (as is described later with the ocular motor system).

THE UPPER MOTOR NEURON SYNDROME

Lesions involving the pyramidal system, especially the pyramidal tract, are common. This is because the pyramidal tract extends through the entire brain and spinal cord, thereby making it susceptible to vascular and traumatic damage at any CNS level. Moreover, the pyramidal tract contains numerous myelinated nerve fibers that make it susceptible to damage in demyelinating diseases such as multiple sclerosis (MS) and amyotrophic lateral sclerosis (ALS).

A lesion of the upper motor neuron is also called a **supranuclear lesion** because damage occurs in the pathway carrying impulses to the lower motor neuron. A lesion of lower motor neurons is called a **nuclear lesion** when the neuronal cell bodies are involved and an **infranuclear lesion** when the lower motor neuron axons are involved. The principal signs of the upper motor neuron syndrome (as given in the introductory case in this chapter) include the absence of volitional movements (paralysis), increased muscle tone, exaggerated myotatic reflexes, and an extensor plantar response—all of these in the contralateral limbs. A comparison of the upper and lower motor neuron syndromes is in Table 6–1.

CAPSULAR STROKE

The most frequent pyramidal system disorder results from a vascular accident in the internal capsule and is called "capsular stroke." Following interruption of the corticospinal and corticobulbar tracts in the internal capsule, there is paralysis of the contralateral upper and lower limbs and the contralateral lower facial muscles. In some cases, a transient weakness may be seen on the contralateral side of the tongue and soft palate due to corticobulbar tract damage.

Immediately after a capsular stroke, volitional movements in the contralateral limbs are absent. With time, movements in the more proximal parts of the limbs recover rather completely, but the recovery of movements in more distal parts is less complete. Rapid individual finger movements such as those used in playing a piano never return. The basis for this partial return of volitional movements is described in Chapter 7.

In addition to the paralysis, the patient has **hypertonia** or increased muscle tone. This is manifested by increased resistance to passive stretch and is especially pronounced in the antigravity muscles, that is, the flexors of the arm and fingers and the extensors of the leg. Severe hypertonia is **spasticity** and this, accompanied by the loss of volitional movements contralaterally, is called spastic hemiplegia (Fig. 6–5). A characteristic of the increased resistance seen in spasticity is the **clasp-knife response** (Fig. 6–6). This response consists of a sudden col-

T A B L E   6 – 1 .   COMPARISON OF UPPER AND LOWER MOTOR NEURON SYNDROMES

	UPPER MOTOR NEURON OR SUPRANUCLEAR LESION	LOWER MOTOR NEURON OR NUCLEAR-INFRANUCLEAR LESION	
Possible locations	CNS only	CNS	PNS
Common causes	CVA, tumors, trauma, demyelinating diseases (MS, ALS), infectious diseases	CVA, polio, tumor, trauma (ruptured disc, gun shot, etc.)	Trauma, metabolic disorders (alcoholism, diabetes)
Structures involved	Upper motor neurons in cerebral cortex or corticospinal and nuclear tracts	Brainstem or spinal α-motoneurons or their intramedullary rootlets	Motor fibers in every cerebrospinal nerve *except* I CN, II CN, and VIII CN
Distribution of abnormalities	Never individual muscles—groups of muscles supplied by motor nuclei below level of lesion Corticonuclear—contralateral lower facial muscles Corticospinal—limb muscles—contralateral if lesion is above decussation, ipsilateral if below	Segmental—limited to muscles innervated by damaged α-motoneurons or their axons	
Status of voluntary movements	Deficient—paralysis or paresis especially of skilled movements	Deficient—paralysis, final common pathway interrupted	
Character of passive stretch (status of muscle tone)	Increased—particularly in antigravity muscles (flexors of upper limbs, extensors of hip and knee, plantar flexors of foot and toes); clasp-knife response may be present	Decreased—loss of final common path produces hypotonicity in affected muscles	
Status of myotatic reflexes	Hyperactive or exaggerated—muscle spindle threshold decreased; clonus may be present	Decreased or absent—efferent limb of reflex interrupted	
Status of cutaneous reflexes	Abnormalities in some—plantar becomes extensor rather than flexor; i.e., extensor plantar or Babinski sign	Decreased or absent—plantar reflex, if present, is of normal flexor type except in infants	
Muscle bulk	Slight atrophy due to disuse	Pronounced atrophy—70–80%	
Classical description	Spastic paralysis	Flaccid paralysis	

lapse of all resistance while a muscle is being rapidly stretched. The clasp-knife effect is due to increased activity of the Golgi tendon organs whose Ib afferent fibers are excitatory to spinal interneurons that inhibit the α-motoneurons responsible for the hypertonia and increased resistance to passive stretch (Fig. 5–14).

In the upper motor neuron syndrome, the myotatic reflexes are most hyperactive or exaggerated in the antigravity muscles; for example, the biceps muscle in the upper limb and the quadriceps muscle in the lower limb. As a result, the biceps and patellar reflexes are exaggerated (Fig. 6–7). Accompanying the severe hyperactive reflexes that occur in spastic hemiplegia is **clonus,** which consists of a rapid series of rhythmical contractions that are elicited by stretching a muscle (Fig. 6–8). Clonus is due to the hyperactive myotatic reflexes; the brisk

contraction of one group of muscles is sufficient to initiate myotatic responses in their antagonists, and so forth.

The most well-known sign associated with the upper motor neuron syndrome is the **extensor plantar** or **Babinski response** (Fig. 6–9). This abnormal cutaneous reflex consists of extension or dorsiflexion of the large toe and fanning of the other toes on stroking the lateral aspect of the sole of the foot with a hard, blunt instrument. When the corticospinal system is normal, this stimulus elicits flexion of all the toes—the flexor plantar response. The Babinski sign is a spinal withdrawal reflex that is normally suppressed directly by the cerebral cortex. It is seen in normal infants before the corticospinal tract is fully myelinated and functional; otherwise, it is almost invariably associated with corticospinal tract damage.

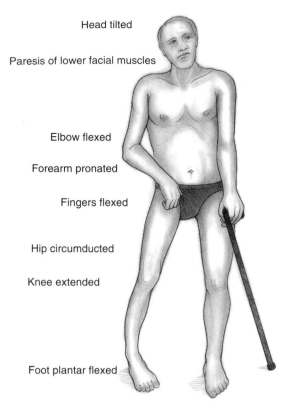

Head tilted

Paresis of lower facial muscles

Elbow flexed

Forearm pronated

Fingers flexed

Hip circumducted

Knee extended

Foot plantar flexed

FIGURE 6-5.   Right spastic hemiplegic. Gait resulting from left capsular lesion.

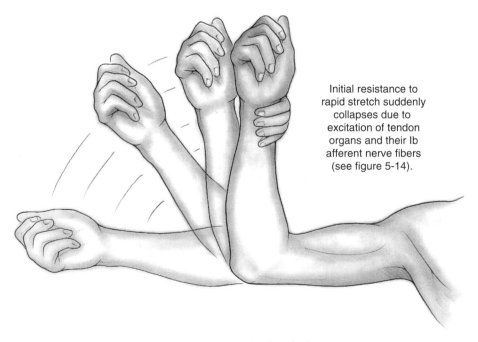

Initial resistance to rapid stretch suddenly collapses due to excitation of tendon organs and their Ib afferent nerve fibers (see figure 5-14).

FIGURE 6-6.   The clasp-knife response.

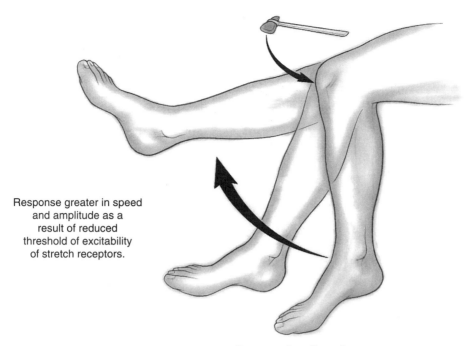

Response greater in speed and amplitude as a result of reduced threshold of excitability of stretch receptors.

FIGURE 6−7.   Exaggerated patellar reflex.

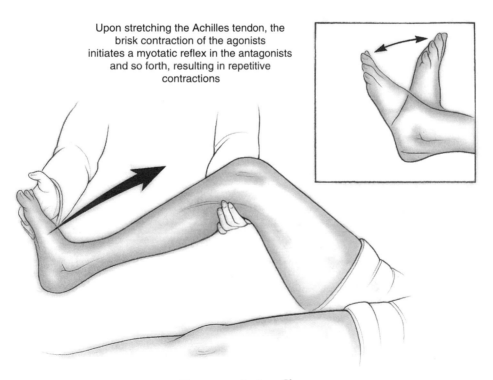

Upon stretching the Achilles tendon, the brisk contraction of the agonists initiates a myotatic reflex in the antagonists and so forth, resulting in repetitive contractions

FIGURE 6−8.   Clonus.

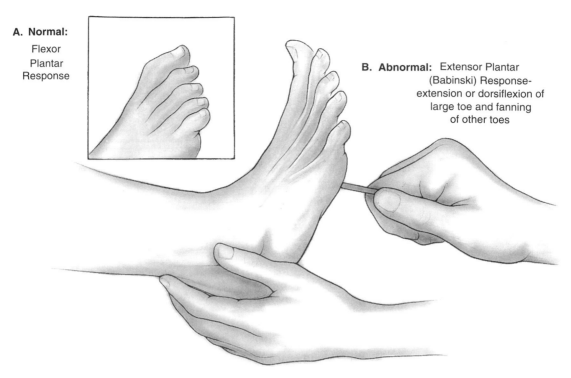

A. Normal:
Flexor Plantar Response

B. Abnormal: Extensor Plantar (Babinski) Response- extension or dorsiflexion of large toe and fanning of other toes

FIGURE 6–9.   Plantar responses. **A.** Normal flexor. **B.** Abnormal extensor or Babinski.

COMBINED UPPER AND LOWER MOTOR NEURON LESIONS

Lesions that damage the pyramidal tract at certain brainstem levels may also involve the intramedullary rootlets of lower motor neurons. These lesions produce combined upper and lower motor neuron signs. The most common of these lesions involves the rootlets of cranial nerves III, VI, or XII, which in their intramedullary courses become closely related to the pyramidal tract (Figs. 6–1, 6–2, 6–3). Due to the pyramidal tract damage, contralateral spastic hemiplegia results in all cases. Because the upper motor neuron deficit is manifested contralaterally and the cranial nerve or lower motor neuron deficit is ipsilateral, these conditions are referred to as **alternating hemiplegia** or crossed paralyses. The conditions are indicative of a brainstem lesion.

Combined upper and lower motor neuron lesions also occur in the spinal cord. In such spinal cord lesions, spasticity and the other upper motor neuron lesion phenomena occur below the level

When a lesion interrupting the pyramidal tract in the cerebral crus extends medially to include the rootlets of the oculomotor nerve, the contralateral spastic hemiplegia is accompanied by ipsilateral ophthalmoplegia with the eye turned down and out, ptosis, and mydriasis (Fig. 5–4). This combination of signs is referred to as alternating oculomotor hemiplegia, superior alternating hemiplegia, or more commonly, **Weber syndrome.** When a lesion of the pyramidal tract in the basilar pons extends laterally to include the rootlets of the abducent nerve, the contralateral spastic hemiplegia is accompanied by an ipsilateral esotropia and paralysis of abduction (Fig. 5–7). This is known as the alternating abducent hemiplegia syndrome or middle alternating hemiplegia. When a lesion of the corticospinal tract in the medullary pyramid extends laterally to include the rootlets of the hypoglossal nerve, the contralateral spastic hemiplegia is accompanied by paralysis of the ipsilateral side of the tongue (Fig. 5–10). This is called the alternating hypoglossal hemiplegia syndrome or inferior alternating hemiplegia.

of the lesion, whereas flaccid paralysis and the other lower motor neuron lesion phenomena occur at the level of the lesion. Both the upper and lower motor neuron signs occur ipsilaterally.

A patient whose spinal cord has been damaged on one side (hemisection) at C8 and T1 would have spasticity, extensor plantar sign, etc. in the ipsilateral lower limb, and flaccid paralysis, atrophy, etc. in the intrinsic muscles of the ipsilateral hand.

SPINAL LESIONS

The pyramidal tracts are frequently damaged in the spinal cord. Such injuries most often occur with fractures or dislocations of cervical or thoracic vertebrae caused by automobile accidents or similar types of impact accidents, although vascular accidents, tumors, and inflammatory diseases may also be causes.

Dislocations and fractures occur most frequently in the lower cervical region and at the thoracolumbar junction. Such injuries usually compress the spinal cord and cause a variable amount of damage. Damage is manifested by a complete loss or a partial loss of function below the level of injury.

When a partial loss of function follows spinal cord trauma, most frequently the damage involves its central part, thus sparing the periphery. In this case, motor activity (and sensations) associated with the lower sacral segments of the spinal cord remain intact even in the acute stage of injury. This phenomenon is called **sacral sparing.**

When sacral sparing is present, the injured person's recovery of other spinal cord functions is much more likely than when sacral sparing is absent. The anatomical basis for sacral sparing is the somatotopic localization in the long ascending and descending paths where fibers carrying impulses to or from the sacral segments are located nearer the surface of the spinal cord, whereas those carrying impulses from more rostral levels are located deeper.

When the spinal cord is completely transected, three functional abnormalities immediately occur in the parts of the body supplied by the spinal cord segments below the lesion:

1. All voluntary movements are lost, completely and permanently.

2. All sensations are lost, completely and permanently.

3. All reflexes involving the isolated spinal cord segments are temporarily abolished.

This areflexia is the result of **spinal shock,** characterized by an absence of neural activity due to the sudden interruption of all supraspinal control. It persists for 1 to 6 weeks; the average is about 3 weeks. Following the shock stage, extensor plantar responses appear initially, followed by heightened reflex activity; eventually the limbs become spastic. Spontaneous and cutaneously provoked spasms may occur; initially these spasms are flexor, but later are both flexor and extensor in nature.

The level of the transection is determined from the clinical picture. With complete transection at C7 or above, the upper and lower limbs are paralyzed (**quadriplegia**). If the lesion is above C5, respiration is also impaired. Transection at the level of C8-T1 results in paralysis of the lower limbs (**paraplegia**) and weakness in both hands. Thoracic and lumbar transections also result in paraplegia. In addition to the paralysis and loss of sensations, autonomic dysfunctions occur in spinal cord injuries. In acute cervical lesions, "sympathetic shock" results in **bradycardia,** hypotension, **miosis,** and difficulties with temperature regulation, (all of which persist for only a few days). The more permanent autonomic disturbances seen with complete spinal cord transection include incontinence and impotence.

CHAPTER REVIEW QUESTIONS

6–1. Give the anatomical basis for the pyramidal tract's high susceptibility to injury.

6–2. What are the chief distinctions between upper and lower motor neuron lesions affecting the facial muscles?

6–3. What abnormalities result from the lesion, appearing as a cross-hatched area in each section below?

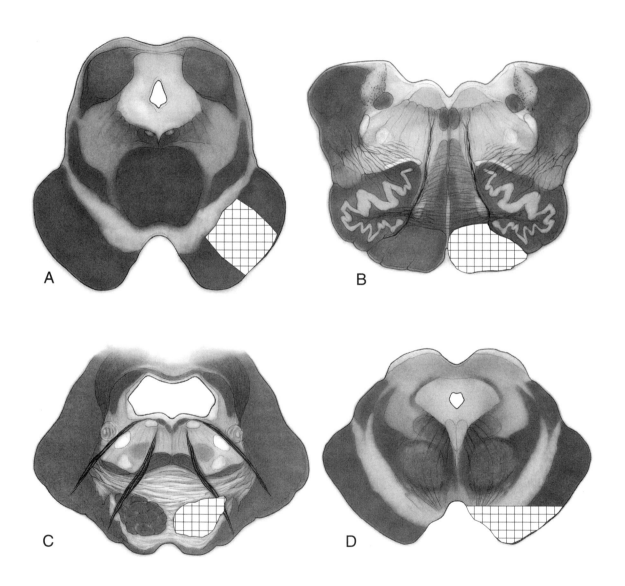

BRAINSTEM MOTOR CENTERS: DECEREBRATE POSTURING AND POSTCAPSULAR LESION RECOVERY

■ **Two comatose patients respond differently to sudden startling auditory or painful stimuli. In one patient, the upper and lower limbs extend; in the other, the lower limbs extend and the upper limbs flex.**

The organization of complex movements that are controlled by the spinal cord involves the activity of neurons at many levels. The spinal lower motor neurons, which are the final common paths for all voluntary movements of the head, neck, trunk, and limbs, are influenced by the pyramidal system upper motor neurons in the cerebral cortex, as well as by centers in the brainstem and in the spinal cord. These supraspinal centers in the brainstem play a major role in the abnormal posturing that occurs in comatose patients and in the partial recovery of volitional movements after lesions in the internal capsule.

BRAINSTEM SUPRASPINAL CENTERS AND THEIR PATHWAYS

The principal brainstem centers that influence spinal motor activity are the vestibular nuclear complex, nuclei in the reticular formation, and the red nuclei.

VESTIBULAR NUCLEI

One of the main functions of the vestibular system is equilibrium or balance. The vestibular system keeps the body on an even keel with the head when the position of the head changes.

The receptors that respond to position of the head, as well as the receptors that respond to rapid rotation of the head and to hearing, are located in the **bony labyrinth** of the internal ear. The bony labyrinth consists of the vestibule, the semicircular canals, and the cochlea. Within the fluid-filled cavity of the bony labyrinth are a series of fluid-filled membranes that form the **membranous labyrinth** (Fig. 7–1): the utricle and saccule in the vestibule, the semicircular ducts in the semicircular canals, and the cochlear duct in the cochlea.

In the walls of each utricle and saccule is a small thickened area called the **macula.** The maculae are the receptors for balance and are oriented at right angles to each other, with that of the utricle being almost in the horizontal plane and that of the saccule in almost the sagittal plane. Hence, changes in position of the head in any direction stimulate a macula on each side. Each macula consists of neuroepithelial hair cells and supporting cells (Fig. 7–1). Overlaying the hair cells is the gelatinous **otolithic membrane** that contains calcium carbonate crystals, the **otoliths** (ear stones) or **otoconia.** When the position of the head changes, gravity causes the otolithic membrane to move, bending the neuroepithelial **stereocilia** embedded in it. This mechanical stimulus is transduced into a receptor potential that then excites the dendrites of the bipolar vestibular ganglion cells, which are in synaptic contact with the hair cells.

The vestibular part of cranial nerve VIII is formed by the central processes of the bipolar cells of the vestibular ganglion (Fig. 7–1). The vestibular nerve enters the brainstem with the

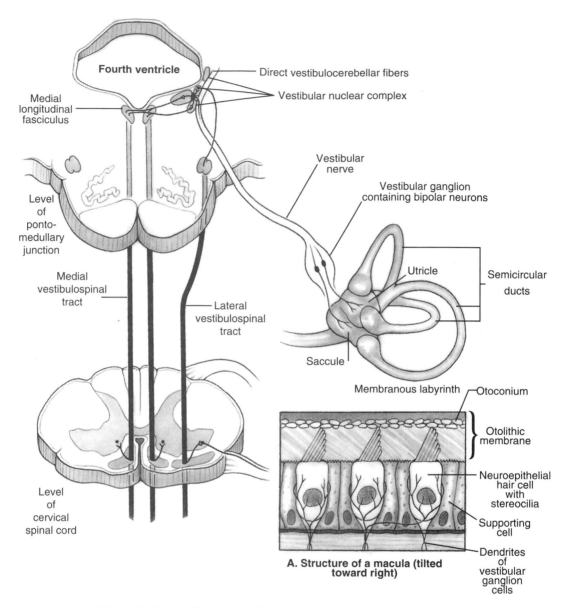

FIGURE 7-1.   Schematic diagram of principal vestibulospinal connections. **A.** Structure of a macula (tilted to right side).

cochlear nerve at the pontomedullary junction, in the area bounded by the pons, medulla, and cerebellum and called the cerebellar angle. The vestibular nerve fibers then pass dorsally to reach the vestibular nuclear complex. Some continue uninterrupted into the cerebellum as the direct vestibulocerebellar fibers, which pass through the **juxtarestiform body** (Fig. 7–2), the most medial part of the inferior cerebellar peduncle.

The vestibular nuclear complex consists pri-

marily of four nuclei located beneath the vestibular area in the floor and wall of the fourth ventricle (Figs. 7–1, 7–2). The inferior vestibular nucleus is in the rostral medulla. The medial vestibular nucleus is located in the lateral part of the floor of the fourth ventricle in the rostral medulla and caudal pons. The lateral vestibular nucleus is limited to the region of the pontomedullary junction and it contains a population of neurons referred to as Deiters nucleus. The superior vestibular nucleus is limited

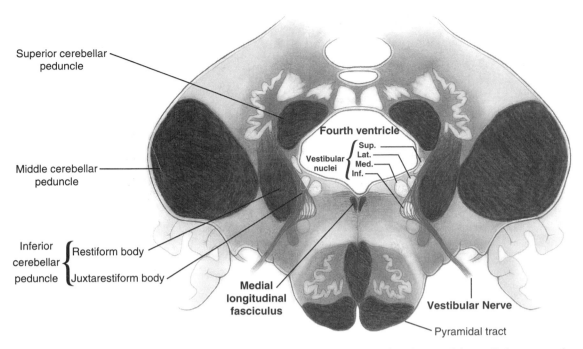

FIGURE 7–2. Section at the level of the pontomedullary junction showing the relations of the vestibular nerve and nuclei.

to the caudal pons where it is located in the wall of the fourth ventricle.

The vestibular nerve fibers carrying input from the maculae synapse in the medial, lateral, and inferior vestibular nuclei. These vestibular nuclei project to the spinal motor nuclei via the lateral and medial vestibulospinal tracts. The lateral vestibulospinal tract, which arises from the lateral vestibular nucleus, strongly facilitates the extensor muscles in the ipsilateral limbs. The medial vestibulospinal fibers arise from the medial and inferior vestibular nuclei; descend bilaterally via the **medial longitudinal fasciculus;** and influence muscles of the head, neck, trunk, and proximal parts of the limbs.

RETICULAR NUCLEI

Two regions of the reticular formation project to spinal motor neurons. From the medullary reticular formation arise lateral reticulospinal fibers, and from the pontine reticular formation arise medial reticulospinal fibers.

Although the reticular formation receives input from many sources, it appears that with respect to its role in voluntary movements, the projections from the cerebral cortex are especially important. Both the pontine and medullary groups of reticulospinal neurons are influenced directly by the cerebral cortex via corticoreticular fibers. In addition to the strong cortical input, these reticular nuclei are also influenced by the cerebellum, the vestibular nuclei, and pain fibers ascending from the spinal cord. In general, the pontine reticular neurons facilitate extensor movements and inhibit flexor movements, whereas the medullary reticular neurons inhibit the extensors and facilitate the flexors. The pontine extensor excitatory area is under inhibitory control of higher centers, whereas the medullary inhibitory area is facilitated by the higher centers.

RUBRAL NUCLEI

The red nucleus is in the tegmentum of the midbrain at the levels of the superior colliculus and pretectum. Its rostral pole overlaps with the thalamus (Fig. 7–3). Input to the red

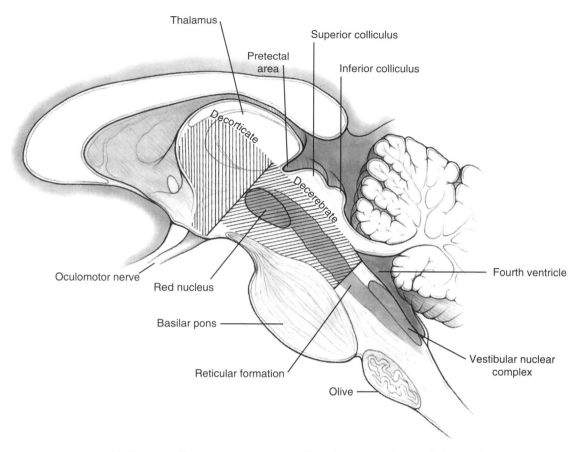

FIGURE 7-3. Median view of brainstem showing levels of impairment associated with abnormal posturing: Rostral to red nucleus—decorticate, midbrain or rostral pons—decerebrate.

nucleus comes from two main sources, the cerebral cortex and the cerebellum. Corticorubral fibers arise mainly from the motor cortex, are uncrossed, and are somatotopically organized. Some are collaterals from the corticospinal tract. Cerebellorubral fibers arise chiefly in the contralateral interposed cerebellar nucleus.

The main outputs of the red nucleus are a large rubrobulbar tract and a small, almost indistinct, rubrospinal tract. Both cross immediately after their origin and descend through the brainstem. The red nucleus facilitates flexor movements in the contralateral upper limb, directly through the small rubrospinal tract and indirectly through connections of the rubrobulbar tract with the flexor areas in the medullary reticular formation.

DECEREBRATE AND DECORTICATE POSTURING

The brainstem motor nuclei and their spinal projections are of limited use in localizing focal lesions. However, their activity (or inactivity) may be used as indicators of the levels of brainstem impairment in comatose patients with brainstem compression, usually caused by herniation.

When brainstem impairment occurs between the levels of the rostral poles of the red nuclei and vestibular nuclei (subthalamus to midpons) (Fig. 7–3), **decerebrate posturing** occurs (Fig. 7–4). In this phenomenon, as exemplified in the case at the beginning of this chapter, the upper and lower limbs extend when a comatose patient receives an appropriate stimulus (startling

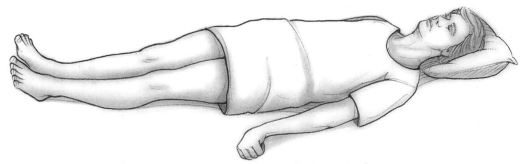

A. Decerebrate : upper and lower limbs extend

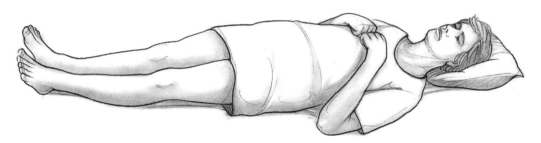

B. Decorticate : upper limbs flex, lower limbs extend

FIGURE 7–4. Abnormal posturing in comatose state. **A.** Decerebrate (upper and lower limbs extend). **B.** Decorticate (upper limbs flex, lower limbs extend).

painful or auditory stimuli). This extensor posturing is thought to occur because of the impairment of the extensor inhibition normally exerted on the reticular formation by the cerebral cortex. As a result, the spinal extensor motoneurons are driven by extensor facilitation parts of the reticular formation, which are activated by the pathways transmitting impulses elicited by the appropriate noxious stimulus. The lateral vestibular nuclei are also intimately involved. As shown in experimental decerebrate animals, the extensor posturing is greatly reduced when the lateral vestibular nuclei are ablated.

If the impairment of brainstem activity is located more rostrally, that is, above the level of the red nuclei, **decorticate posturing** occurs (Fig. 7–4). In this case, the lower limbs extend

but the upper limbs flex when the comatose patient receives an appropriate stimulus. This phenomenon is a manifestation of activity in brainstem flexor facilitation centers such as the red nuclei, which most strongly influence flexion in the upper limbs.

Decorticate posturing signifies a higher or more rostral level of brainstem impairment than decerebrate posturing. Hence, in comatose patients whose condition alters from decerebrate to decorticate posturing, the prognosis is better than in those patients who pass from decorticate to decerebrate. In the former, brainstem impairment is receding from caudal to rostral levels, whereas in the latter, impairment is proceeding from rostral to caudal levels and may become life threatening because of the vital respiratory and cardiovascular centers located in the medulla.

POSTCAPSULAR LESION RECOVERY

Following a lesion of the pyramidal tract, such as occurs in a vascular accident in the internal capsule, severe paralysis of the contralateral limbs occurs. As time passes, however, there may be a gradual and variable recovery of volitional movements. This recovery is thought to occur through the actions of the brainstem supraspinal motor centers and the relation of their projections to spinal cord motor and **propriospinal neurons.**

SPINAL MOTONEURONS

The spinal α-motoneurons innervating an individual muscle or a particular group of muscles are arranged in longitudinal columns extending for various distances in a specific part of the anterior horn. The medial cell column extends the entire length of the spinal cord and innervates the paravertebral or axial muscles. The lateral cell column, which is found at the spinal cord enlargements, innervates the muscles of the limbs. Within the lateral cell column further

somatotopic organization exists: the proximal limb muscles are represented medially and the distal muscles laterally (Figs. 5–11, 5–12, 7–5). The most distal muscles (in the fingers and toes) are represented most dorsolaterally and are limited to the most caudal segments of the cervical and lumbosacral enlargements, respectively.

THE PROPRIOSPINAL SYSTEM OF NEURONS

All movements require the activity of lower motor neurons in more than one spinal cord segment. The number of segments involved in a movement varies. Because axial movements depend on the activity of muscles that extend for great distances along the vertebral column, the paravertebral muscles are innervated by numerous spinal nerves. In contrast, individual finger movements are controlled by the intrinsic muscles of the hand that are innervated by only spinal nerves C8 and T1.

The intersegmental activity required for any particular movement is integrated by the pro-

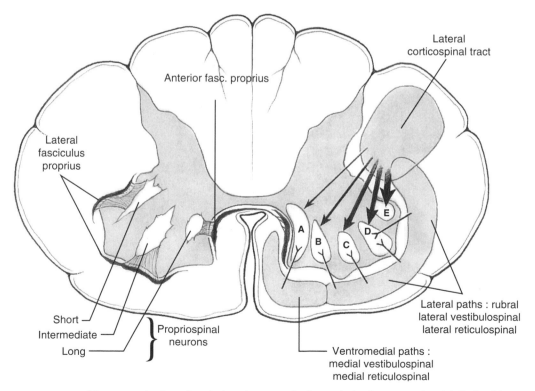

FIGURE 7–5.   Motor organization of a spinal cord segment in the cervical enlargement. A=axial, B=shoulder, C=arm, D=forearm, E=hand.

priospinal system of neurons. The propriospinal system includes three groups of intraspinal neurons whose axons influence homologous areas of the spinal cord gray matter at different levels by traveling through the fasciculi proprii bordering the gray matter (Fig. 7–5):

1. The long propriospinal neurons have axons that ascend and descend in the anterior fasciculus proprius to all levels of the spinal cord. These neurons have a bilateral influence on the more medial motor neurons subserving movements of the axial muscles.

2. The intermediate propriospinal neurons have axons that extend for shorter distances in the ventral part of the lateral fasciculus proprius and influence the motor neurons that innervate the more proximal muscles of the limbs.

3. The short propriospinal neurons are limited to the cervical and lumbosacral enlargements. Their axons travel in the lateral fasciculus proprius and terminate within several segments of their origin. These propriospinal neurons influence the motor neurons that innervate the more distal muscles of the limbs.

SPINAL CORD ARRANGEMENT OF SUPRASPINAL PATHS

The motor paths descending through the spinal cord from higher centers are divided into three groups: ventromedial, lateral, and cortical (Fig. 7–5). The ventromedial group is located in the anterior funiculus and includes the medial vestibulospinal fibers and medial reticulospinal fibers that chiefly influence the long propriospinal and lower motor neurons in the more medial parts of the anterior horn. The ventromedial group strongly influences movements of the axial muscles.

The lateral group of supraspinal paths is located in the lateral funiculus and includes the rubrospinal tract and any other axons carrying impulses from the red nucleus, as well as other fibers descending in the ventral part of the lateral funiculus (e.g., lateral reticulospinal and lateral vestibulospinal). This group synapses in the central and lateral parts of the anterior horn, strongly influencing proximal and distal muscles of the limbs.

The cortical group consists of the lateral corticospinal tract, which synapses throughout the intermediate zone and in the dorsolateral part of the anterior horn. Many of its fibers terminate directly on lower motor neurons, especially those innervating the most distal muscles of the limbs. In fact, the α-motoneurons supplying the intrinsic muscles of the hand are not influenced by any other descending path. Thus, the location of supraspinal fibers within the white matter of the spinal cord is closely related to their areas of termination and ultimately to the muscles and movements that they influence.

CLINICAL IMPLICATIONS OF SPINAL MOTOR ORGANIZATION

Spinal cord somatotopic organization holds not only for the α-motoneurons but also for the γ-motoneurons, the interneuronal pools, the propriospinal neurons, and the terminations of the supraspinal paths. Thus, the most medial part of the anterior horn controls the bilateral axial movements associated with posture. These movements are most strongly influenced by the supraspinal paths located in the ventromedial parts of the spinal cord, chiefly the medial vestibulospinal and reticulospinal tracts. Because postural adjustments of the vertebral column require muscular activity bilaterally and at multiple levels, intersegmental communication is necessary. This occurs through the long propriospinal neurons whose axons pass bilaterally to reach homologous regions in the anterior horn at far rostral and caudal levels. Although movements by the paravertebral muscles can be commanded by the corticospinal tracts, the influence of the cortex is relatively small and occurs only through interneurons.

Movements of proximal limb muscles are represented in the more central and ventral parts of the anterior horn. The motoneurons here are influenced most strongly by the lateral reticulospinal and vestibulospinal tracts and less strongly by the corticospinal tracts. Because these movements are chiefly unilateral and may be limited to a single limb, intersegmental connections are ipsilateral and more limited. These occur through intermediate propriospinal neurons.

Movements of more distal muscles, especially the flexors of the upper limb, are most strongly influenced by the corticospinal and rubral tracts. Intersegmental connections occur via the short propriospinal neurons.

Movements in the most distal parts of the limbs, e.g., the fingers, are under direct control of the cerebral cortex. The α-motoneurons supplying the intrinsic muscles of the hand are located in the retrodorsolateral cell column of segments C8 and T1, and these motoneurons are innervated solely by large numbers of corticospinal fibers that synapse directly on them.

Therefore, three groups of descending paths regulate movements. The ventromedial group (medial vestibulospinal and reticulospinal tracts) has the strongest influence on the axial muscles. The lateral group (lateral vestibulospinal and reticulospinal tracts) strongly influences the proximal and distal limb muscles. The cortical group weakly reinforces the ventromedial paths for axial movements, more strongly reinforces the lateral paths for proximal and distal limb movements, and is solely responsible for the very skilled movements of the individual fingers.

The clinical relevance of this organization is best exemplified in the recovery of function after a pyramidal tract lesion occurs in the internal capsule. The patient readily recovers neck and trunk movements because the dependence of such movements on the pyramidal tract is very meager. The main supraspinal control of neck and trunk movements is via the ventromedial descending paths. Recovery of function occurs more slowly and less completely from the proximal to the distal parts of the limbs because of the increased influence exerted by the corticospinal tract. Nevertheless, due to the strong influences on the proximal and distal limb muscles by the lateral descending paths, some recovery does occur. It is only in the movements that are solely dependent on the corticospinal tract that no recovery occurs. Thus, rapid and independent finger movements are permanently lost.

CHAPTER REVIEW QUESTIONS

7–1. Describe the pathway that causes extension of the left limbs on falling toward the left.

7–2. Locate the level of impairment in each of the comatose patients shown below.

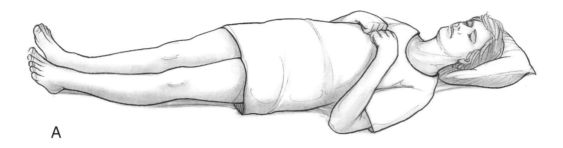

A

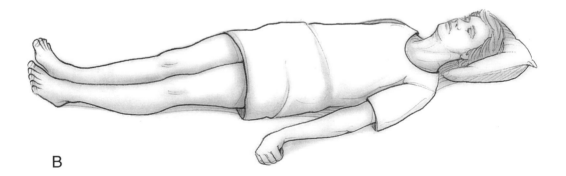

B

THE BASAL GANGLIA: MOVEMENT DISORDERS

■ **A 63-year-old man has been bothered by the shaking of his hands and generalized body stiffness that have become progressively worse over the past 3 years. He moves slowly and deliberately, shuffling his feet as he walks. His shoulders and trunk stoop forward, and his arms hang at his sides. His face remains mask-like with no changes of expression. In both hands, a resting tremor of the pill-rolling type stops only when the patient performs a voluntary movement such as picking up a pencil. Examination reveals a generalized hypertonicity with greatly increased resistance to passive stretch in all directions. Although the patient moves his limbs infrequently, examination reveals no paralysis or sensory disturbances in any part of the body.**

The term "basal ganglia" refers to the large, strongly interconnected nuclear masses deep within the cerebral hemispheres, diencephalon, and midbrain that are instrumental in the initiation of voluntary movements and the control of the postural adjustments associated with voluntary movements. Abnormalities of the basal ganglia result in movement disorders such as **Parkinson** and **Huntington diseases.** The basal ganglia are the corpus striatum (in the cerebral hemisphere), the subthalamic nucleus (in the diencephalon), and the substantia nigra (in the midbrain).

CORPUS STRIATUM

The **corpus striatum** is subdivided anatomically into the caudate and lentiform nuclei. These two large nuclear masses are deep within the cere-

bral hemisphere, with the comma-shaped caudate nucleus located in the wall of the lateral ventricle (Fig. 8–1). The caudate nucleus is divided into three parts: head, body, and tail. The head is the largest part and protrudes into the anterior horn of the lateral ventricle. Posteriorly, the head tapers and, at the level of the interventricular foramen, it becomes the body. The tail of the caudate nucleus continues from the body and arches downward and forward into the temporal lobe where it eventually becomes continuous with the amygdaloid nucleus (Fig. 8–2**A**).

The lentiform nucleus is wedge-shaped and consists of several segments that form the putamen and the globus pallidus (Figs. 8–2**B,C** 8–3). The putamen is in the most lateral position and is located between the external capsule and globus pallidus. The globus pallidus is located between the putamen and the internal capsule and is divided into lateral (outer) and medial (inner) segments.

The lentiform nucleus is separated from the thalamus by the posterior limb of the internal capsule (Figs. 8–2–8–4) and superiorly it is separated from the head of the caudate nucleus by the **anterior limb of the internal capsule.** Inferiorly, the putamen fuses with the caudate nucleus by thin strands of gray matter that span the anterior limb of the internal capsule (Figs. 8–2**B,** 8–4). In brain slices, the alternate strands of gray and white matter provide the striated appearance for which the corpus striatum was named.

Because of numerous morphologic and physiologic similarities, the caudate nucleus and putamen are referred to as the striatum. The globus pallidus, however, is morphologically

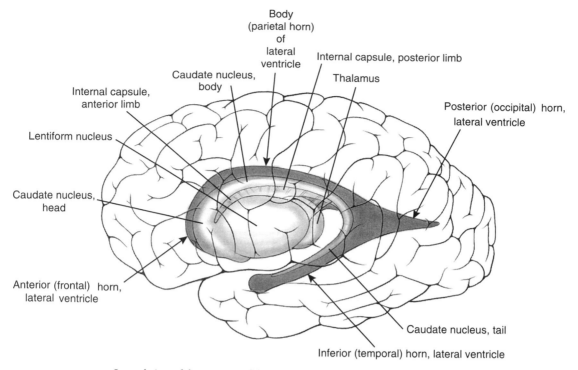

FIGURE 8–1. Lateral view of the position of the corpus striatum and its relations in the left cerebral hemisphere.

and physiologically dissimilar from the rest of the corpus striatum. It is referred to as the pallidum. As a result, the corpus striatum consists of the caudate nucleus, the putamen, and the globus pallidus structurally, but the striatum and pallidum functionally (Fig. 8–5).

SUBTHALAMIC NUCLEUS

The subthalamic nucleus is the largest nuclear mass in the subthalamus, the wedge-shaped subdivision of the diencephalon located ventral to the thalamus and lateral to the hypothalamus. The subthalamus contains three nuclei: (1) the zona incerta dorsolaterally, (2) the prerubral field dorsomedially, and (3) the subthalamic nucleus ventrally (Fig. 8–3). The subthalamic nucleus appears as a prominent biconvex structure nestled in the arm of the most rostral part of the cerebral crus, often referred to as the peduncular part of the internal capsule.

SUBSTANTIA NIGRA

The substantia nigra is the largest nuclear mass of the midbrain (Fig. 8–6), extending

throughout its length and even overlapping with the subthalamus rostrally (Fig. 8–3). It consists of two parts: a more dorsal part that is compact and a more ventral part that is reticular. The compact part contains neurons filled with **melanin,** which accounts for the black color of the substantia nigra. The reticular part intermingles with the fiber bundles of the cerebral crus and extends more rostrally than does the compact part (Fig. 8–3).

CONNECTIONS OF THE BASAL GANGLIA

The connections of the basal ganglia (Fig. 8–7A) are extremely complex and for description purposes are divided into

1. Input from sources outside the basal ganglia;

2. Interconnections between the nuclear masses that form the basal ganglia;

3. Output from the basal ganglia to motor centers elsewhere in the brain.

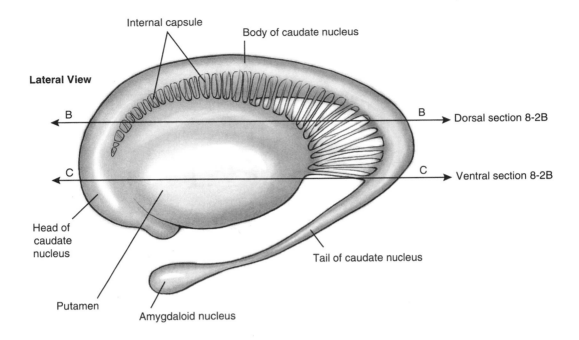

Internal capsule

Body of caudate nucleus

Lateral View

B   B → Dorsal section 8-2B

C   C → Ventral section 8-2B

Head of
caudate
nucleus

Tail of caudate nucleus

Putamen

Amygdaloid nucleus

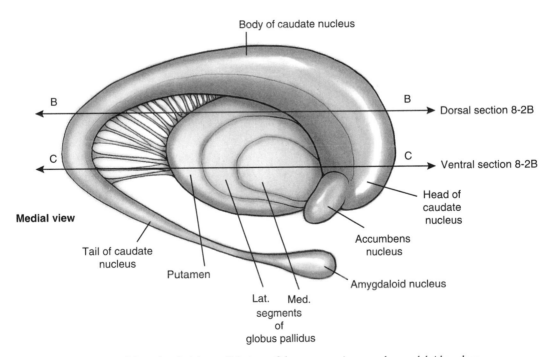

Body of caudate nucleus

B   B → Dorsal section 8-2B

C   C → Ventral section 8-2B

Head of
caudate
nucleus

Medial view

Accumbens
nucleus

Tail of caudate
nucleus

Putamen

Amygdaloid nucleus

Lat.   Med.
segments
of
globus pallidus

FIGURE 8–2. **A.** Left lateral and right medial views of the corpus striatum and amygdaloid nucleus.

INPUT

The basal ganglia receive input mainly from the cerebral cortex (Fig. 8–7A). Virtually all areas of the cerebral cortex project in an orderly manner to the striatum. These corticostriate projections reach the caudate nucleus and putamen directly from the adjacent white matter, most via the anterior limb of the internal capsule and the external capsule. A thalamic input to the

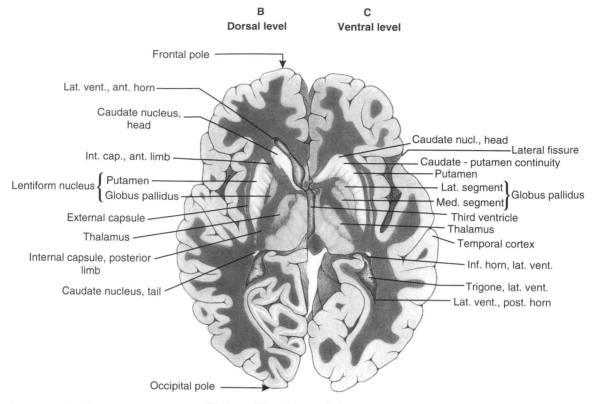

B — Dorsal level **C** — Ventral level

Frontal pole

Lat. vent., ant. horn

Caudate nucleus, head

Int. cap., ant. limb

Lentiform nucleus { Putamen, Globus pallidus }

External capsule

Thalamus

Internal capsule, posterior limb

Caudate nucleus, tail

Caudate nucl., head

Lateral fissure

Caudate - putamen continuity

Putamen

Lat. segment } Med. segment } Globus pallidus

Third ventricle

Thalamus

Temporal cortex

Inf. horn, lat. vent.

Trigone, lat. vent.

Lat. vent., post. horn

Occipital pole

FIGURE 8-2 (CONTINUED). Horizontal lines B-B and C-C in part A indicate levels of **B** and **C**. **B.** Horizontal section through dorsal level of corpus striatum. **C.** Horizontal section through ventral level of corpus striatum.

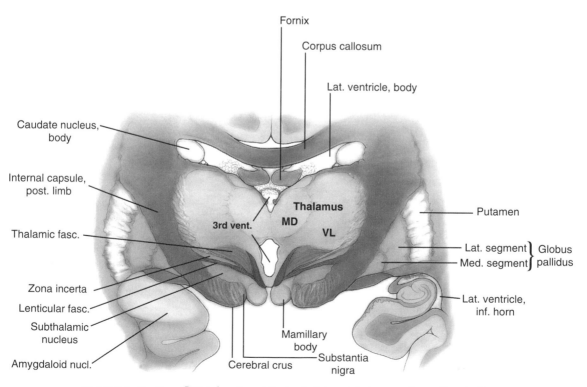

Fornix

Corpus callosum

Lat. ventricle, body

Caudate nucleus, body

Internal capsule, post. limb

Thalamic fasc.

Zona incerta

Lenticular fasc.

Subthalamic nucleus

Amygdaloid nucl.

Cerebral crus

Mamillary body

Substantia nigra

Thalamus
MD
3rd vent.
VL

Putamen

Lat. segment } Med. segment } Globus pallidus

Lat. ventricle, inf. horn

FIGURE 8-3. Coronal section at the level of the subthalamus and mamillary bodies.

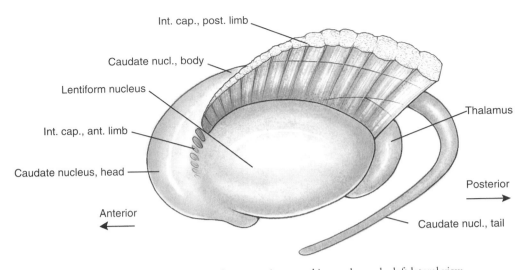

FIGURE 8-4.   Relation of corpus striatum and internal capsule, left lateral view.

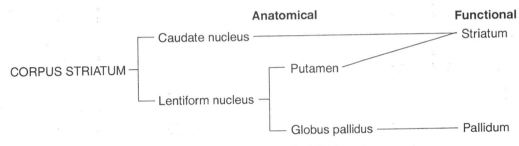

FIGURE 8-5.   Anatomical and functional subdivisions of corpus striatum.

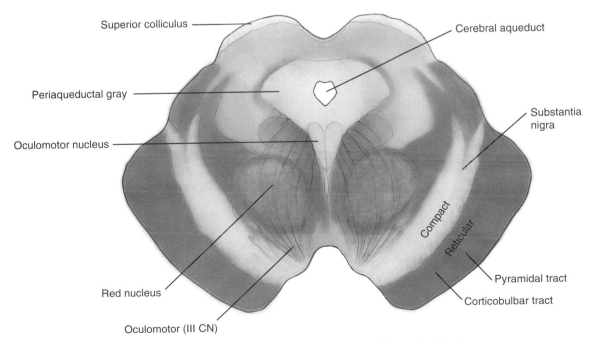

FIGURE 8-6.   Transverse section at the level of the rostral midbrain.

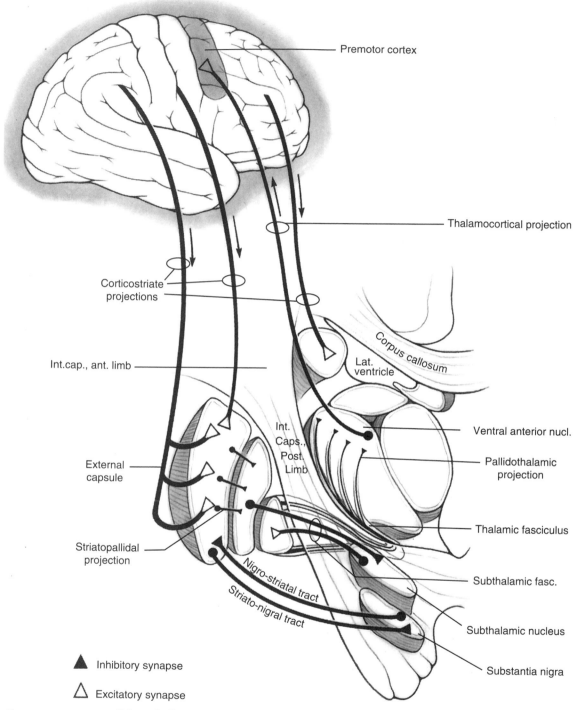

Premotor cortex

Thalamocortical projection

Corticostriate projections

Corpus callosum

Int.cap., ant. limb

Lat. ventricle

Int. Caps., Post. Limb

Ventral anterior nucl.

External capsule

Pallidothalamic projection

Thalamic fasciculus

Striatopallidal projection

Nigro-striatal tract

Striato-nigral tract

Subthalamic fasc.

Subthalamic nucleus

Substantia nigra

▲ Inhibitory synapse

△ Excitatory synapse

FIGURE 8–7A. Schematic diagram of principal connections of basal ganglia. Excitatory synapses (*white triangles*); inhibitory synapses (*black triangles*). (See Fig. 8–7B for position of pallidothalmic projections and additional labelling of basal ganglia).

striatum arises in the intralaminar nuclei. A direct cortical projection also passes from the motor and premotor areas to the subthalamic nucleus.

INTERCONNECTIONS

The most important connections between individual nuclei of the basal ganglia are:

1. Reciprocal connections between the striatum and substantia nigra;

2. Reciprocal connections between the pallidum and subthalamic nucleus;

3. A massive striatopallidal projection.

A topographically organized striatonigral projection arises from all parts of the striatum and terminates mainly in the reticular part of the substantia nigra. From the compact part of the substantia nigra arises the nigrostriatal projection, which terminates in the caudate nucleus and putamen in a manner reciprocal to the striatonigral projections.

The pallidum and subthalamic nucleus are interconnected by the subthalamic fasciculus, a small bundle that intersects with the internal capsule, where it separates these two nuclei. The pallidosubthalamic fibers arise chiefly from the lateral segment of the globus pallidus, whereas the subthalamopallidal fibers project chiefly to the medial pallidal segment (Fig. 8–7A).

Extending from all parts of the striatum to all parts of the pallidum are abundant striatopallidal fibers. The corticostriate and striatopallidal projections are topographically organized; hence, specific areas of the cerebral cortex influence specific parts of the globus pallidus via the corticostriatopallidal pathway.

OUTPUT

The chief output nucleus of the basal ganglia is the pallidum, which exerts a strong influence on the thalamus. Pallidothalamic fibers arise from the medial segment and are gathered in two bundles—the lenticular fasciculus and the ansa lenticularis. The lenticular fasciculus arises

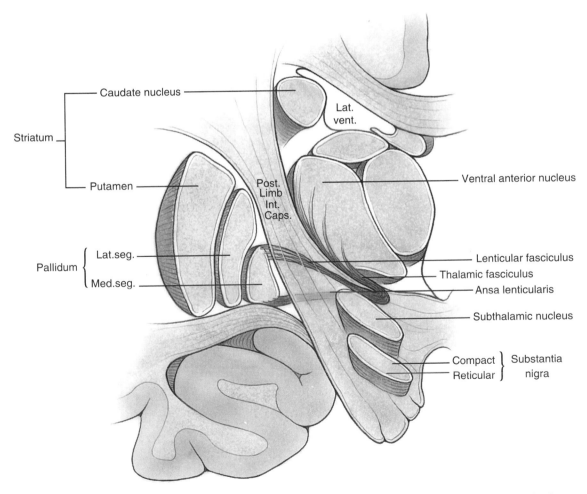

FIGURE 8–7B. Schematic diagram of principal output of basal ganglia. Position of pallidothalamic projections.

from the dorsal surface of the pallidum (Fig. 8–7B), passes medially initially through the posterior limb of the internal capsule, and then through the subthalamus where it is located between the subthalamic nucleus and zona incerta (Fig. 8–3). The ansa lenticularis arises from the ventral surface of the pallidum (Fig. 8–7B) and loops anterior to the internal capsule to enter the subthalamus. Both bundles join and travel in the thalamic fasciculus (Fig. 8–3, 8–7A, 8–7B) chiefly to the ventral anterior nucleus. From this nucleus, the pallidal influences are carried via thalamocortical projections to the premotor area of the cerebral cortex which, in turn, projects to the motor cortex and its upper motor neurons. Thus, ultimately the basal ganglia influence movements through the pyramidal system.

In addition to these conspicuous pallidothalamic connections, the reticular part of the substantia nigra also projects directly to the thalamus. These nigrothalamic fibers also terminate chiefly in the ventral anterior nucleus.

MANIFESTATIONS OF BASAL GANGLIA DISORDERS

The abnormalities associated with malfunctions of the basal ganglia are the result of the loss of control normally exerted on the striatum by the substantia nigra or on the pallidum by the striatum and subthalamic nucleus. In primates, and particularly in humans, the cerebral cortex is the "supreme" motor center. In humans, the cerebral cortex receives the sensory input, and its association areas generate the will to move. In order to relieve the cortex from involvement in all of the events leading to a movement, the striatum stores the necessary programs and, when a movement is desired, the striatum is activated by association areas. The striatum initiates and controls the movement through the chief efferent nucleus of the basal ganglia, the pallidum, which projects to the premotor cortex via the ventral anterior nucleus of the motor thalamus. The premotor cortex programs complex voluntary movements through connections with the motor cortex and its upper motor neurons. Honing of striatal and pallidal output occurs through reciprocal connections with the substantia nigra and the subthalamic nucleus, respectively.

Abnormalities of the basal ganglia result in negative and positive signs. The negative signs are actions the patient wants to perform but cannot; the positive signs are actions the patient does not want to perform but cannot prevent. The negative signs occur because the abnormal neurons can no longer elicit an activity. The positive signs occur because of the loss of control or the release of other parts of the motor system, thereby producing an abnormal pattern of movement.

NEGATIVE SIGNS

Negative signs of basal ganglia disease include akinesia, bradykinesia, and abnormal postural adjustments. Akinesia refers to the hesitancy in starting a movement and bradykinesia to the slowness with which the movement is executed. Neither occurs because of **paresis** or paralysis; these signs do not exist in basal ganglia disorders. Abnormal postural adjustments take the form of head and trunk flexion and the incapacity to make appropriate adjustments when falling or tilting or when attempting to stand after sitting or reclining. A form of abnormal postural adjustments is seen in dystonia, in which unusual fixed postures occur spontaneously. Such abnormalities occur with bilateral lesions of the globus pallidus in which the patient is unable to keep the head and trunk upright: the neck is flexed so that the chin rests on the chest, and when the patient is walking, the body bends at the waist so that the trunk is almost horizontal.

POSITIVE SIGNS

Positive signs of basal ganglia disease include alterations in muscle tone and various forms of **dyskinesia.** Both are manifestations of the "release" phenomena. Alterations in muscle tone in basal ganglia disorders usually take the form of hypertonicity. In severe cases, there is **rigidity** in which the tone in all of the muscles acting on a joint is increased. In such cases, the increased resistance to passive stretch is bidirectional and occurs throughout the range of the movement. It is described as **lead-pipe rigidity.** If severe tremor is present, the resistance to passive stretch exhibits intermittent jerkiness with a ratchet-like characteristic. The frequency of the jerks corresponds to the frequency of the tremors. The hypertonicity in this case is termed **cogwheel rigidity.**

DYSKINESIA

Dyskinesia take the form of tremors, **chorea, athetosis, ballismus,** and tics. Tremors are rhythmical or oscillatory movements in the distal parts of the limbs, such as the hands. Chorea is rapid, jerky movements in the more distal parts of the limbs and in the face. Athetosis is slow, writhing, or snake-like movements of the limbs. Ballismus is violent flinging movements of the entire limb as a result of contractions of the more proximal muscles. Tics are stereotypical and repetitive movements involving several muscle groups simultaneously.

The hallmark of basal ganglia disorders is that various forms of dyskinesia occur "at rest," i.e., in the absence of a command. These abnormal movements occur against the will of the patient and can neither be prevented from starting nor interrupted once they do start.

PARKINSON DISEASE

The combination of tremor, rigidity, akinesia, bradykinesia, and abnormal postural adjustments occurs in Parkinson disease, also called **paralysis agitans,** the best-known basal ganglia disease and the disease described in the case at the beginning of this chapter. The tremor consists of rhythmical movements in the thumbs and fingers at the rate of three to six per second that resemble pill-rolling movements and diminish during voluntary movement. The rigidity is more prominent in the advanced stages of the disease. The akinesia and bradykinesia are so severe that movements are initiated and carried out very slowly; in fact, the patient appears almost paralyzed. The akinesia accompanied by the tremor was the basis of the term "paralysis agitans." Characteristically, the Parkinsonian patient has a mask-like facial expression and when attempting to walk is stooped over (Fig. 8–8), shuffles the feet, does not swing the arms, and, on gaining momentum, is unable to stop and falls if not caught. In advanced

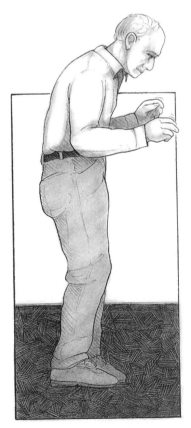

Mask-like facial expression

Pill-rolling tremor

Flexion of trunk

Slow, shuffling feet movements

FIGURE 8–8. Parkinson disease posture. Mask-like facial expression, pill-rolling tremor, trunk flexed, slow shuffling gait.

stages, handwriting becomes small and speech is reduced to a whisper.

Parkinson disease is associated with degeneration of the dopamine neurons in the substantia nigra. The resulting dopamine deficiency in the striatum is treated by the administration of levodopa (Dopar, Procter & Gamble, Norwich, NY), a dopamine precursor that can be transported through the blood-brain barrier. Transplantation of fetal dopamine-producing tissue, such as the suprarenal medulla, is being used in the treatment of advanced Parkinson disease. Surgical procedures such as bilateral ablations of the medial pallidum or implantation of self-stimulating electrodes into the motor thalamus are being used with some success to treat severe tremors in advanced Parkinsonian patients. Both procedures interrupt the abnormal basal ganglia output that results in the severe tremors.

HUNTINGTON DISEASE

The most well-known disease associated with the striatum is Huntington chorea (Fig. 8–9). This progressive disorder is acquired by inher-iting a dominant gene and is caused by degeneration of striatal neurons. Neuronal degeneration may also occur in the cerebral cortex; such patients suffer progressive dementia. Athetosis may also occur in Huntington disease. In fact, athetosis and chorea, or intermediate forms of the two (choreoathetosis), are frequently encountered. Athetosis has been associated primarily with abnormalities in the striatum, although pathologic changes in the pallidum have also been found. The gene associated with Huntington disease has recently been identified.

LESIONS OF THE SUBTHALAMIC NUCLEUS

A contralateral hemiballismus is associated with abnormalities of the subthalamic nucleus. Such abnormalities are usually vascular in nature, and it is fortunate that these extremely violent conditions are most often of short duration. If they are long lasting and cannot be controlled by medication, the motor parts of the thalamus (ventral anterior and ventral lateral nuclei) may be ablated cryosurgically as a

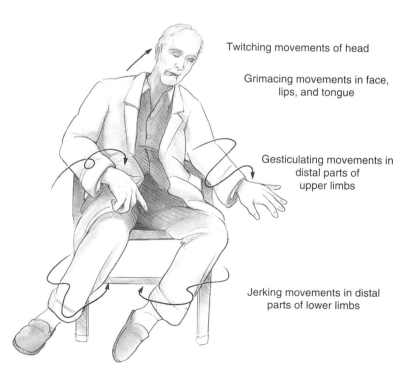

Twitching movements of head

Grimacing movements in face, lips, and tongue

Gesticulating movements in distal parts of upper limbs

Jerking movements in distal parts of lower limbs

FIGURE 8–9.   Huntington chorea posture. Jerking of head, smacking of lips and tongue, gesticulation of distal parts of upper and lower limbs.

last resort. This procedure was also the treatment of choice of severe Parkinson disease before the advent of levodopa. In both cases, the motor thalamus is ablated in order to interrupt the abnormal influence of the basal ganglia on the motor areas of the cortex.

TARDIVE DYSKINESIA

Tardive dyskinesia is a basal ganglia disorder that involves the face, lips, and tongue and is manifested by involuntary chewing movements accompanied by smacking of the lips and tongue. It is often seen in workers exposed to manganese and in patients who have undergone long-term treatment with drugs such as chlorpromazine. This disorder is thought to result from a hypersensitivity to dopamine and its agonists.

CEREBRAL PALSY

Cerebral palsy is a nonprogressive neonatal CNS disorder that affects the motor system and sometimes impairs mental function. The cortical neurons giving rise to the pyramidal tract and the basal ganglia are most often involved, the cerebellum much less frequently. Hence, spasticity or dyskinesia are seen commonly, and **ataxia** is found only occasionally. Lesions may be found in the cerebral cortex, hemispheric white matter, striatum, and thalamus and rarely in the cerebellar cortex or white matter. A common etiologic factor seems to be hypoxemia, and the majority of cases are due to birth injury.

FUNCTIONAL CONSIDERATIONS

Knowledge is gradually being revealed about the physiologic influences of the various parts of the basal ganglia and also that of the principal neurotransmitters (Fig. 8–10). Cortical influences on the striatum and subthalamic nucleus are excitatory, with **glutamate** acting as the neurotransmitter. The dopaminergic nigrostriatal connection appears to have excitatory ef-

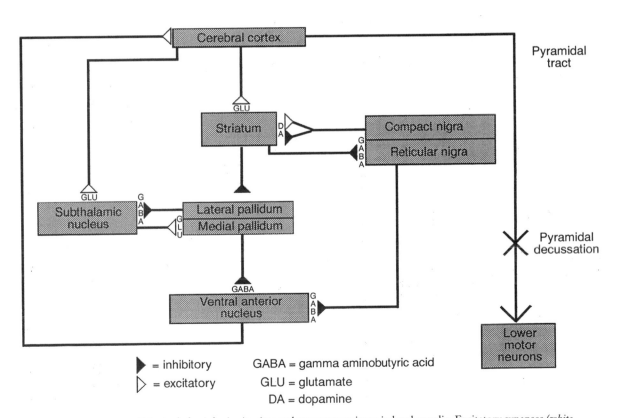

FIGURE 8–10. Principal physiologic circuitry and neurotransmitters in basal ganglia. Excitatory synapses (*white triangles*); inhibitory synapses (*black triangles*).

fects on some striatal neurons and inhibitory effects on others. Striatal output to the reticular part of the substantia nigra and to the pallidum is inhibitory, with **GABA** as the neurotransmitter. Excitatory impulses reach the subthalamic nucleus from the cerebral cortex and reach the pallidum from the subthalamic nucleus, with glutamate being the probable neurotransmitter in both cases. The pallidum and the reticular part of the substantia nigra inhibit the ventral anterior thalamic nucleus, with GABA as the neurotransmitter. The ventral anterior nucleus activates the premotor cortex with glutamate as the probable neurotransmitter.

HYPERKINESIA AND SUBTHALAMIC NUCLEUS

The **hyperkinetic disorders** exemplified by chorea, athetosis, ballismus, and tics appear to result from impairment of the strong excitatory influence exerted by the subthalamic nucleus on the medial pallidum. This impairment may

occur because of damage to the nucleus itself (Fig. 8–11), as seen in ballismus. More commonly, however, it occurs because of damage to the striatal neurons that inhibit the neurons of the lateral pallidum which, in turn, inhibit the subthalamic nucleus (Fig. 8–12). In both cases, the ultimate effect is a decrease in the inhibition exerted on the motor thalamus by the pallidum. Hence, the connections between the motor thalamus and the motor areas of the cortex are hyperactive.

HYPOKINESIA AND DOPAMINE

In Parkinson disease, the akinesia, bradykinesia, and impaired postural reflexes, sometimes referred to as **hypokinetic disorders,** result from decreased dopamine in the striatum. This deficiency apparently causes increased activity of striatal inhibitory connections to the inhibitory pallidosubthalamic circuit, and decreased activity of striatal inhibition of the pallidal and perhaps nigral projections to the mo-

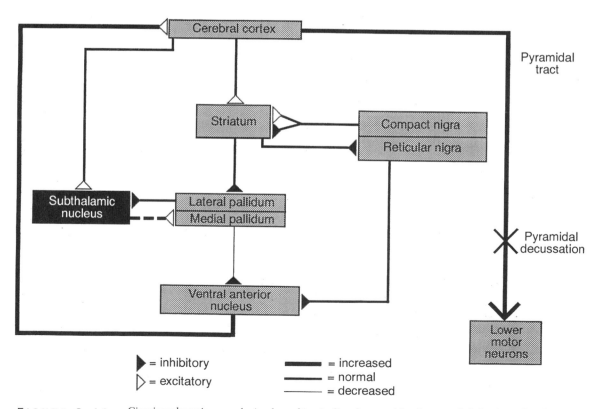

FIGURE 8–11. Circuitry alterations producing hyperkinetic disorders resulting from a subthalamic nucleus lesion. Excitatory synapses (*white triangles*); inhibitory synapses (*black triangles*); increased activity (*thick rule*); normal activity (*medium rule*); decreased activity (*thin rule*).

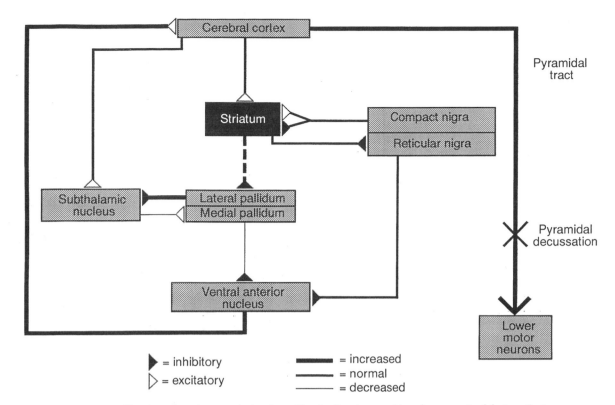

FIGURE 8-12. Circuitry alterations producing hyperkinetic disorders resulting from a striatal lesion. Excitatory synapses (*white triangles*); inhibitory synapses (*black triangles*); increased activity (*thick rule*); normal activity (*medium rule*); decreased activity (*thin rule*).

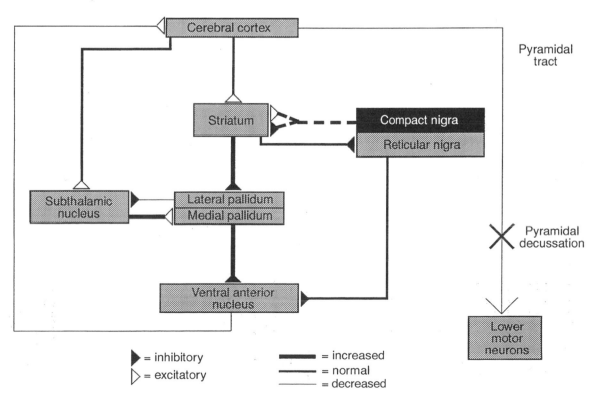

FIGURE 8-13. Circuitry alterations producing hypokinetic disorders resulting from decreased dopamine. Excitatory synapses (*white triangles*); inhibitory synapses (*black triangles*); increased activity (*thick rule*); normal activity (*medium rule*); decreased activity (*thin rule*).

tor thalamus. In both cases, the ultimate effect is increased inhibition of the motor thalamus. Hence, the connections between the motor thalamus and motor areas of the cortex are underactive (Fig. 8–13). Because decreased dopamine in the striatum results in decreased activity of other striatal inhibitory neurons, the hyperkinetic disorder of rigidity also occurs in Parkinson disease.

COGNITION

In addition to their well-known roles in the initiation and control of voluntary movements, parts of the basal ganglia appear to be intimately involved in the cognitive aspects of behavior. The two components of the striatum may subserve different functions. It appears that the putamen may be more associated with motor activity, whereas the caudate nucleus may be associated with cognitive functions. Although both exert their influence through the pallidum mainly to the ventral anterior nucleus, those parts of the ventral anterior nucleus that project to the premotor cortex are influenced by the putamen. However, those parts of the ventral anterior nucleus and other thalamic nuclei that project to the prefrontal cortex appear to be influenced by the caudate nucleus. It, therefore, appears likely that the striatum receives input from all parts of the cerebral cortex thereby accessing what is going on and programming what needs to be done next.

CHAPTER REVIEW QUESTIONS

8–1. What are the anatomical and functional subdivisions of the corpus striatum?

8–2. What is the chief input to the basal ganglia?

8–3. What are the cardinal manifestations of basal ganglia disorders?

8–4. What structures are involved, what abnormalities result, and how are the circuitries altered by the lesion or lesions in each section below?

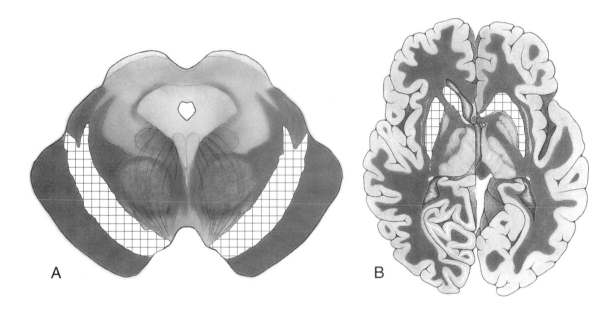

A

B

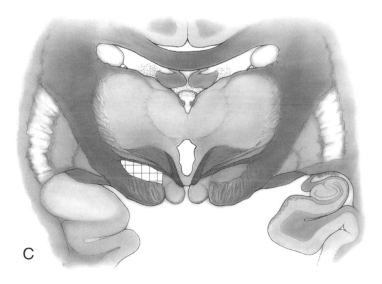

C

THE CEREBELLUM: ATAXIA

■ **A 56-year-old woman, who was a heavy cigarette smoker for 35 years, is experiencing difficulties in walking and in using her right arm. Both symptoms became progressively worse over a period of 4 months. Examination shows an intention tremor and dysmetria in her right upper and lower limbs while she performs the finger-to-nose and heel-to-shin tests. In addition, she has difficulty with heel-to-toe walking and tends to veer toward the right. She is unable to supinate and pronate her right arm repetitively even for a short time.**

The cerebellum is the large, bilaterally symmetrical "little brain" in the posterior cranial fossa. Through its afferent and efferent connections, the cerebellum influences the timing and force of contractions of voluntary muscles that result in smooth, coordinated move-ments.

Three is the key number associated with the cerebellum. The cerebellum is divided sagittally into three areas and horizontally into three lobes. The cerebellum is also connected to the brainstem by three pairs of peduncles, its cortex is composed of three layers, its output occurs through three nuclei, and three cerebellar syndromes can be identified.

ANATOMICAL SUBDIVISIONS

The surface of the cerebellum is thrown into numerous parallel folds, the folia, oriented in the transverse plane, i.e., in an ear-to-ear direction. In the sagittal plane, the cerebellum consists of a median part, the **vermis,** and lateral expansions of the vermis, the hemispheres (Fig. 9–1). Each hemisphere is divided into paravermal or intermediate and lateral parts.

In the transverse plane, two major fissures separate groups of folia into the three lobes of the cerebellum (Fig. 9–1). Each lobe is named anatomically, phylogenetically, and functionally (Fig. 9–2). The small flocculonodular lobe is most inferior and lies posterior to the posterolateral fissure. The flocculonodular lobe is phylogenetically the most ancient part of the cerebellum, and it receives its major input from the vestibular apparatus; hence, it is referred to as the **archicerebellum** or the vestibulocerebellum. The anterior lobe is most superior and lies anterior to the primary fissure. It appeared somewhat later in evolution than the vestibulocerebellum, and its main input is from the limbs via their spinal connections; hence, the anterior lobe is called the paleocerebellum or the spinocerebellum. Between the posterolateral and primary fissures is the largest part of the cerebellum, the posterior lobe. It is the newest part and has very strong connections with the cerebral cortex; hence, it is called the neocerebellum or the **cerebrocerebellum.**

CEREBELLAR PEDUNCLES

Three pairs of cerebellar peduncles, containing input and output fibers, connect the cerebellum and brainstem (Figs. 9–3, 9–4). The inferior cerebellar peduncle arches dorsally from the dorsolateral surface of the medulla. Its composition is chiefly input fibers, although

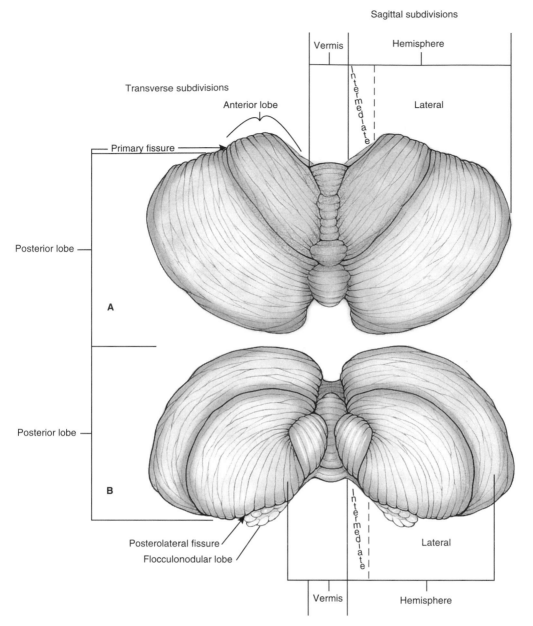

FIGURE 9—1. Drawings of the superior and inferior surfaces of cerebellum showing its sagittal and transverse subdivisions. **A.** Superior surface, **B.** Inferior surface.

Anatomical	Phylogenetic	Functional
Anterior lobe	Paleocerebellum	Spinal cerebellum
Primary fissure		
Posterior lobe	Neocerebellum	Cerebral cerebellum
Posterolateral fissure		
Flocculonodular lobe	Archicerebellum	Vestibular cerebellum

FIGURE 9—2. Anatomical, phylogenetic, and functional subdivisions of cerebellum.

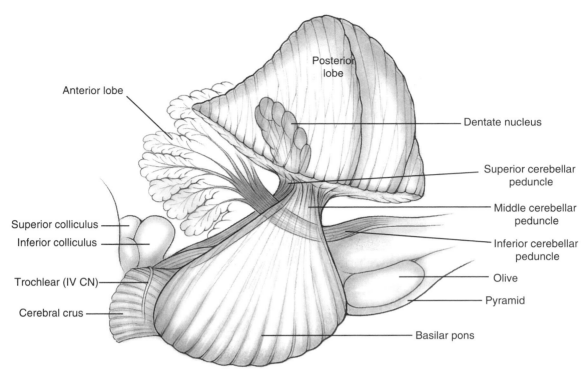

FIGURE 9–3. Three-dimensional drawing of the relation of cerebellar peduncles. (Left lateral view of dissected specimen).

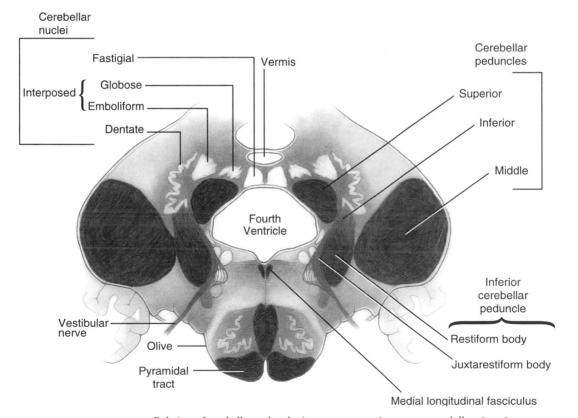

FIGURE 9–4. Relation of cerebellar peduncles in transverse section at pontomedullary junction.

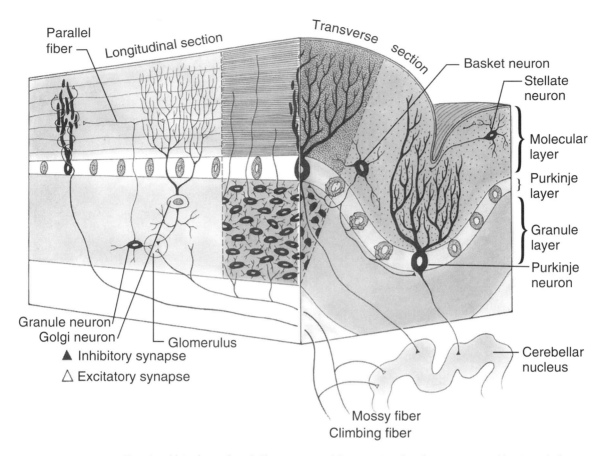

FIGURE 9-5. Functional histology of cerebellar cortex in a folium sectioned in the transverse and horizontal planes. Black synapses inhibitory; white synapses excitatory.

it does contain some output fibers. It consists of a large lateral part, the restiform body, and a small medial part, the juxtarestiform body.

The middle cerebellar peduncle, or brachium pontis, is the largest peduncle and connects the basilar part of the pons to the cerebellum. Its fibers are entirely input.

The superior cerebellar peduncle or brachium conjunctivum connects the cerebellum to the midbrain. Although it contains a limited number of input fibers, its most abundant and most important components are output fibers.

CEREBELLAR CORTEX

HISTOLOGY

The cytoarchitecture of the cerebellar cortex is of uniform structure throughout. Each **folium** is composed of an internal part consisting of white matter, and an external part that forms the cortical gray matter (Fig. 9–5). The cortex has three layers, which from external to internal are:

1. The molecular layer, characterized by few neurons;

2. The Purkinje cell layer, a single row of huge neurons unique to the cerebellum;

3. The granular layer, composed of numerous densely packed, small **granule cells.**

The molecular layer contains chiefly the massive dendritic trees of the **Purkinje neurons** interspersed with stellate and basket neurons and a profusion of axons oriented parallel to the surface of the cerebellum. The stellate neurons are found in the superficial part of the molecular layer, the **basket cells** in the deep part. In addition to myriads of granule cells in the internal cortical layer, the cell bodies of the **Golgi neurons** are also located here.

The cerebellar cortex receives information from many parts of the nervous system, both central and peripheral. Hence, the cerebellum has numerous afferent connections; in fact, it is said to have three times as many afferent fibers as efferent. The cerebellar cortex is dissimilar to the cerebral cortex in many ways, the most important of which are:

1. None of its activity contributes directly to consciousness.

2. Its hemispheres possess ipsilateral representation of the body parts, whereas the motor areas of the cerebral hemispheres possess contralateral representation.

CIRCUITRY OF THE CEREBELLAR CORTEX

There are two major types of input fibers to the cerebellar cortex: climbing and mossy. The **climbing fibers** arise from the olivocerebellar afferents from the inferior olivary nucleus. The inferior olivary complex consists of the large convoluted principal or main nucleus (Fig. 9–4) and two accessory nuclei, the dorsal and medial.

The massive olivocerebellar projections pass medially, decussate, sweep through the opposite inferior olive nucleus and medullary tegmentum, and enter the cerebellam through the inferior cerebellar peduncle. The **mossy fibers** arise from all of the other cerebellar afferent fibers, which are described later in this chapter.

On entering the cerebellar cortex, the climbing fibers pass through the granule cell layer and climb on the Purkinje cell body and its main dendrites (Fig. 9–5), where they make multiple excitatory synapses. The climbing fibers are extremely active while the cerebellar cortex is adapting to a new movement.

Unlike the climbing fibers, which have virtually no branches, the mossy fibers branch repeatedly in the cerebellar white matter and even after

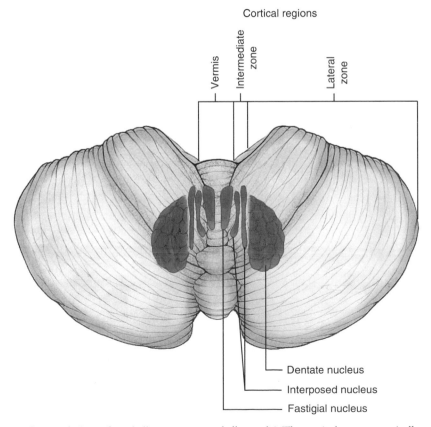

FIGURE 9-6. Input relations of cerebellar cortex to cerebellar nuclei. The cortical area anatomically related to each nucleus is the principal source of Purkinje neuron input to the nucleus.

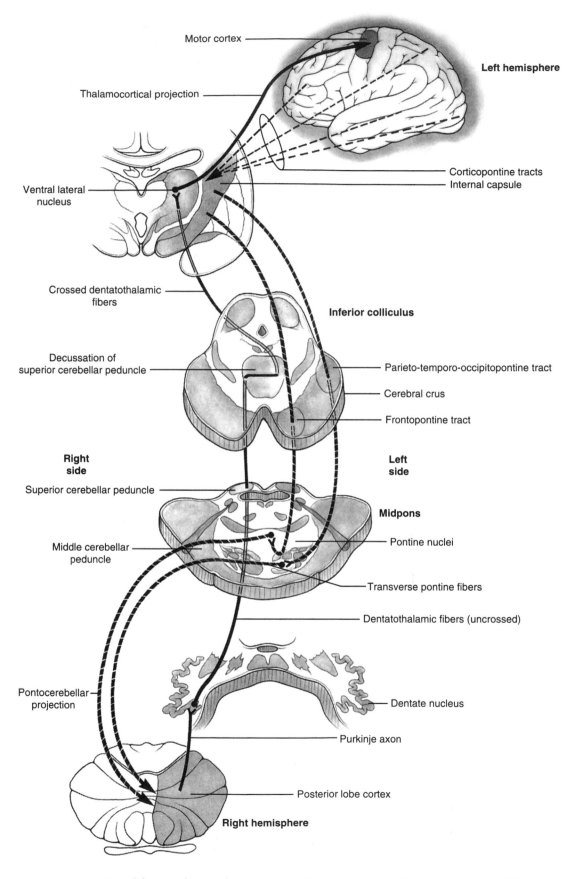

Motor cortex

Left hemisphere

Thalamocortical projection

Corticopontine tracts
Internal capsule

Ventral lateral
nucleus

Crossed dentatothalamic
fibers

Inferior colliculus

Decussation of
superior cerebellar peduncle

Parieto-temporo-occipitopontine tract

Cerebral crus

Frontopontine tract

**Right
side**

**Left
side**

Superior cerebellar peduncle

Midpons

Middle cerebellar
peduncle

Pontine nuclei

Transverse pontine fibers

Dentatothalamic fibers (uncrossed)

Pontocerebellar
projection

Dentate nucleus

Purkinje axon

Posterior lobe cortex

Right hemisphere

FIGURE 9–7. Schematic diagram showing posterior lobe circuitry. Input (*broken lines*); output (*solid lines*).

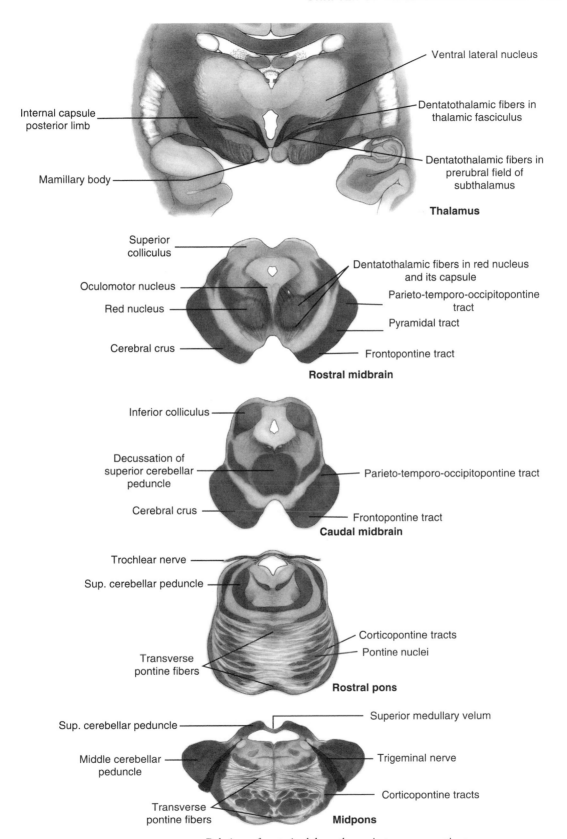

FIGURE 9-8.   Relations of posterior lobe pathways in transverse sections.

entering the granule cell layer. Each mossy fiber terminal is large and lobulated, synapses with dendrites of about 20 granule cells, and is also in contact with axons of Golgi neurons. Surrounded by a glial cell layer this entire mass is called a glomerulus. The mossy fiber system initiates the release of cerebellar cortical programs by its diffuse excitatory synapses on the granule cells.

The granule cells give rise to axons that enter the molecular layer and bifurcate, forming the parallel fibers. These parallel fibers synapse on the Purkinje dendrites, as well as the dendrites of the stellate, basket, and Golgi neurons.

The *only* excitatory neuron in the cerebellar cortex is the granule cell. The stellate and basket neurons inhibit the Purkinje neurons, and the Golgi neurons inhibit the granule cells. The Purkinje neurons, the sole output neurons of the cerebellar cortex, inhibit the neurons in the cerebellar nuclei, which give rise to the output fibers of the cerebellum. Because the neurons of the cerebellar nuclei are excited by collateral branches of the climbing and mossy fibers, the output of the cerebellar nuclei is regulated and fine-tuned by cortical inhibitory impulses from the Purkinje neurons.

CEREBELLAR NUCLEI

The cerebellum influences motor centers at various levels almost exclusively through the cerebellar nuclei. These paired neuronal masses, embedded in the medullary white matter near the roof of the fourth ventricle, are, from medial to lateral, the fastigial, interposed (composed of globose and emboliform parts), and dentate (Fig. 9–4). Cells in each nucleus receive excitatory impulses from collateral branches of the mossy and climbing fibers and inhibitory impulses from Purkinje cells in topographically defined parts of the cerebellar cortex. Purkinje neurons in the vermis project to the fastigial nuclei (Fig. 9–6), whereas those in the intermediate parts of the hemisphere project to the interposed nuclei. The lateral parts of the hemispheres project to the dentate nuclei. Each of the cerebellar nuclei, in turn, exerts its influence on motor activity via certain parts of the brainstem and the motor thalamus.

POSTERIOR LOBE

The lateral parts of the cerebellar hemispheres are chiefly concerned with the learning and storage of all of the sequential components of skilled movements. The major input to the lateral parts of the cerebellar hemispheres originates in the association areas of the cerebral cortex where the desire to perform a volitional movement occurs, and the major output of the cerebellar hemisphere is directed to the motor cortex where skilled movements are represented. It has been shown that activity in this part of the cerebellum and in its nucleus, the dentate, precedes the activity in the motor cortex that ultimately commands a particular movement.

CONNECTIONS OF THE POSTERIOR LOBE

The posterior lobe, by far the largest of the cerebellar lobes, has massive reciprocal connections with the cerebral cortex (Fig. 9–7). It receives by far the largest group of cerebellar mossy fiber afferents, the corticopontocerebellar projections. Most of the corticopontine fibers arise from the sensorimotor part, premotor part, and posterior parietal parts of the cerebral cortex, although the association areas of all the lobes contribute heavily. The corticopontine fibers reach the ipsilateral pontine nuclei by coursing through the internal capsule and cerebral crus (Fig. 9–8). The pontine nuclei give rise to the transverse pontine fibers, which, after crossing and proceeding through the contralateral basilar pons, form the massive middle cerebellar peduncles that project chiefly to the posterior lobe.

Axons from Purkinje neurons in the lateral parts of the posterior lobe project to the dentate nucleus. Dentatofugal fibers pass to the contralateral ventral lateral nucleus of the thalamus, from whence there is a thalamocortical projection to the motor cortex. The dentatofugal fibers pass rostrally in the superior cerebellar peduncle. This prominent bundle arises mainly from the dentate nucleus, although it also contains a considerable number of fibers from the interposed nucleus and a small contribution from the fastigial nucleus.

The superior cerebellar peduncle courses initially in the roof of the fourth ventricle (Fig. 9–8), then moves into the ventricular wall, and, in the rostral pons, enters the tegmentum. At the level of the inferior colliculus, it decussates before continuing rostrally through the red nucleus and the prerubral field of the subthalamus. Here, it is joined by pallidothalamic fibers, and the two groups of fibers form the thalamic fasciculus, which passes to the motor thalamus.

POSTERIOR LOBE SYNDROME

The neocerebellar or **posterior lobe syndrome,** commonly resulting from cerebral vascular accidents, tumors, trauma, or degenerative diseases, is manifested by a loss of coordination of voluntary movements (ataxia) and decreased muscle tone, the latter being most prominent in acute lesions. The rate, range, and force of movements are abnormal; thus, the ataxic patient is unable to direct the limb to a target without its progression being interrupted by a swaying to and fro that is perpendicular to the direction of the movement (Fig.

> Various degrees of intention tremor occur with neocerebellar damage, but the most severe tremors are associated with damage to the dentatothalamic tract that occurs in multiple sclerosis (MS) or midbrain infarctions.

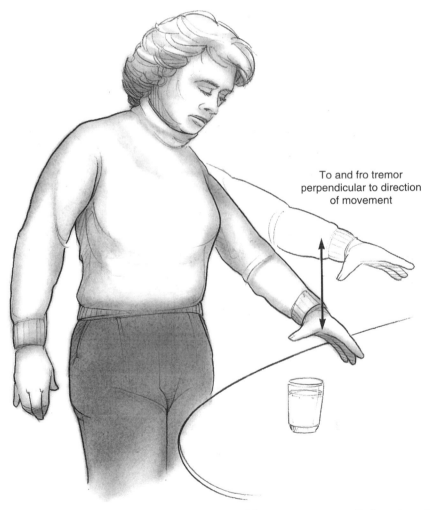

To and fro tremor
perpendicular to direction
of movement

FIGURE 9–9. Posterior lobe syndrome: Intention tremor. To and fro movements perpendicular to intended direction of movement.

9–9). This is referred to as **intention tremor** because it occurs only when a volitional movement is being performed; it is not present at rest.

Other manifestations of posterior lobe lesions, as described in the case at the beginning of this chapter, are **dysmetria,** in which the patient overshoots or undershoots when attempting to touch a target, and **dysdiadochokinesia,** the inability to perform rapid alternating movements such as repetitive hand pronation and supination. In unilateral lesions, ataxia is found ipsilateral; in bilateral lesions both sides are involved. Speech, too, may be affected; the normal rhythm and flow of words is disrupted and words are slurred or broken into their individual syllables. The patient may attempt to compensate by uttering words with great force (explosive speech).

ANTERIOR LOBE

The vermal and paravermal parts of the anterior lobe chiefly maintain coordination of

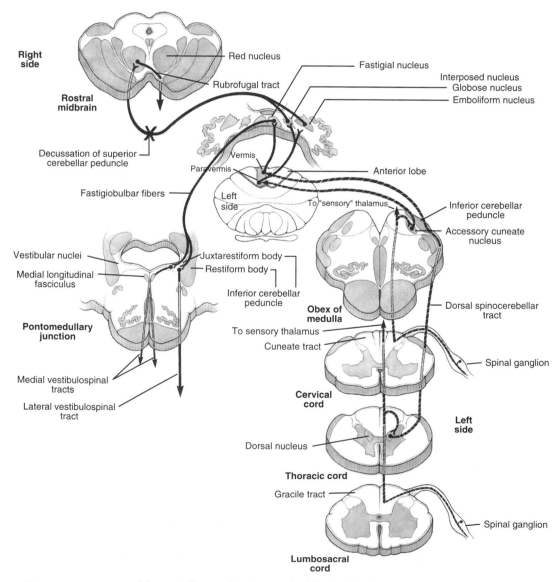

FIGURE 9–10.   Schematic diagram showing anterior lobe circuitry. Input (*broken lines*); output (*solid lines*).

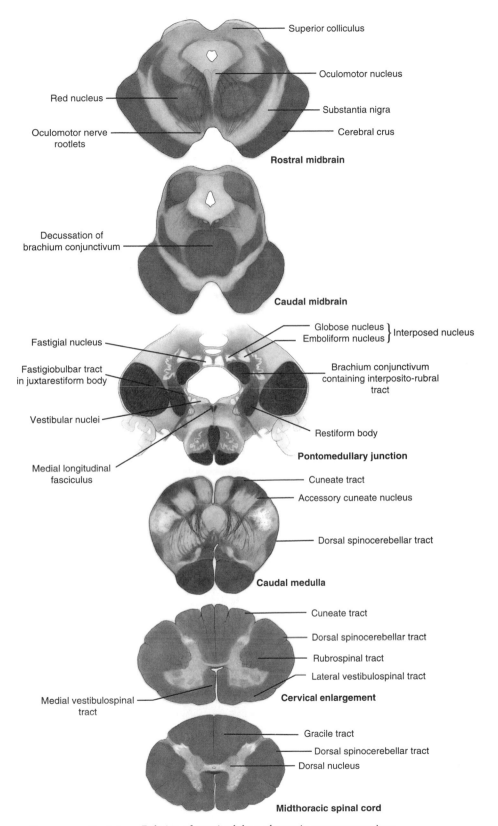

FIGURE 9-11.   Relation of anterior lobe pathways in transverse sections.

limb movements while the movements are being executed, and, hence, the anterior lobe has strong connections with the spinal cord (Fig. 9–10). In the anterior lobe, the lower limb seems to be represented more anteriorly, and the upper limb and then the head are represented more posteriorly.

CONNECTIONS OF THE ANTERIOR LOBE

Discrete information chiefly from muscle spindles and tendon organs of individual lower limb muscles reaches the cerebellum through the dorsal spinocerebellar tract. This tract arises from the dorsal nucleus of Clarke (nucleus thoracicus), which forms a column of neurons in the medial part of lamina VII from spinal cord levels C8 to L2. The dorsal nucleus receives input directly from collaterals ascending from the lumbosacral parts of the gracile tract. The axons of the dorsal nucleus of Clarke ascend ipsilaterally as the dorsal spinocerebellar tract and enter the cerebellum via the inferior cerebellar peduncle (Fig. 9–11).

> The dorsal spinocerebellar tract may be damaged in demyelinating diseases such as MS and Friedreich ataxia. When damaged, cerebellar input from the ipsilateral lower limb is impaired. As a result, lower limb ataxia occurs.

Equivalent types of information from the upper limb ascend in the cuneate tract to the accessory cuneate nucleus. Its neurons, which resemble those of Clarke column, give rise to the cuneatocerebellar tract that also enters the cerebellum through the inferior cerebellar peduncle.

Information of the ongoing influences of the descending motor pathways on the spinal gray matter, reaches the cerebellum through the ventral spinocerebellar tract. This tract differs from the dorsal spinocerebellar tract not only because of its different function, but also because it

1. Originates from neurons scattered in the intermediate zone and anterior horn, and

along the border of the anterior horn at lumbosacral levels;

2. Decussates in the spinal cord and carries impulses from the contralateral side;

3. Enters the cerebellum through the superior cerebellar peduncle and decussates to its original (ipsilateral) side;

4. Appears to be extremely small in the human.

Its medical importance rivals that of the "rostral spinocerebellar tract," which carries similar information from the forelimbs of lower animals, but has not been identified in humans.

Information pertaining to activity in the motor cortex and its pyramidal tract neurons reaches the anterior lobe via the pontine nuclei. This information comes from collaterals of the pyramidal tract fibers. From the pontine nuclei, pontocerebellar fibers cross and enter the cerebellum through the contralateral middle cerebellar peduncle to reach the lateral parts of the anterior lobe. Through these connections, the anterior lobe receives information about the impending influence of the corticospinal fibers on an ongoing movement.

Through the spinal cord and, to a certain extent, the brainstem, the cerebellum receives voluminous information from general sensory receptors throughout the body. Much of this information is from muscular, joint, and cutaneous **mechanoreceptors** that project monosynaptically via the spinocerebellar, cuneocerebellar, and trigeminocerebellar tracts to the vermal and paravermal parts of the anterior lobe chiefly. The trigeminocerebellar fibers carry information from the temporomandibular joint, masticatory and external ocular muscles, etc. Sensory information also reaches the cerebellum via the reticular formation that receives input from the spinal cord and brainstem.

Axons from Purkinje neurons in the anterior lobe, especially its vermal and paravermal parts, influence the fastigial nuclei and interposed nuclei, and the lateral vestibular nucleus. Through the fastigial nucleus and its connections with the vestibular nuclei and reticular formation, the vermis of the anterior lobe has a strong influence

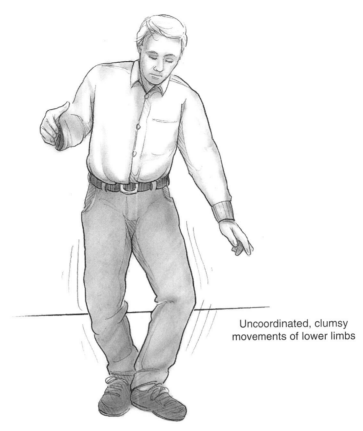

Uncoordinated, clumsy
movements of lower limbs

FIGURE 9-12. Anterior lobe syndrome: Gait ataxia. Clumsy movements of lower limbs.

on the proximal muscles of the limbs. Through the interposed nucleus and its connections with the contralateral red nucleus and reticular formation, which occur via the superior cerebellar peduncle and its decussation (Fig. 9–8), the paravermal part of the anterior lobe influences the more distal muscles of the limbs.

ANTERIOR LOBE SYNDROME

The most common lesions of the anterior lobe result from the malnutrition accompanying chronic alcoholism, which results in damage to the Purkinje neurons—initially damage to those more anterior. Patients with **anterior lobe syndrome** suffer the loss of coordination chiefly in the lower limbs; they have marked gait instability (Fig. 9–12) and walk as if drunk, staggering and reeling in a somewhat stiff-legged manner. Sliding the heel of one foot smoothly down the shin of the other leg (the heel-shin test) is extremely difficult, if not impossible, for the patient to do. If the degeneration progresses posteriorly, the upper limbs and speech may also be affected.

FLOCCULONODULAR LOBE

The flocculonodular lobe, or vestibular part of the cerebellum, is responsible for coordination of the paraxial muscles associated with equilibrium.

CONNECTIONS OF THE FLOCCULONODULAR LOBE

Direct and indirect impulses from the vestibular apparatus in the inner ear carry in-

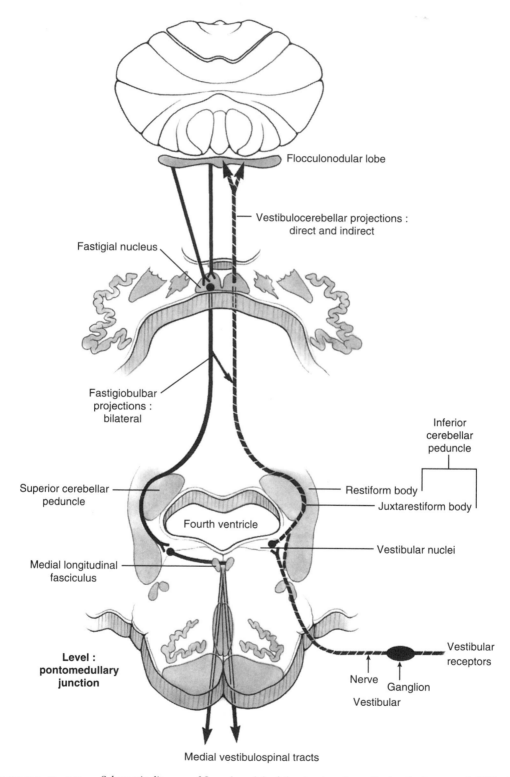

Flocculonodular lobe

Vestibulocerebellar projections :
direct and indirect

Fastigial nucleus

Fastigiobulbar
projections :
bilateral

Inferior
cerebellar
peduncle

Superior cerebellar
peduncle

Restiform body

Juxtarestiform body

Fourth ventricle

Vestibular nuclei

Medial longitudinal
fasciculus

Level :
pontomedullary
junction

Vestibular
receptors

Nerve

Ganglion

Vestibular

Medial vestibulospinal tracts

FIGURE 9-13. Schematic diagram of flocculonodular lobe circuitry. Input (*broken lines*); output (*solid lines*).

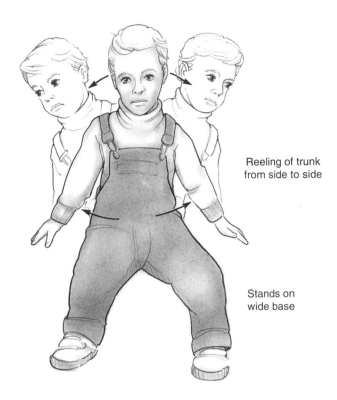

Reeling of trunk
from side to side

Stands on
wide base

FIGURE 9-14. Flocculonodular lobe syndrome: Truncal ataxia. Standing on wide base and reeling from side to side.

formation about position and movements of the head. The direct vestibulocerebellar impulses reach the cerebellum via central projections of the vestibular nerve without synapsing (Fig. 9–13). The indirect vestibulocerebellar impulses come from the vestibular nuclei. Both groups enter the cerebellum in the medial part of the inferior cerebellar peduncle, the juxtarestiform body (Fig. 9–3), and pass chiefly to the flocculonodular lobe and the adjacent parts of the vermis.

Axons from Purkinje neurons in the flocculonodular lobe influence the vestibular nuclei and the adjacent reticular formation indirectly through the fastigial nuclei and directly from the Purkinje cells. The fastigiobulbar projections as well as the direct flocculonodular pro-

jections reach the vestibular nuclei through the juxtarestiform body. Vestibulospinal projections and vestibulo-ocular projections then descend and ascend in the medial longitudinal fasciculus (MLF) to reach the motor neurons innervating the axial muscles and the external ocular muscles, respectively.

FLOCCULONODULAR LOBE SYNDROME

Lesions of the flocculonodular lobe and posterior vermis cause disturbances of balance manifested chiefly by a lack of coordination of the paraxial muscles, a condition referred to as **truncal ataxia** (Fig. 9–14). The patient has no control over the axial muscles and, hence, attempts to walk on a wide base with the trunk constantly reeling and swaying. In severe cases, it is impossible for the patient to sit or stand without falling. This condition is most often seen in young children with **medulloblastomas** arising in the roof of the fourth ventricle, although it may be encountered in older children and adults with other types of tumors in the same region.

Although the precise function of the inferior olivary complex is unknown, unilateral lesions of this structure in experimental animals result in abnormalities similar to destruction of the contralateral half of the cerebellum. In humans, olivary lesions virtually always include the adjacent pyramid whose injury overshadows the cerebellar signs. An exception occurs in cases of olivocerebellar degeneration, a disorder that usually begins at 40 to 50 years of age, in which atrophy of the inferior olive results in progressive ataxia of the upper and lower limbs. In addition to the gait ataxia and intention tremor, dysarthria may develop.

CHAPTER REVIEW QUESTIONS

9–1. Name the cerebellar peduncles and give the principal components of each.

9–2. Name the cerebellar nuclei and give their chief excitatory and inhibitory inputs.

9–3. Give the cardinal manifestations of the three cerebellar syndromes.

9–4. What structures are involved and what abnormalities result from the lesions, appearing as cross-hatched areas in the sections below?

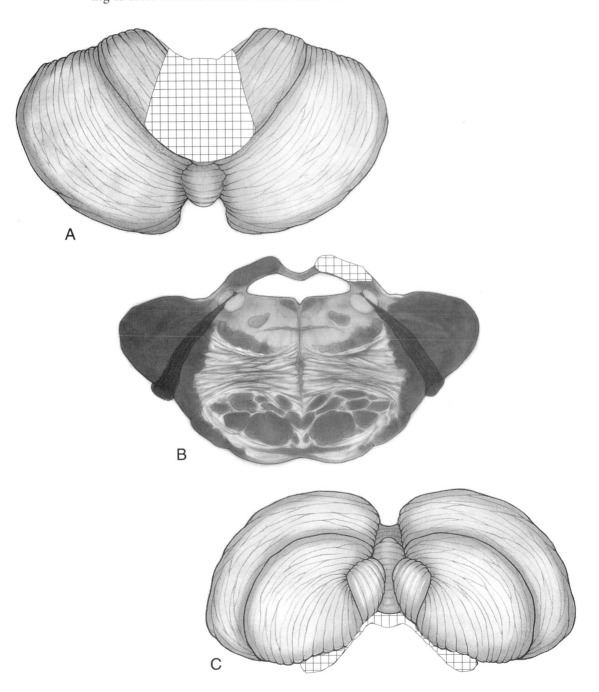

The Ocular Motor System: Vestibulo-ocular Reflex and Conjugate Gaze

■ **On irrigation of the right external auditory canal with cold water in one comatose patient, the eyes turn toward the right and remain in that position until the irrigation is stopped. Similar irrigation in a second comatose patient results in one eye turning up and out and the other eye turning down and in.**

Our sense of vision depends on intact visual pathways that transmit information from receptors in the eyes to the brain. For normal vision to occur, the eyes must move in such a way that an object in the visual field is focused precisely on the visual receptors in the binocular zone of each eye. Otherwise, double vision (diplopia) occurs. Eye movements are controlled by complex and well-organized CNS connections involving centers in the brainstem and cerebral cortex.

Ocular Motor Nuclei

The movement of each eye is controlled by the coordinated action of six muscles: four recti (superior, medial, lateral, inferior) and two obliques (superior and inferior). The muscles are innervated by three cranial nerves: the oculomotor, trochlear, and abducent. The clinical testing of the individual muscles is given in Figure 10–1. Their innervations, actions, and the abnormalities that occur after nerve lesions are shown in Table 10–1.

Vestibulo-Ocular Reflex

One of the two main functions of the vestibular system is to keep the eyes fixed on a target when the head is in motion. Thus, the eyes always reflexly turn opposite to the direction of rotation of the head. The anatomical basis for this phenomenon is the very strong **vestibulo-ocular reflex,** which includes three groups of neurons (Fig. 10–2):

1. Afferent neurons in the vestibular ganglion;

2. Interneurons in the vestibular nuclei;

3. Efferent or lower motor neurons in the oculomotor, trochlear, and abducent nuclei.

Receptors

The receptors for the vestibulo-ocular reflex are located in the ampullae of the three semicircular ducts of the internal ear (Fig. 10–2). The anterior and posterior ducts are oriented vertically but at right angles to each other, whereas the lateral duct is oriented horizontally. Thus, rotation of the head in any direction stimulates the receptors in functional pairs of semicircular ducts. At one end of each duct is an enlargement, the ampulla. In each ampulla, a part of the wall is thickened and projects into the cavity of the duct as the **ampullary crest.** The ampullary crest is a vestibular receptor organ composed of sensory neuroepithelial hair cells and supporting cells (Fig. 10–2A). Overlying each ampullary crest is a gelatinous substance, the **cupula,** in which are embedded the free ends of the stereocilia of the hair cells of the cristae. One of the hairs in each hair cell is longer and is called the **kinocilium.**

When the head begins to rotate, the endolymph in the semicircular duct lags behind

TABLE 10–1. THE EXTRAOCULAR MUSCLES: CLINICAL TESTING, NERVE SUPPLY, AND EYE POSITION AFTER NERVE INJURY.

MUSCLE	CLINICAL TEST	NERVE SUPPLY	EYE POSITION AFTER NERVE INJURY
Medial rectus	Adduction		
Superior rectus	Elevation after abduction		
Inferior rectus	Depression after abduction	Oculomotor	Abducted and depressed
Inferior oblique	Elevation after adduction		
Superior oblique	Depression after adduction	Trochlear	Extorted
Lateral rectus	Abduction	Abducent	Adducted

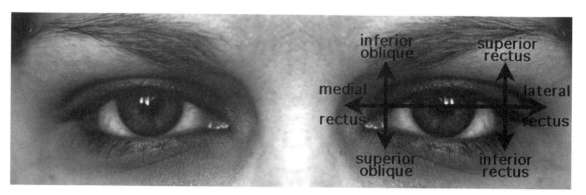

FIGURE 10–1. Clinical testing of extraocular muscles.

and prevents the cupula from moving. As a result, the stereocilia embedded in the cupula are bent in the direction opposite that of the rotation. The hair cells are polarized so that when the stereocilia are bent toward the kinocilium they are depolarized, whereas when they are bent away from the kinocilium they are hyperpolarized. In this way, the receptors in the right and left semicircular ducts work in pairs: when one side is excited, the other is inhibited. The hair cells are in synaptic contact with the dendrites of the bipolar vestibular ganglion cells (Fig. 10–2). Through these synapses, the vestibular ganglion cells are excited as receptor potentials occur in the hair cells when the stereocilia are bent.

NUCLEI

The axons of the vestibular ganglion cells form the vestibular nerve, which enters the brainstem at the pontomedullary junction in the cerebello-pontine angle. The fibers proceed dorsally and terminate in the superior and medial vestibular nuclei (Figs. 10–**2B**, 10–3).

Vestibulo-ocular fibers then pass to the ocular motor nuclei chiefly via the medial longitudinal fasciculus (MLF). The vestibulo-ocular reflex connections for horizontal rotation to the right are shown in Figure 10–4.

The vestibulo-ocular reflex can be used to assess levels of brainstem damage in a comatose patient. When a comatose patient's head is briskly turned to one side or the other, or is tilted up or down, the eyes turn in the opposite direction. This phenomenon, referred to as the **oculocephalic reflex** or **doll's eye movement,** is indicative of an intact pathway subserving the vestibulo-ocular reflex. Normally these reflex movements are suppressed by the cerebral cortex. In the comatose patient, however, the reflex is disinhibited and its presence shows that the central parts of the tegmentum of the midbrain and pons are intact.

Likewise, the oculocephalic reflex can be induced in comatose patients by irrigating the external auditory canal with warm or cold water, as described in the case that introduced the chapter. With cold water irrigation, both eyes turn toward the side irrigated, whereas with warm water irrigation they turn toward the opposite side. These movements are also manifestations of the

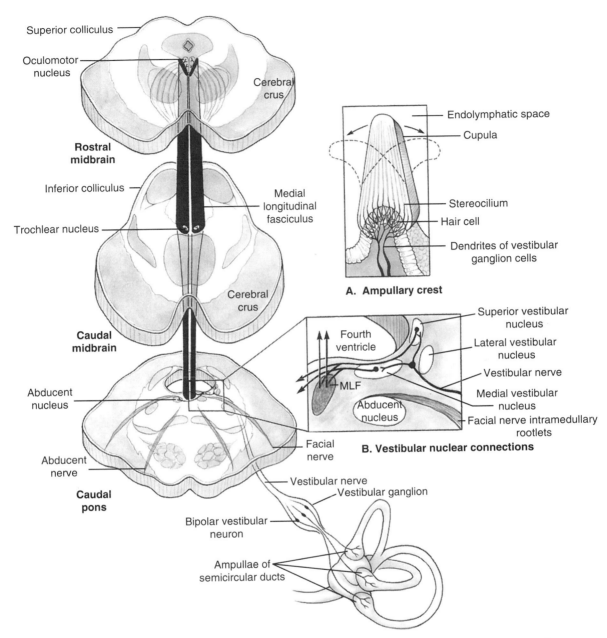

FIGURE 10-2. Schematic diagram of vestibulo-ocular reflex principal connections. **A.** Histology of ampullary crest. **B.** Connections of vestibular nuclei.

vestibulo-ocular reflex and are comparable to the slow phase of the **nystagmus** induced by caloric stimulation in normal individuals.

Nystagmus refers to involuntary rhythmical movements of the eyes that include two components: a slow drifting away from the target and a fast return to the target. Nystagmus can also be induced by stimulating the vestibular apparatus either by rotating the head (vestibular nystagmus) or by placing cold or warm water in the ear (caloric nystagmus). Both methods induce currents in the en-

dolymphatic fluid in the semicircular ducts, the rotation because of the fluid inertia and the thermal because of convection currents. Both stimulate the hair cells of the cristae and initiate the powerful vestibulo-ocular reflex. The slow phases of the vestibular and caloric nystagmus are caused by this vestibulo-ocular path, whereas the fast phases are triggered by the cerebral cortex. In all cases, nystagmus is described according to the fast phase because it is more obvious than the slow phase.

Rostral midbrain

Superior colliculus

Cerebral aqueduct

Periaqueductal gray

Oculomotor nucleus
Medial longitudinal fasc.

Red nucleus

Substantia nigra

Pyramidal tract

Oculomotor (IIICN)

Caudal midbrain

Inferior colliculus

Cerebral aqueduct

Periaqueductal gray

Trochlear nucleus

Medial longitudinal fasc.

Decussation of superior cerebellar peduncle

Substantia nigra

Pyramidal tract

Cerebral crus

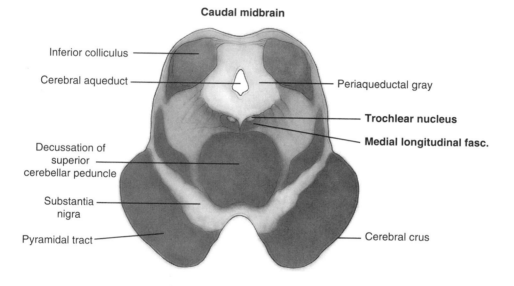

Caudal pons

Inferior } Cerebellar peduncles
Superior }

Fourth ventricle

Abducent nucleus

Superior } Vestibular nuclei
Medial }

Medial longitudinal fasciculus

Paramedian pontine reticular formation

Spinal trigeminal tr.

Middle cerebellar peduncle

Facial nucleus

Facial (VIICN)

Corticospinal tract

Abducent (VICN)

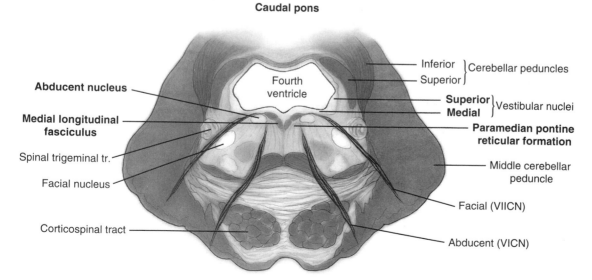

FIGURE 10-3. Relations of vestibulo-ocular paths in transverse section (bolded terms relate to ocular motor paths).

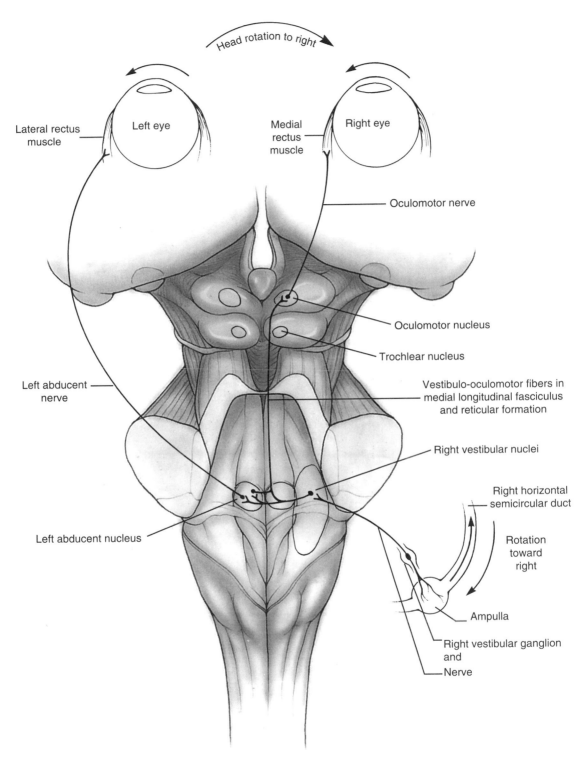

Head rotation to right

Lateral rectus muscle

Left eye

Medial rectus muscle

Right eye

Oculomotor nerve

Oculomotor nucleus

Trochlear nucleus

Vestibulo-oculomotor fibers in medial longitudinal fasciculus and reticular formation

Left abducent nerve

Right vestibular nuclei

Right horizontal semicircular duct

Rotation toward right

Left abducent nucleus

Ampulla

Right vestibular ganglion and Nerve

FIGURE 10-4. Schematic drawing of dorsal aspect of brainstem showing the vestibulo-ocular reflex on rotation to right.

VOLUNTARY EYE MOVEMENTS

Voluntary eye movements are of two types: vergence and conjugate. Vergence movements occur when eyes shift between distant and near objects. When the shift is from distant to near objects, the eyes converge; when from near to distant, they diverge. Conjugate movements occur when the eyes move in the same direction, i.e., to the right, left, up, or down. The six pairs of external ocular muscles responsible for keeping both eyes focused on the same object are controlled by gaze centers, highly specialized groups of neurons in the brainstem and cerebral cortex.

BRAINSTEM GAZE CENTERS

There are three centers in the brainstem that control eye movements. The horizontal gaze center is in the pons, and the vertical gaze and vergence centers are in the midbrain.

HORIZONTAL CENTER

The **horizontal gaze center** is located in the paramedian pontine reticular formation (PPRF) (Fig. 10–3). The center on each side is responsible for conjugate movements toward that side; hence, a unilateral lesion results in paralysis of gaze toward the ipsilateral side. From each center, nerve impulses pass to the ipsilateral abducent nucleus and, via the contralateral medial longitudinal fasciculus (MLF), to the lower motor neurons in the oculomotor nucleus innervating the medial rectus muscle (Fig. 10–5). In this way, the lateral rectus muscle of the ipsilateral eye and the medial rectus muscle of the contralateral eye contract

---

Clinical evidence supports the contralateral MLF route to the oculomotor nucleus. A unilateral lesion of the MLF rostral to the abducent nucleus results in paralysis of adduction in the eye ipsilateral to the lesion when the patient attempts to gaze toward the opposite side. The affected eye does adduct during convergence; hence, the medial rectus muscle and its innervation are functional. This phenomenon is referred to as **internuclear ophthalmoplegia.** If present bilaterally, it is almost invariably associated with MS.

---

simultaneously. It is currently thought that the connection to the oculomotor nucleus occurs via interneurons in the abducent nucleus whose axons cross and ascend in the contralateral MLF.

VERTICAL CENTER

The **vertical gaze center** resides in the periaqueductal gray matter of the rostral midbrain (Fig. 10–3). This gaze center is bilateral and is thought to influence the ocular nuclei through accessory oculomotor nuclei located at this level. Clinical evidence indicates that upward movements are represented more dorsally; with pressure on the tectum, such as that caused by a pineal tumor, upward gaze becomes paralyzed before downward. Paralysis of downward gaze is seen with lesions located more deeply.

VERGENCE CENTER

A brainstem center controlling convergence and divergence of the eyes, as when directing vision from far to near or near to far objects, is thought to be located in the rostral midbrain near the vertical gaze center. Evidence for this location is derived from clinical cases in which vergence is paralyzed when pressure is exerted on the roof of the midbrain by an expanding pineal tumor.

CORTICAL GAZE CENTERS

Within the cerebral cortex are several centers associated with eye movements. The two most well known are the **frontal eye field** and the **occipital eye field.** Anatomical and physiological information concerning similar centers in the parietal and temporal lobes is meager.

FRONTAL EYE FIELD

A center in the cerebral cortex for voluntary eye movements is located chiefly in the posterior part of the middle frontal gyrus and called the frontal eye field (Fig. 10–6). Stimulation of this area results in aversive eye movements in the form of **saccade** (rapid voluntary searching movements). The frontal eye field chiefly influ-

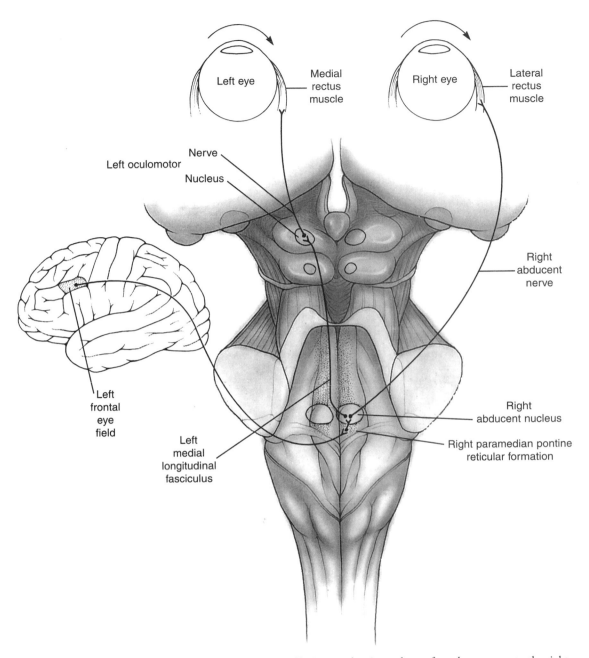

FIGURE 10-5. Schematic drawing of dorsal view of brainstem showing pathways for voluntary gaze to the right.

ences the contralateral horizontal gaze center. Recent evidence suggests that additional areas in the frontal and parietal lobes also influence voluntary eye movements.

Lesions affecting horizontal gaze and the resulting abnormalities are given in Figure 10–7.

Acute lesions of the frontal eye field result in conjugate deviation of the eyes toward the side of the lesion and paralysis of voluntary gaze toward the contralateral side (Fig. 10–7). This paralysis is transient because of the bilateralism of these cortical connections with the brainstem gaze centers.

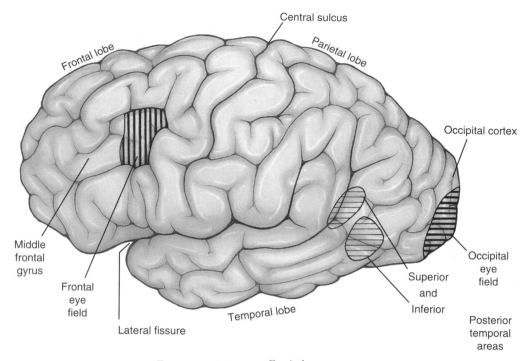

FIGURE 10-6.   Cortical gaze centers.

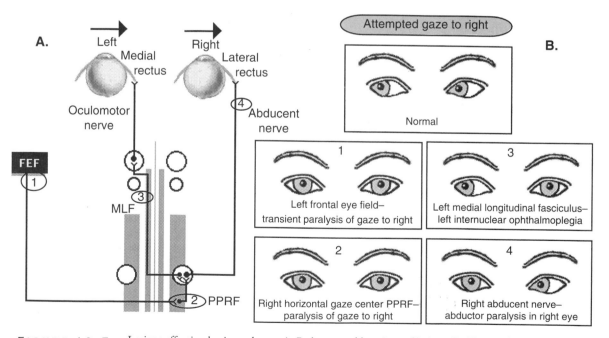

FIGURE 10-7.   Lesions affecting horizontal gaze. **A.** Pathways and locations of lesions. **B.** Abnormalities with attempted gaze to the right.

OCCIPITAL EYE FIELD

The occipital eye field is located in the primary visual and perhaps the visual association parts of the occipital cortex. It functions as a cortical reflex center and plays a role in optokinetic and smooth pursuit (tracking) movements. An example of the former occurs in an individual in a moving vehicle watching an object in the passing landscape. The eyes will automatically follow the particular object in the landscape until it disappears from view, at which time the eyes move rapidly in the opposite direction and fix on a new object in the landscape. A similar phenomenon occurs when vision is directed at vertical black and white stripes on a slowly rotating drum. The eyes will fix on a particular stripe, follow it until it disappears from view, and then move rapidly in the opposite direction to fix on a new stripe on the drum. These slow drifting and fast return movements are referred to as **optokinetic nystagmus.** Smooth pursuit movements occur when the observer is stationary and an object in the environment is reflexly followed by the eyes. Conjugate reflex movements are also associated with cortical areas in the posterior parts of the temporal lobe (Fig. 10–6) because lesions here disrupt smooth pursuit movements.

Optokinetic nystagmus is the result of deep-seated tracking mechanisms and is thought to involve several cortical phenomena. An absence or a decrease in the amplitude of optokinetic nystagmus occurs after a lesion in the parieto-occipital region. The absence or decrease is manifested only when an object is rotating toward the side of the lesion.

Vergence movements are also controlled by the occipital eye field. Occipitofugal fibers pass to the superior colliculus and midbrain vergence centers, which then influence the medial rectus muscles and lateral rectus muscles via the oculomotor and abducent nuclei. The connections to the abducent nucleus are made through the reticular formation, not the MLF, because vergence is not impaired by MLF lesions.

SUPERIOR COLLICULUS

It is well-known that the superior colliculus is responsible for reflex turning of the head and eyes in response to startling pain and auditory stimuli; however, the role of the superior colliculus in the control of ordinary eye movements is not entirely clear. Because of the input it receives from the retina and cortical eye fields and its output to the brainstem gaze centers, this structure undoubtedly plays a role as a visuomotor integration center. Lesions of the superior colliculi do not result in major eye movement abnormalities, however, probably due to the diversity of the connections between the cortical and brainstem gaze centers. For instance, the frontal eye field projects bilaterally to the brainstem gaze centers via (*a*) corticonuclear paths that travel with the corticospinal tracts to the levels of the gaze centers, where the fibers then enter the tegmentum to reach these centers, and (*b*) a transtegmental route that descends through the tegmentum of the midbrain and pons. Thus, focal lesions in the brainstem interrupt only a small portion of the total input to the gaze centers.

Programming of eye movements appears to occur not only in the frontal eye field but also in the basal ganglia. Input reaches the basal ganglia via corticostriate projections from the frontal eye field, prefrontal cortex, and the posterior parietal cortex. Outputs from the globus pallidus and substantia nigra (reticular part) pass to the ventral anterior thalamic nuclei and medial dorsal thalamic nuclei, which, in turn, directly influence the frontal eye field and adjacent parts of the prefrontal cortex. In basal ganglia disorders such as Parkinson disease, normal spontaneous ocular movements are lacking or seldom occur. This phenomenon, along with slightly widened palpebral fissures and infrequent blinking, gives the eyes a staring appearance.

Cerebellar coordination of eye movements occurs via connections of the flocculonodular lobe and fastigial nuclei with the vestibular nuclei. Vestibulo-ocular connections then carry the cerebellar influences to the nuclei of the ocular motor nerves. Unilateral cerebellar lesions result in a conspicuous nystagmus, especially when the eyes are directed toward the side of the lesion.

CHAPTER REVIEW QUESTIONS

Locate the lesion in each of the following:

10–1. Cold water irrigation of the left external auditory canal in a comatose patient results in:

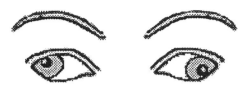

10–2. Attempted gaze to the left results in:

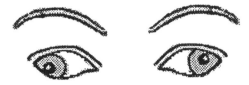

10–3. Attempted gaze to the right results in:

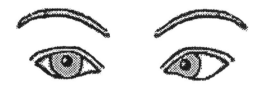

10–4. Attempted gaze to the left results in:

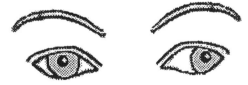

10–5. Attempted gaze to the right results in:

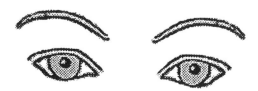

The Somatosensory System: Anesthesia and Analgesia

■ The following three sets of neurologic symptoms are indicative of lesions involving the somatosensory pathways at three different levels in the central nervous system (CNS):

1. **The first patient has loss of general sensations below the umbilicus, such that on the right side only the touch, pressure, and limb position senses are lost whereas on the left side only the pain and temperature senses are lost.**

2. **The second patient has loss of pin prick and temperature sensations on the left side in the limbs, trunk, neck, and back of the head and on the right side on the face and anterior part of the scalp.**

3. **The third patient has total left hemianesthesia, that is, loss of pin prick, temperature, touch, pressure, and limb position senses on the left side of the entire body.**

All sensations arising from skin, connective tissues, voluntary muscles, periosteum, teeth, etc., belong to the general somatic sensory system, more commonly referred to as the **somatosensory system.**

General Senses

The general senses include light touch or tactile discrimination and sensations of pressure or deep touch, vibration, limb position and motion, pain, and temperature. The somatosensory pathways consist of three neurons: number 1 in the sensory ganglia, number 2 in the spinal cord or brainstem or both, and number 3 in the thalamus.

Light Touch

Light touch is also called tactile sense and refers to the awareness and precise location of very delicate mechanical stimuli such as stroking the hairs on the skin or, in hairless areas, stroking the skin with a wisp of cotton or a feather. Light touch includes three other phenomena: two-point sense, **stereognosis,** and **graphesthesia.** Two-point sense is the ability to distinguish stimulation by one or two points applied to the skin. The minimal distance between the two points that can be felt separately varies considerably on different parts of the body. Two points can be distinguished as close as 1 mm on the tip of the tongue and 2 to 4 mm on the finger tips, whereas on the dorsum of the hand two points closer than 20 to 30 mm cannot be distinguished from one another. Stereognosis is the ability to recognize objects by touch alone, using the object's size, shape, texture, weight, etc. Graphesthesia is the ability to recognize numbers or letters drawn on the skin. Both stereognosis and graphesthesia require intact light touch pathways and memory; in other words, the objects, numbers, or letters must be known to the individual being tested.

Pressure

The perception of pressure involves stimuli applied to subcutaneous structures. Pressure sense is tested by firmly pressing on the skin with a blunt object and by squeezing subcutaneous structures and muscles. Pressure sensations are often referred to as deep touch.

VIBRATION SENSE

When the shaft of an oscillating high-frequency (256 vibrations per second) tuning fork is gently applied to the skin overlying bony prominences, vibrations in the subcutaneous tissues are perceived. **Vibration sense,** therefore, requires intact pathways from deep structures such as subcutaneous connective tissue, periosteum, and muscle.

When an oscillating low-frequency (128 vibrations per second) tuning fork is used, the sensation is described as "flutter" or fine vibrations in the skin itself. Flutter sensations are associated with the light touch pathways.

LIMB POSITION AND MOTION SENSE

Position or posture sense is the awareness of the position of the skeletal parts of the body. Motion sense is the awareness of active or passive movements of the skeletal parts of the body. Motion sense can be tested by passively flexing and extending individual fingers and toes, the hand and foot, the forearm and leg, etc. With eyes closed, the subject should be able to recognize the direction, speed, and range of the movement. Position sense can be tested by passively moving a limb or one of its parts to a certain position and having the subject move the opposite limb to the same position. A patient who can stand with the feet together and the eyes open, but who sways and falls when the eyes are closed, has the **Romberg sign,** which indicates an absence of position sense in the lower limbs.

PAIN

There are two types of pain sensations: fast and slow. **Fast pain** is of the sharp, pricking type and is well localized. The ability to feel fast pain is tested by alternately touching the tip and head of a safety pin to the surface of the skin. The patient should be able to readily distinguish the sharpness of the tip of the pin from the dullness of the head. **Slow pain** is of the dull, burning type and is diffuse rather than localized. It results from tissue injury.

TEMPERATURE

Temperature sensations range from cold to hot and can be tested by touching the skin with test tubes filled with either cold or warm water.

PERIPHERAL COMPONENTS

The peripheral fibers of the somatosensory system are the branches of unipolar neurons in the dorsal root (spinal) ganglia and the homologous ganglia of cranial nerves V, VII, IX, and X. These are the first neurons in the paths and, hence, are referred to as the primary somatosensory neurons or first order neurons. Each possesses only one process, the axon, which bifurcates into a peripheral branch and a central branch. The central branch enters the dorsal root of the spinal nerve or the sensory root of the appropriate cranial nerve, and passes to the spinal cord or brainstem, respectively. The peripheral branch enters the spinal or cranial nerve and eventually terminates as an ending that responds to a specific type of stimulus. These endings are called sensory receptors.

SOMATOSENSORY RECEPTORS

The receptors for general sensations can conveniently be divided into three groups: mechanoreceptors, **nociceptors,** and thermoreceptors. Mechanoreceptors respond to information of the receptor itself or the tissue surrounding it and are associated with the touch, pressure, vibration, and limb position and motion sensations. Nociceptors (noci means noxious) respond to pain, and thermoreceptors respond to warm or cold stimuli. All of these receptors possess the property of converting a change in the environment, the stimulus, into an electrical signal, the receptor potential, which can then trigger an impulse or action potential in the nerve fiber. The principal somatosensory receptors and their functions are given in Table 11–1.

TABLE 11–1. CLASSIFICATION OF SOMATOSENSORY RECEPTORS

CATEGORY	NAME	FUNCTION
Mechanoreceptors	Meissner corpuscles	Tactile (in hairless skin)
	Hair follicle receptors	Tactile (in hairy skin)
	Merkel discs	Pressure
	Ruffini endings	Pressure
	Pacinian corpuscles	Vibration
	Muscle spindles	Limb position and motion
Nociceptors	A-delta mechanical (encapsulated)	Pin prick
	C-polymodal (free nerve ending)	Tissue damage
Thermoreceptors	Free nerve endings	Cold or warmth

TABLE 11–2. CLASSIFICATION OF SOMATOSENSORY NERVE FIBERS

NUMERICAL CLASS	MYELINATED	DIAMETER (μM)	CONDUCTION VELOCITY (M/SEC)	LETTER CLASS	TYPES OF SENSATIONS
I	Yes	12–20	75–120	A_α	Limb position and motion
II	Yes	6–12	30–75	A_β	Tactile, pressure, vibration
III	Yes	1–6	5–30	A_d	Fast pain, cold
IV	No	<1.5	0.5–2	C	Slow pain, warmth

SOMATOSENSORY NERVE FIBERS

The nerve fibers conducting general sensations vary in their sizes or diameters and in their conduction velocities. In general, the larger the fiber, the faster the conduction velocity. The velocity at which a nerve fiber conducts impulses is important because the faster the conduction the quicker the impulses reach the CNS where a response can be elicited. The nerve fibers conducting tactile, pressure, vibratory, and limb position and motion sensations are larger and faster conducting than those nerve fibers conducting pain and temperature impulses.

Nerve fibers are classified in two ways, by conduction velocity and by diameter. Nerve fibers are classified according to conduction velocity as type A, B, or C, with A indicating the fastest conduction velocity and C the slowest. Nerve fibers are classified according to diameter into groups I, II, III, and IV. Groups I, II, and III consist of myelinated fibers of decreasing size, whereas group IV consists of unmyelinated fibers. The classifications of the various types of somatosensory fibers are given in Table 11–2.

> The differences in the size and conduction velocity of the larger touch fibers and smaller pain fibers in peripheral nerves allow the selective electrical stimulation of one group and not the other. This phenomenon is the basis for the selective stimulation of the larger touch fibers by **transcutaneous electrical nerve stimulation (TENS)**, a current clinical treatment for the relief of some forms of chronic pain.

DERMATOMES

The area of skin supplied by the somatosensory fibers from a single spinal nerve is called a **dermatome** (Fig. 11–1). Although there is overlap between the dermatomes, they are very useful in localizing the levels of lesions. The dermatomes essential to know for neuroanatomy problem solving are: C2, back of the head; C5, tip of the shoulder; C6, thumb; C7, middle finger; C8, small finger; T4 or T5, nipple; T10, umbilicus; L1, inguinal ligament; L4 or L5, big toe; S1, small toe; and S5, perianal region.

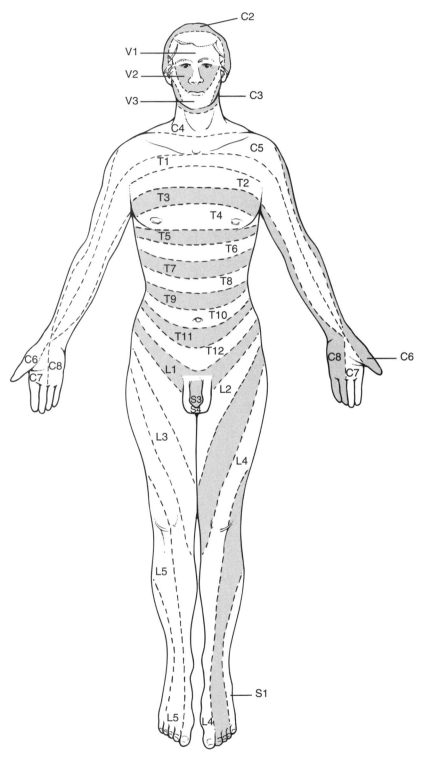

FIGURE 11-1.   Dermatomes. **A.** Anterior surface.

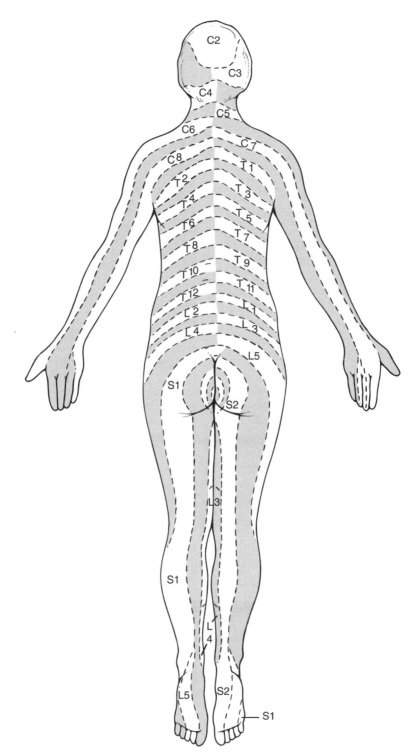

FIGURE 11-1 (CONTINUED). **B.** Posterior surface.

SPINAL TACTILE, VIBRATION, AND LIMB POSITION AND MOTION PATHWAYS

A series of three neurons transmits the touch system impulses from the mechanoreceptors in the periphery to the cerebral cortex, where these sensations are perceived (Figs. 11–2, 11–3).

FIRST ORDER NEURONS

The larger, fast conducting unipolar neurons in the dorsal root or spinal ganglia are the primary touch, vibration, and limb position neurons. The central branches enter the spinal cord through the more medial parts of the dorsal roots (Fig. 2–4) and are funneled medially into the dorsal funiculus or column where they immediately turn and ascend. As the entering touch and limb position fibers turn to ascend, they give branches that enter the spinal gray matter for reflex and pain modulation purposes. (The role of muscle spindle afferent fibers in the myotatic reflex is described in Chapter 5, and the role of touch afferent fibers in pain modulation is described later in this chapter.) Those entering below midthoracic levels form the gracile tract and those entering above midthoracic levels form the cuneate tract. In the cervical segments of the spinal cord, the two tracts are partially separated by the posterior intermediate septum.

Because new fibers are added to the dorsal columns at their lateral surfaces, a precise somatotopic localization exists, i.e., fibers conducting impulses from the sacral dermatomes are most medial, whereas those from the lumbar, thoracic, and cervical dermatomes are located progressively more laterally. Some shifting occurs in the rostral half of the spinal cord because the sacral fibers here occupy most of the dorsal part of the dorsal column and hence tend to be spared when the central part of the spinal cord is damaged.

> Because the gracile and cuneate tracts ascend to the brain without crossing, their unilateral interruption at any level of the spinal cord results in the loss of the tactile, pressure, vibration, and limb position sensations in the dermatomes on the ipsilateral (same) side below the level of the lesion.

SECOND ORDER NEURONS

The axons of the gracile and cuneate tracts terminate at the secondary somatosensory neurons located in the gracile and cuneate nuclei, the dorsal column nuclei, within the caudal medulla. Axons from the dorsal column nuclei form small bundles of myelinated fibers termed **internal arcuate fibers** (Figs. 11–2–11–4), which pass anteromedially as they arch toward the midline. The axons from the dorsal column nuclei cross the midline as the "sensory decussation" and immediately begin to ascend in a large bundle located next to the midline, the **medial lemniscus.**

> The level of the dorsal column nuclei and sensory decussation is of medical significance because a unilateral lesion that interrupts the impulses before they decussate, that is, a lesion in the dorsal columns or their nuclei, results in losses of the tactile, vibration, and limb position senses on the ipsilateral side below the level of the lesion. However, a unilateral lesion beyond the sensory decussation, that is, a lesion in the medial lemniscus or subsequent structures in the path, results in the loss of these sensations contralaterally.

The medial lemniscus borders the midline in the medulla and contains axons from the gracile nucleus in its anterior half and from the cuneate nucleus in its posterior half (Figs. 11–2–11–4). Thus, in the medulla, the medial lemniscus contains impulses from the contralateral lower limb anteriorly and from the contralateral upper limb posteriorly. In the pons, the medial lemniscus gradually shifts laterally and becomes oriented horizontally. At this point, the lower limb is represented laterally and the upper limb medially.

THIRD ORDER NEURONS

The medial lemniscus passes without interruption to the ventral posterolateral (VPL) nucleus of the thalamus. The VPL nucleus is somatotopically organized, so that the contralateral lower limb is represented laterally and the contralateral upper limb medially.

Axons from tertiary somatosensory neurons within the VPL nucleus pass laterally as thalamocortical fibers and enter the posterior limb of the internal capsule where they are located in its more posterior part. They terminate in the

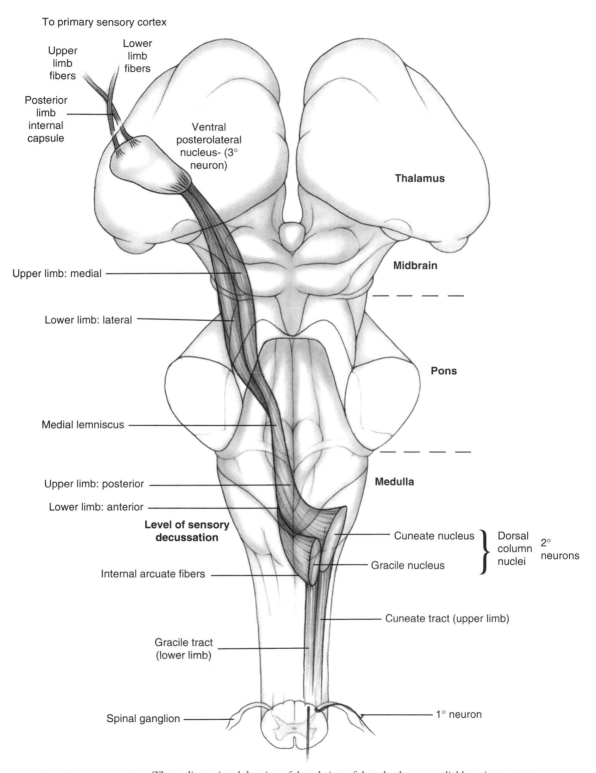

To primary sensory cortex

Upper limb fibers

Lower limb fibers

Posterior limb internal capsule

Ventral posterolateral nucleus- (3° neuron)

Thalamus

Upper limb: medial

Midbrain

Lower limb: lateral

Pons

Medial lemniscus

Medulla

Upper limb: posterior

Lower limb: anterior

Cuneate nucleus

Gracile nucleus

Dorsal column nuclei } 2° neurons

Level of sensory decussation

Internal arcuate fibers

Cuneate tract (upper limb)

Gracile tract (lower limb)

Spinal ganglion

1° neuron

FIGURE 11–2.   Three-dimensional drawing of dorsal view of dorsal column–medial lemniscus system.

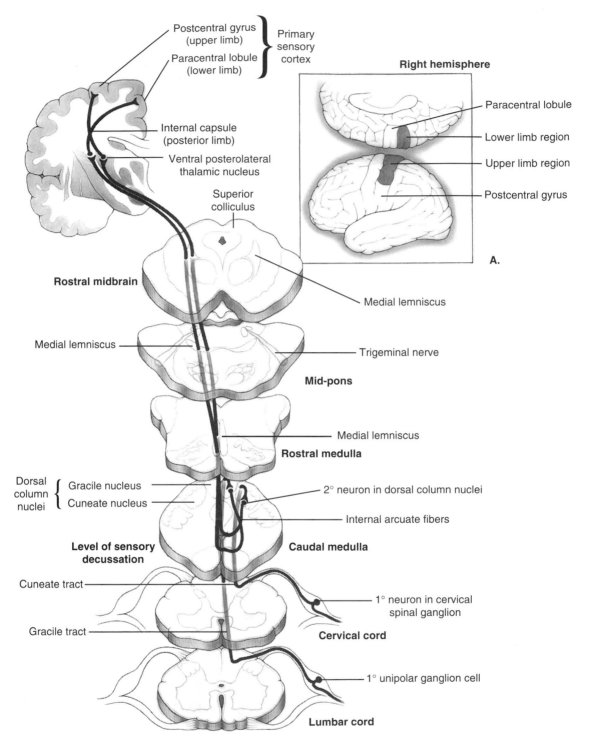

F I G U R E   1 1 – 3 .   Schematic diagram showing the touch system pathway from spinal nerves. **A.** Distribution in primary sensory cortex.

primary somatosensory (SI) cortex, which is located in the postcentral gyrus and the adjacent posterior part of the paracentral lobule. The contralateral upper limb is represented approx-

imately in the dorsal half of the postcentral gyrus, and the contralateral lower limb is represented in the posterior part of the paracentral lobule (Fig. 11–3).

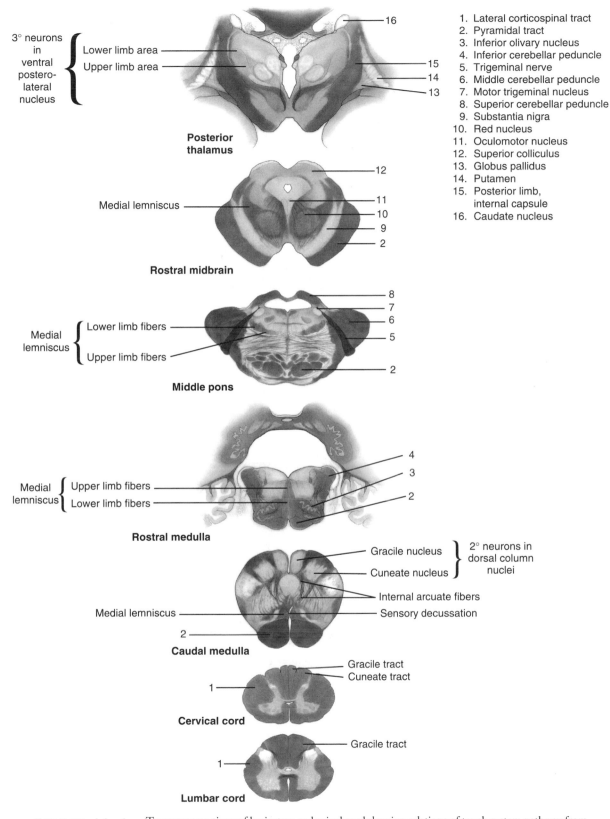

3° neurons in ventral posterolateral nucleus
{
Lower limb area
Upper limb area
}

16

15
14
13

Posterior thalamus

1. Lateral corticospinal tract
2. Pyramidal tract
3. Inferior olivary nucleus
4. Inferior cerebellar peduncle
5. Trigeminal nerve
6. Middle cerebellar peduncle
7. Motor trigeminal nucleus
8. Superior cerebellar peduncle
9. Substantia nigra
10. Red nucleus
11. Oculomotor nucleus
12. Superior colliculus
13. Globus pallidus
14. Putamen
15. Posterior limb, internal capsule
16. Caudate nucleus

Medial lemniscus

12
11
10
9
2

Rostral midbrain

8
7
6
5
2

Medial lemniscus {
Lower limb fibers
Upper limb fibers
}

Middle pons

4
3
2

Medial lemniscus {
Upper limb fibers
Lower limb fibers
}

Rostral medulla

Gracile nucleus
Cuneate nucleus
}
2° neurons in dorsal column nuclei

Internal arcuate fibers

Medial lemniscus

Sensory decussation

2

Caudal medulla

Gracile tract
Cuneate tract

1

Cervical cord

Gracile tract

1

Lumbar cord

FIGURE 11–4. Transverse sections of brainstem and spinal cord showing relations of touch system pathway from spinal nerves.

SPINAL PAIN AND TEMPERATURE PATHWAYS

Recent anatomical and clinical evidence indicates that the fast and slow pain paths are dissimilar. It is now thought that the fast pain associated with pin prick is carried by a phylogenetically newer pathway often referred to as the **neospinothalamic system.** Slow pain, however, is transmitted by phylogenetically older neurons that form the **paleospinothalamic** and spinoreticulothalamic systems. The anatomical differences in these systems are described later.

A series of three neurons transmits fast pain and temperature impulses from the receptors in the periphery to the cerebral cortex where these sensations are perceived (Figs. 11–5, 11–6).

FIRST ORDER NEURONS

The smaller, slower conducting unipolar neurons in the dorsal root or spinal ganglia are the primary neurons for the pain and temperature impulses carried by the spinal nerves. The central branches of their axons enter the spinal cord through the more lateral parts of the dorsal rootlets (Fig. 2–4), which funnel them into the **dorsolateral fasciculus** or tract of Lissauer. On entering this tract, each axon bifurcates into an ascending and a descending branch. These branches extend for one or two segments

> The entrance and termination of primary pain fibers in the dorsal horn form the anatomical basis for the relief of pain in neurosurgical destruction of the **dorsal root entry zone (DREZ).** This procedure is especially useful in cases of chronic pain resulting from avulsion of spinal nerves from the cord and in cancer-related pain syndromes.
>
> In some cases of **dorsal rhizotomy,** that is, cutting the dorsal roots to relieve chronic pain, the pain persists. In such cases, the persisting pain can be relieved by a second operation that removes the spinal ganglia. The obvious explanation for this phenomenon is the entrance of pain fibers via the ventral roots. Such aberrant routes have been shown to exist in humans.

and give off collateral branches along their entire length. The collaterals enter the gray matter and synapse chiefly in the dorsal horn (laminae I–VI) (Figs. 11-6, 11-7).

SECOND ORDER NEURONS

Secondary nociceptive neurons are widely distributed in the spinal gray matter. Those carrying fast pain impulses, and probably temperature impulses also, are located primarily in the marginal nucleus (lamina I), although some are also found as deep as the proper sensory nucleus (laminae IV and V). The axons from the secondary pain and temperature neurons pass ventromedial and decussate in the ventral white commissure, which is just anterior to the central canal.

> The proximity of the ventral white commissure to the central canal is a relation that can become clinically important in cases of pathologic cavitation of the spinal cord, termed **syringomyelia.** When the cavitation extends ventrally and interrupts this commissure, bilateral loss of pain and temperature sensations in the dermatomes at the levels of the lesion occurs—the **commissural syndrome** (Fig. 11–8).

After crossing to the contralateral side, the secondary pain and temperature axons pass to the anterior part of the lateral funiculus, the anterolateral quadrant, where they ascend in the spinothalamic tract. Because fibers are added to this tract at its medial surface, somatotopic localization results: the sacral fibers are located laterally, that is, near the surface of the anterolateral quadrant. The lumbar, thoracic, and cervical dermatomes are located successively most medially (Fig 11–8).

> Surgical interruption of the anterolateral quadrant of the spinal cord (**anterolateral cordotomy**) results in the loss of all pain and temperature sensations contralaterally in dermatomes below the level of the lesion. The procedure is mostly used for the relief of pain associated with terminal cancer because these patients will unlikely survive long enough to suffer the intense chronic pain that eventually occurs after most injuries to the CNS pain pathways.

THIRD ORDER NEURONS

The spinothalamic tract ascends in the lateral parts of the medulla and pons and intermingles

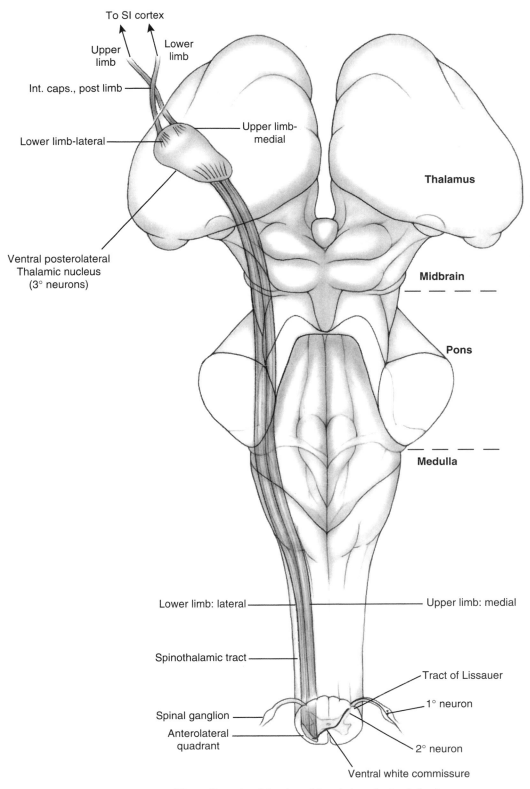

To SI cortex

Upper limb

Lower limb

Int. caps., post limb

Upper limb-medial

Lower limb-lateral

Thalamus

Ventral posterolateral Thalamic nucleus (3° neurons)

Midbrain

Pons

Medulla

Lower limb: lateral

Upper limb: medial

Spinothalamic tract

Tract of Lissauer

1° neuron

Spinal ganglion

Anterolateral quadrant

2° neuron

Ventral white commissure

FIGURE 11-5.   Three-dimensional drawing of dorsal view of spinothalamic system.

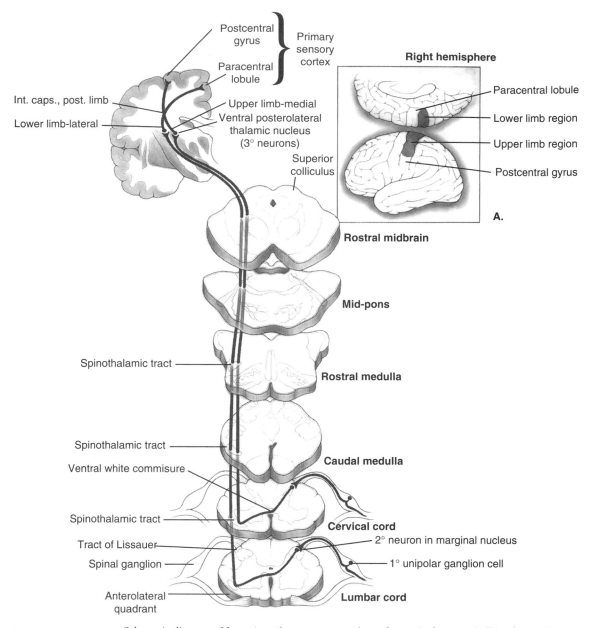

FIGURE 11–6. Schematic diagram of fast pain and temperature pathway from spinal nerves. **A.** Distribution in primary sensory cortex.

with the medial lemniscus in the rostral midbrain. Both tracts terminate in the VPL. The tertiary fast pain and temperature neurons in the VPL give off thalamocortical fibers that pass laterally and enter the posterior limb of the internal capsule where they intermingle with the tactile and limb position axons. Like the tertiary touch system fibers, the tertiary fast pain and temperature fibers terminate in those parts of the postcentral gyrus and paracentral lobule associated with the contralateral upper and lower limbs. On reaching these parts of the SI cortex, the fast pain and temperature impulses are precisely localized, and the sharpness and intensity of the pin prick stimuli and the warmth or coldness of the temperature sensations are perceived.

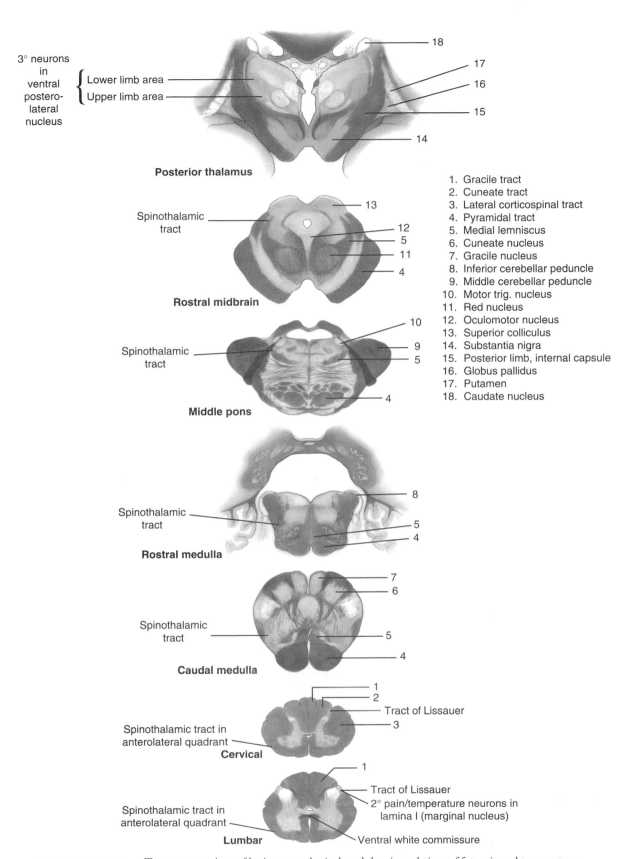

3° neurons in ventral postero-lateral nucleus { Lower limb area — Upper limb area —

Posterior thalamus

18

17
16
15
14

Spinothalamic tract

13
12
5
11
4

Rostral midbrain

1. Gracile tract
2. Cuneate tract
3. Lateral corticospinal tract
4. Pyramidal tract
5. Medial lemniscus
6. Cuneate nucleus
7. Gracile nucleus
8. Inferior cerebellar peduncle
9. Middle cerebellar peduncle
10. Motor trig. nucleus
11. Red nucleus
12. Oculomotor nucleus
13. Superior colliculus
14. Substantia nigra
15. Posterior limb, internal capsule
16. Globus pallidus
17. Putamen
18. Caudate nucleus

Spinothalamic tract

10
9
5

4

Middle pons

Spinothalamic tract

8

5
4

Rostral medulla

7
6

Spinothalamic tract

5

4

Caudal medulla

1
2
Tract of Lissauer
3

Spinothalamic tract in anterolateral quadrant

Cervical

1

Tract of Lissauer
2° pain/temperature neurons in lamina I (marginal nucleus)

Spinothalamic tract in anterolateral quadrant

Lumbar

Ventral white commissure

FIGURE 11–7. Transverse sections of brainstem and spinal cord showing relations of fast pain and temperature pathway from spinal nerves.

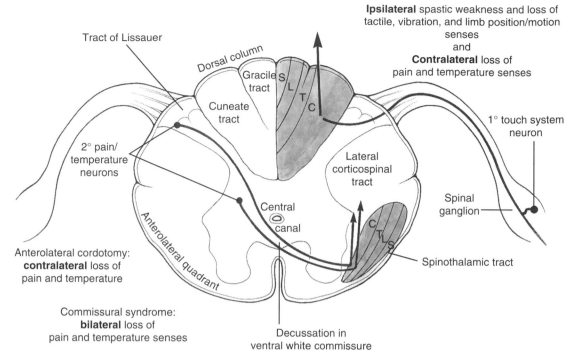

FIGURE 11-8.   Spinal cord somatosensory and motor pathways and their clinical syndromes.

CLINICAL SIGNIFICANCE OF SPINAL SOMATOSENSORY PATHWAYS

Within the spinal cord, the somatosensory paths are located in the dorsal columns and the anterolateral quadrants. Axons in the dorsal columns transmit the tactile, pressure, vibration, and limb position and motion impulses (Table 11–3). The more medial gracile tract conducts these types of discriminative impulses from the spinal nerves below midthoracic levels (Fig. 11–8), i.e., chiefly from the lower limb. The more lateral cuneate tract conducts the discriminative impulses from the spinal nerves above midthoracic levels, i.e., chiefly from the upper limb. The axons of both of these dorsal column tracts arise from large, first order neurons in the dorsal root or spinal ganglia on the same side. Hence, a unilateral lesion of the dorsal column results in an ipsilateral loss of tactile, pressure, vibration, and limb position and mo-

tion sensations in the parts of the body supplied by the spinal nerves below the level of the lesion.

> Severe degeneration of the dorsal columns accompanied by loss of the discriminative touch, vibratory, and limb position and motion senses commonly occurs in **tabes dorsalis,** a syndrome resulting from syphilitic infection of the large diameter axons and their ganglion cells. The dorsal column degeneration and sensory losses also occur in cases of pernicious anemia. Degeneration of the more medial parts of the gracile tract, i.e., the sacral and lower lumbar portions, occurs in lesions involving the dorsal roots in the cauda equina.

The anterolateral quadrants contain the spinothalamic tracts that transmit pain and temperature impulses (Table 11–3). The axons of the spinothalamic tract arise from second order neurons in the contralateral dorsal horn. As a result, the spinothalamic tract transmits pain and temperature impulses from the opposite side.

TABLE 11–3. COMPARISON OF DORSAL COLUMNS AND ANTEROLATERAL QUADRANTS OF SPINAL CORD

	DORSAL COLUMNS	ANTEROLATERAL QUADRANTS
Sensory Components	Tactile, vibration, and limb position and motion	Pain and temperature
Major Tracts	Gracile and cuneate	Spinothalamic
Origins of Tracts	Ipsilateral 　Spinal ganglia 　　Below midthoracic: Gracile 　　Above midthoracic: Cuneate	Contralateral 　Dorsal horn at all levels
Results of Damage	Ipsilateral loss—tactile, vibration, limb position and motion	Contralateral loss—pain and temperature
Medical Importance	Hemisected cord (Brown-Séquard syndrome): Below level of lesion- 　Contralateral pain and temperature 　Ipsilateral tactile, vibration, and limb position senses Also, ipsilateral lower limb spastic paralysis, Babinski sign, etc. 　(due to lateral corticospinal tract interruption)	

The **Brown-Séquard** syndrome results from a lesion involving either the right or left half of the spinal cord. The cardinal manifestation of this spinal cord hemisection is alternating somatosensory loss below the level of the lesion. The touch, vibration, and limb position and motion senses are lost on the same side, and pain and temperature senses are lost on the opposite side (Fig. 11–8).

GENERAL SENSATIONS FROM THE HEAD

General sensations from the face, anterior scalp, orbit, oral and nasal cavities, sinuses, teeth, and supratentorial dura are conducted chiefly in the trigeminal nerve. The facial, glossopharyngeal, and vagus nerves contain small numbers of somatosensory fibers that are distributed to the external ear, the posterior part of the tongue, and the tonsillar region. The primary somatosensory neurons are unipolar ganglion cells in the trigeminal ganglion of CN V, the geniculate ganglion of CN VII, the superior (petrosal) ganglion of CN IX, and the superior (jugular) ganglion of CN X. The central connections of all the cranial nerve somatosensory fibers are made with the trigeminal sensory nuclei.

TRIGEMINAL SENSORY NUCLEI

A continuous nuclear column related to somatosensory impulses extends from the level of

the superior colliculus caudad through the brainstem and the entire spinal cord. At spinal levels, this nuclear column is represented by the dorsal horn laminae and nuclei that conduct pain and temperature sensations. In the brainstem, this nuclear column is represented by the sensory trigeminal nuclei (Fig. 11–9).

At midpontine levels, where the trigeminal nerve enters, the principal trigeminal nucleus is located. Extending caudally from this nucleus is the spinal trigeminal nucleus, which becomes continuous with the dorsal horn of the spinal cord. The spinal trigeminal nucleus consists of three parts: oral, interpolar, and caudal. The oral and interpolar parts are chiefly associated with trigeminal reflexes related to blinking, lacrimation, and salivation. The caudal part is associated primarily with pain and temperature impulses from the face.

The primary neurons for proprioceptive reflexes from the muscles of mastication, teeth, periodontal membrane, and the external ocular muscles form the mesencephalic trigeminal nucleus. This nucleus extends rostrally from the principal trigeminal nucleus to the level of the superior colliculus as a slender column of unipolar ganglion cells located in the lateral part of the periaqueductal gray matter. Accompanying it is the mesencephalic trigeminal tract, formed by the axons of this nucleus, which emerge from the brainstem in the motor root of the trigeminal nerve. The central con-

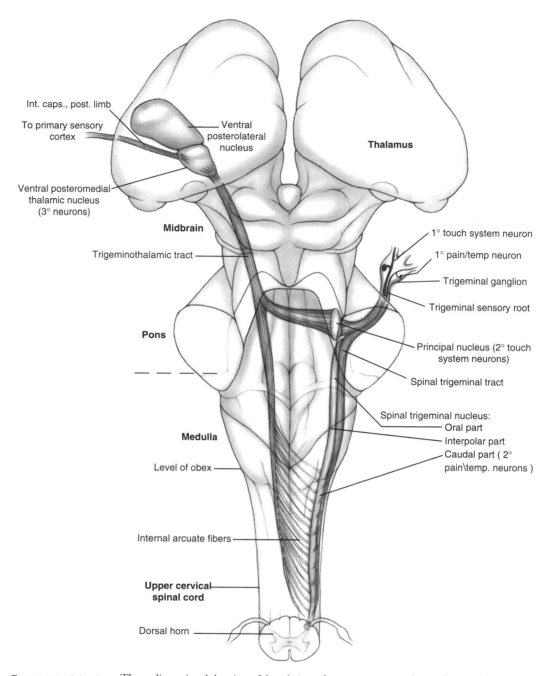

FIGURE 11-9.   Three-dimensional drawing of dorsal view of somatosensory pathways from cranial nerves.

nections of the mesencephalic trigeminal nucleus are primarily with the motor trigeminal nucleus and form monosynaptic reflexes associated with control of the force of bite and chewing.

CRANIAL TOUCH PATHWAYS

Touch impulses from mechanoreceptors in the head are conducted centrally, chiefly in the trigeminal nerve. Central connections are

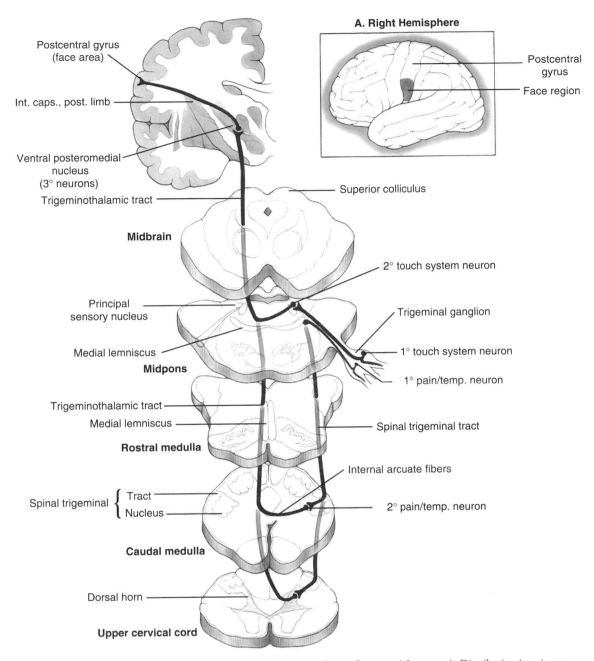

A. Right Hemisphere

Postcentral gyrus (face area)

Int. caps., post. limb

Ventral posteromedial nucleus (3° neurons)

Trigeminothalamic tract

Midbrain

Principal sensory nucleus

Medial lemniscus

Midpons

Trigeminothalamic tract

Medial lemniscus

Rostral medulla

Spinal trigeminal { Tract / Nucleus

Caudal medulla

Dorsal horn

Upper cervical cord

Postcentral gyrus

Face region

Superior colliculus

2° touch system neuron

Trigeminal ganglion

1° touch system neuron

1° pain/temp. neuron

Spinal trigeminal tract

Internal arcuate fibers

2° pain/temp. neuron

FIGURE 11–10.   Schematic diagram of somatosensory pathways from cranial nerves. A. Distribution in primary sensory cortex.

made with trigeminal nuclei, and the impulses ascend via the trigeminothalamic system. Three neurons transmit the impulses from the receptor to the cerebral cortex (Figs. 11–9, 11–10).

FIRST ORDER NEURONS

The primary trigeminal touch system neurons are large unipolar cells in the trigeminal (CN V) ganglion. The central branches of their

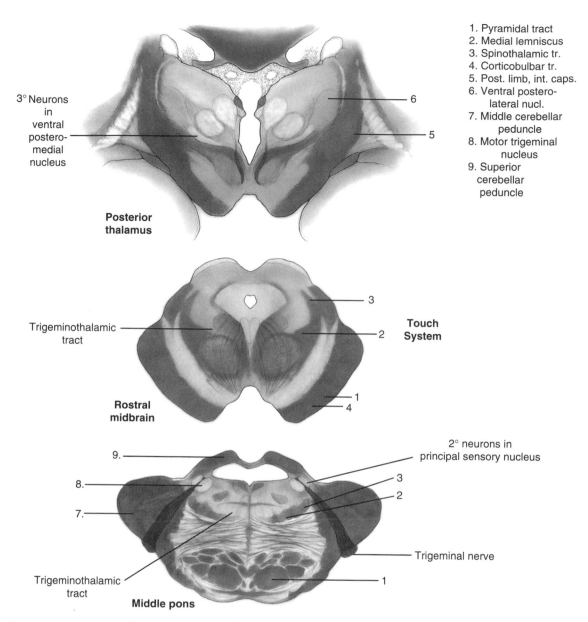

1. Pyramidal tract
2. Medial lemniscus
3. Spinothalamic tr.
4. Corticobulbar tr.
5. Post. limb, int. caps.
6. Ventral postero-
   lateral nucl.
7. Middle cerebellar
   peduncle
8. Motor trigeminal
   nucleus
9. Superior
   cerebellar
   peduncle

3° Neurons in ventral postero-medial nucleus

Posterior thalamus

Trigeminothalamic tract

Touch System

Rostral midbrain

2° neurons in principal sensory nucleus

Trigeminal nerve

Trigeminothalamic tract

Middle pons

FIGURE 11–11.   Transverse sections of brainstem showing relations of somatosensory pathways from cranial nerves. **A.** Touch system.

axons approach the pons in the sensory root of the trigeminal nerve and pass dorsomedially toward the pontine tegmentum (Fig. 11–11A).

SECOND ORDER NEURONS

The primary trigeminal touch system axons terminate on secondary neurons in the principal trigeminal nucleus. Axons from most of these secondary somatosensory neurons cross at midpontine levels and ascend in the contralateral trigeminothalamic tract, commonly called the ventral trigeminal tract. A small number of axons that ascend ipsilaterally from the second order neurons in the principal trigeminal nucleus form the dorsal trigeminal tract. The clinical significance of this tract is not known.

THIRD ORDER NEURONS

The secondary trigeminothalamic fibers terminate in the ventral posteromedial (VPM) nucleus. Tertiary trigeminal touch system neurons here send thalamocortical axons via the posterior limb of the internal capsule to the ventral part of the postcentral gyrus, the SI cortex face area, where the type of sensation and its precise localization are perceived.

CRANIAL PAIN AND TEMPERATURE PATHWAYS

A series of three neurons transmit fast pain and temperature impulses from the cranial nerve nociceptors and thermoreceptors to the cerebral cortex where they are perceived (Figs. 11–9, 11–10).

FIRST ORDER NEURONS

Smaller unipolar neurons in the trigeminal ganglion transmit pain and temperature impulses. The central branches of the axons of these unipolar trigeminal ganglion cells enter the pons via the sensory root of the trigeminal nerve and pass dorsomedial at the junction of the middle cerebellar peduncle and basilar part of the pons (Fig. 11–11B). On reaching the pontine tegmentum, they form a conspicuous bundle, the spinal trigeminal tract, which descends through the pons and medulla and intermingles with the dorsolateral tract of Lissauer in the upper cervical segments of the spinal cord.

Pain and temperature impulses from the facial, glossopharyngeal, and vagus nerves have as their primary neurons small unipolar cells in their respective ganglia, namely, the geniculate of cranial nerve VII, the superior (petrosal) of cranial nerve IX, and the superior (jugular) of cranial nerve X. The central branches of their axons enter the brainstem with their respective nerves and join the spinal trigeminal tract.

SECOND ORDER NEURONS

The primary pain and temperature fibers descending in the spinal trigeminal tract terminate in the caudal part of the spinal trigeminal nucleus. This caudal subnucleus extends from

the level of the obex to the spinal cord, where it becomes continuous with the dorsal horn. Interruption of the spinal trigeminal tract anywhere from its origin in the midpons inferiorly to the level of the obex results in complete loss of pain and temperature sensations on the ipsilateral side of the face and anterior scalp.

> Spinal trigeminal tractotomy has been used for the relief of the spontaneous, excruciating pain that occurs in cases of **trigeminal neuralgia** or **tic douloureux.** The advantage of surgically transecting the tract in the medulla at the level of the obex is that the facial pain is alleviated and the **corneal reflex** is spared. In the absence of the corneal reflex, which moistens and cleanses the cornea, infection and ulceration of the cornea may occur. The corneal reflex comprises an afferent limb, the trigeminal nerve, and an efferent limb, the facial nerve. This reflex is elicited when the cornea is touched with a wisp of cotton, thereby stimulating nociceptors whose cell bodies are in the trigeminal ganglion. The afferent corneal reflex impulses descend as pain fibers in the spinal trigeminal tract, which, at levels rostral to the obex, give collateral branches that synapse in the oral or interpolar part of the spinal trigeminal nucleus. Connections are then made, via the reticular formation, with the facial nuclei bilaterally. The efferent limb consists of the facial nerve fibers that supply the orbicularis oculi muscles.

> A small unilateral lesion in the lateral parts of the medulla or caudal half of the pons at any level may interrupt the spinal trigeminal and spinothalamic tracts. In such cases, the patient loses pain and temperature sensations on the ipsilateral side in the face and on the contralateral side in the limbs, trunk, neck, and back of the head.

Second order pain and temperature neurons in the caudal part of the spinal trigeminal nucleus and the adjacent reticular formation give rise to axons that cross the midline and ascend in the trigeminothalamic tract. This tract is located in the reticular formation near the upper limb part of the medial lemniscus at medullary, pontine, and mid-

> Caudal to midpontine levels, the trigeminothalamic tract is almost exclusively conducting pain and temperature impulses from the contralateral side of the face. At more rostral levels, the trigeminothalamic tract conducts all types of somatosensory impulses from the contralateral face.

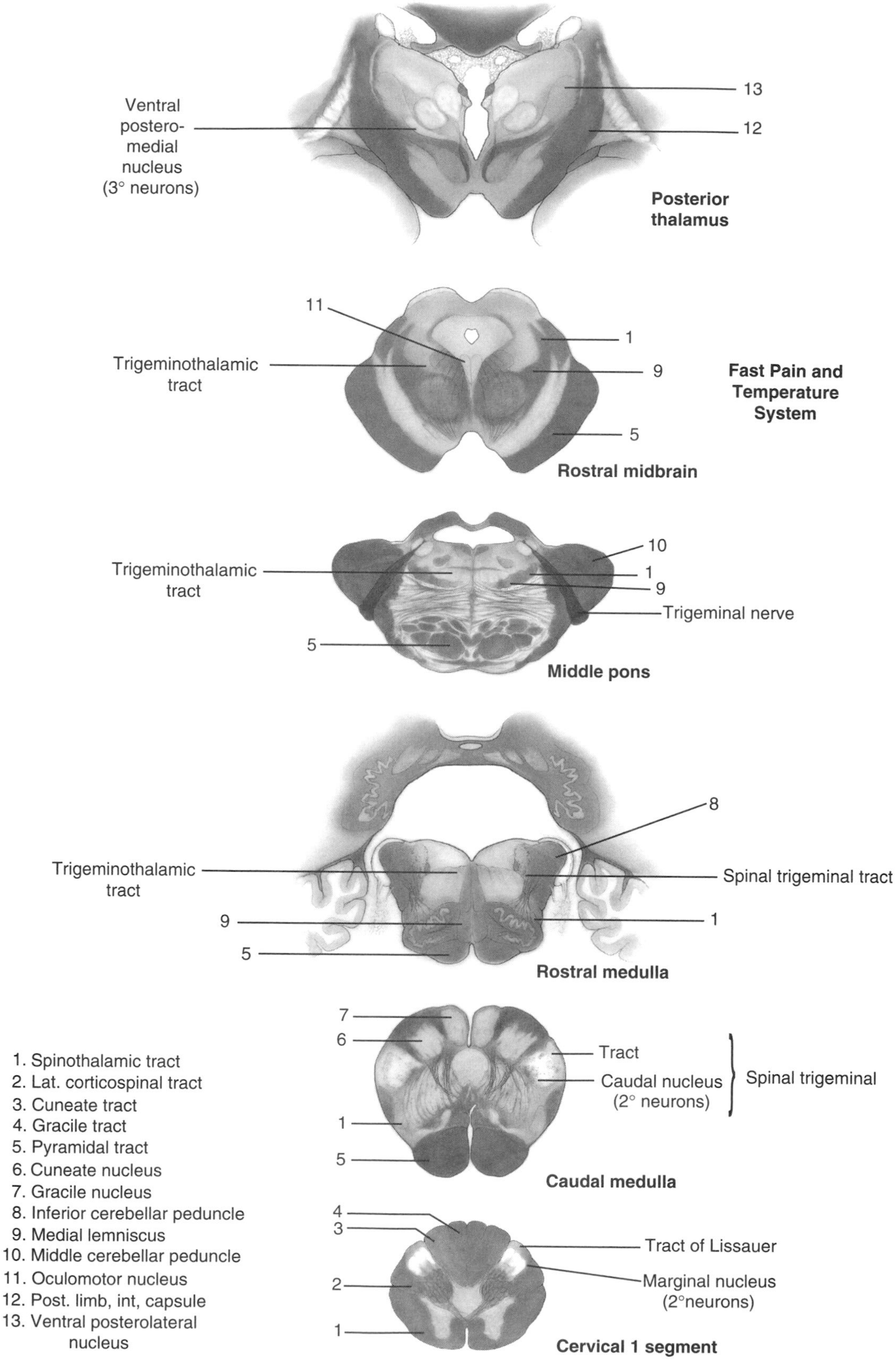

Ventral postero-medial nucleus (3° neurons)

13

12

Posterior thalamus

11

Trigeminothalamic tract

1

9

5

Fast Pain and Temperature System

Rostral midbrain

10

1

9

Trigeminothalamic tract

Trigeminal nerve

5

Middle pons

8

Trigeminothalamic tract

Spinal trigeminal tract

9

1

5

Rostral medulla

7

6

Tract

Caudal nucleus (2° neurons)

} Spinal trigeminal

1

5

Caudal medulla

1. Spinothalamic tract
2. Lat. corticospinal tract
3. Cuneate tract
4. Gracile tract
5. Pyramidal tract
6. Cuneate nucleus
7. Gracile nucleus
8. Inferior cerebellar peduncle
9. Medial lemniscus
10. Middle cerebellar peduncle
11. Oculomotor nucleus
12. Post. limb, int, capsule
13. Ventral posterolateral nucleus

4

3

Tract of Lissauer

2

Marginal nucleus (2°neurons)

1

Cervical 1 segment

FIGURE 11-11 (CONTINUED). **B.** Fast pain and temperature system.

brain levels and is commonly called the ventral trigeminal tract.

THIRD ORDER NEURONS

The secondary fast pain and temperature axons in the trigeminothalamic tract terminate in the VPM nucleus. Tertiary VPM neurons send thalamocortical axons via the posterior limb of the internal capsule to the facial region of the SI cortex, which is located in the ventral part of the postcentral gyrus.

CLINICAL IMPLICATIONS OF SOMATOSENSORY PATHWAYS

As exemplified in the three sets of somatosensory signs described at the beginning of this

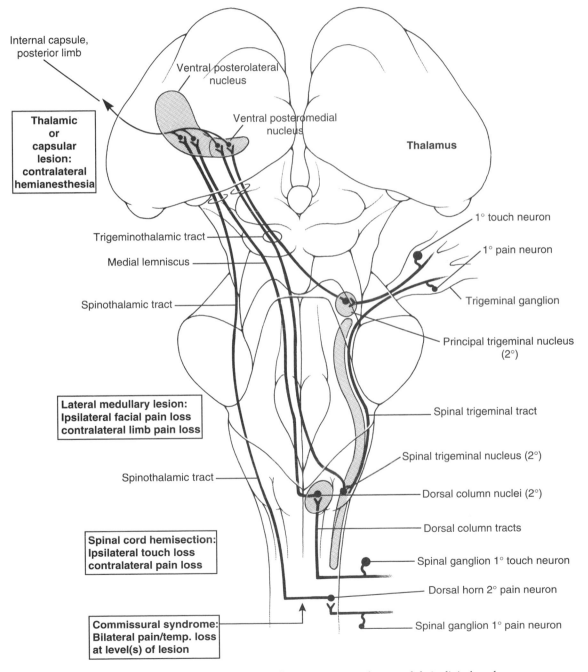

FIGURE 11–12. Schematic synopsis of somatosensory pathways and their clinical syndromes.

chapter, unilateral lesions at various CNS levels can frequently be localized by the somatosensory abnormalities that result (Fig. 11–12).

In the first patient, an alternating somatosensory loss is located below the umbilicus: touch, pressure, and limb position of the right side and pain and temperature on the left side. These losses result from interruption of the dorsal column and anterolateral quadrant, respectively, on the right side at the T10 spinal cord level. Only in the spinal cord can a unilateral lesion result in this alternating somatosensory loss.

The second patient has loss of pin prick and temperature sensations on the left side in the limbs, trunk, neck, and back of the head, and on the right side in the face and anterior part of the scalp. These losses result from interruption of the spinothalamic tract and spinal trigeminal tract, respectively, on the right side at some level between midpons and the obex in the medulla. Only in the lateral parts of the caudal pons and rostral medulla can a unilateral lesion result in an alternating pain and temperature loss.

In the third patient, left hemianesthesia (ex-cluding slow pain) manifests as a result of interruption of the somatosensory structures on the right side. The spinal and trigeminal somatosensory systems intermingle with each other in the forebrain paths. Thus, the paths are together in the ventral posterior thalamic nucleus. As a result, a unilateral lesion in this structure results in a contralateral hemianesthesia. Likewise, a capsular lesion involving the posterior limb will result in contralateral hemianesthesia, but this will be accompanied by contralateral spastic hemiplegia due to involvement of the adjacent pyramidal tract.

CENTRAL CONNECTIONS OF SLOW PAIN

Slow pain from spinal nerves is transmitted within the CNS by the phylogenetically older and more diffuse pathways commonly referred to as the "paleospinothalamic" and "spinoreticulothalamic" systems (Fig. 11–13).

Most paleospinothalamic neuronal cell bodies are in lamina V. Most nociceptive neurons in

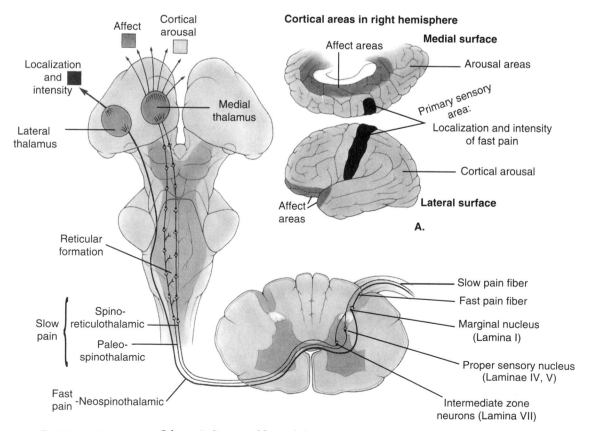

FIGURE 11–13.   Schematic diagram of fast and slow pain pathways. **A.** Distribution in cerebral cortex.

TABLE 11–4.   SUMMARY OF SPINAL PAIN PATHS

		FAST PAIN		SLOW PAIN	
PNS	Nociceptors	A-delta mechanical (pinprick)		C-polymodal (tissue damage)	
	Nerve Fibers	Small myelinated (5–30 m/sec)		Unmyelinated (0.5–2 m/sec)	
CNS	Tracts	Neospinothalamic		Paleospinothalamic	Spinoreticulothalamic
	Origins	Marginal nucleus (I) Proper nucleus (V)		Proper nucleus (V) Marginal nucleus (I) (also VII and VIII)	Intermediate zone (VII) Anterior horn (VIII)
	Thalamic Terminations	VPL	Posterior thalamic nuclei	Medial thalamus	Medial thalamus Hypothalamus
	Cortical Terminations	SI area	Parietal lobe	Frontal lobe	Limbic lobe
	Functions	Localization and sharpness	Sensation of pain	Cortical arousal	Affect

laminae VII and VIII, especially in the upper cervical segments, give rise to the spinoreticulothalamic system of slow pain impulses. In the spinal cord, the paleospinothalamic and spinoreticulothalamic tracts are located in the anterolateral quadrants where they intermingle with the fast pain fibers of the "neospinothalamic" system.

In the brainstem, the slow pain fibers are located more medially than the fast pain fibers. The paleospinothalamic fibers have collateral axons that synapse in the medullary reticular formation where they overlap with the synapses of large numbers of spinoreticular fibers. These two inputs to the reticular formation form a massive multisynaptic reticulothalamic system that chiefly projects nociceptive impulses to more medial parts of the thalamus, which then project to widespread regions of the cerebral cortex.

There is no perception of the pain associated with tissue damage in the SI cortex. The perception of slow pain in other cortical areas accounts for the awareness of pain in contralateral parts of the body in patients with internal capsule or SI cortex damage. Although specific nociceptive functions cannot be located in the cerebral cortex, other than the SI area where the localization and intensity of fast pain occurs, the function of other cortical areas can be postulated on the basis of their thalamocortical connections. Thus, it appears that

1. Projections from posterior thalamic nuclei (at the junction of the midbrain and diencephalon) to parietal cortical areas can define nociceptive stimuli as painful.

2. Intralaminar nuclear connections to widespread cortical areas play a role in cortical arousal and attention.

3. Medial and midline nuclear projections to the orbitofrontal cortex and other parts of the brain associated with behavior and emotions, the **limbic system,** are responsible for the affective responses to pain (anguish, depression, fear, anger, etc.).

In general, therefore, the cortical areas receiving nociceptive impulses from the lateral part of the thalamus perceive the sensory discriminative aspects of pain, whereas those areas receiving nociceptive impulses from the medial part of the thalamus are for the arousal, attention, affective, and motivational aspects of pain. The peripheral nervous system (PNS) and CNS structures and their functional roles in fast and slow pain systems are summarized in Table 11–4. Although information on the central connections and paths of cranial slow pain

---

The immediate result of anterolateral cordotomy is complete loss of all pain (and temperature) senses contralaterally and below the level of the lesion. This complete loss occurs because both the fast and the slow pain fibers are located in the anterolateral quadrants of the spinal cord. Such is not the case in the brainstem where the fast pain fibers ascend in the spinothalamic tract, which is located laterally, whereas the slow pain fibers ascend more medially. Therefore, interruption of the spinothalamic tract in the brainstem results in decreased sensitivity and localization of fast pain, i.e., pin prick (and temperature sense), but not the loss of slow pain. In fact, discrete lesions in the spinothalamic tract in the brainstem may result in agonizing intractable chronic pain of the so-called "thalamic" type.

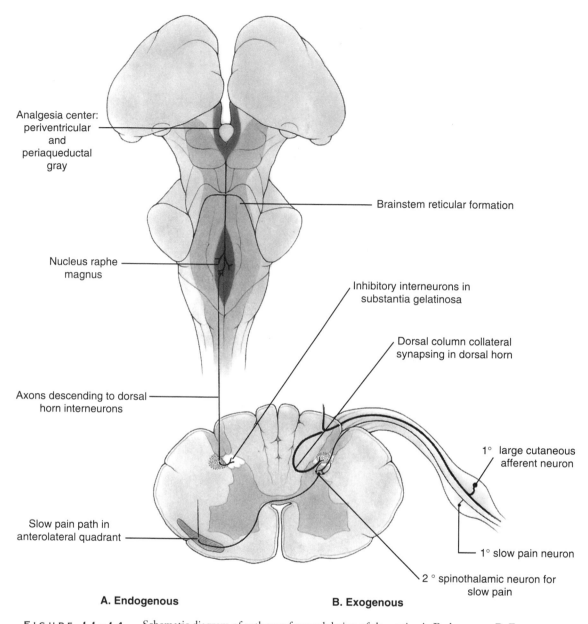

Analgesia center: periventricular and periaqueductal gray

Brainstem reticular formation

Nucleus raphe magnus

Inhibitory interneurons in substantia gelatinosa

Dorsal column collateral synapsing in dorsal horn

Axons descending to dorsal horn interneurons

1° large cutaneous afferent neuron

Slow pain path in anterolateral quadrant

1° slow pain neuron

2° spinothalamic neuron for slow pain

A. Endogenous   **B. Exogenous**

FIGURE 11-14.   Schematic diagram of pathways for modulation of slow pain. **A.** Endogenous; **B.** Exogenous.

is meager, it is reasonable to assume that they are similar to those of the paleospinothalamic and spinoreticulothalamic systems, i.e., reticular formation to medial thalamus and then to widespread areas of the cerebral cortex.

PAIN MODULATION

The anatomical features of exogenous and endogenous modulation of the spinal pain paths are fairly well known. In both cases, the interneurons that form the substantia gelatinosa (lamina II) and more ventral laminae (III, IV, V) of the dorsal horn play a key role (Fig. 11–14). These interneurons act on secondary slow pain neurons, and, through their action, the excitability of the secondary slow pain neurons can be altered to prevent the transmission of pain impulses to higher centers.

EXOGENOUS CONTROL

Large cutaneous afferent nerve fibers conducting touch impulses are able to modulate pain through massive connections with substantia gelatinosa and other dorsal horn neurons. These connections occur via branches of the touch fibers ascending in the dorsal columns. This phenomenon is the basis for the clinical control of chronic pain by TENS. The treatment produces selective activation of the larger cutaneous touch fibers that result in **analgesia** due to activation of the spinal interneurons that inhibit the secondary slow pain neurons.

ENDOGENOUS CONTROL

Groups of neurons in the periaqueductal gray of the rostral midbrain and the periventricular gray of the adjacent diencephalon, on electrical or neural stimulation or the administration of opiates, produce analgesia. Such modulation of pain occurs through connections of this analgesia center with neurons of the nucleus raphe magnus and other reticular formation neurons near the pontomedullary junction. Axons descend from these reticular formation nuclei to the region of the substantia gelatinosa and secondary spinal pain neurons and inhibit the transmission of ascending pain impulses.

This endogenous pain modulation system is used clinically for the relief of some types of chronic pain. The procedure involves the surgical implantation of a stimulating electrode into the analgesia center. The stimulation is controlled by the patient through the use of a battery-powered stimulation unit. The duration of the chronic pain relief is extremely variable, but, through this procedure, the patient can obtain relief as often as necessary.

CHAPTER REVIEW QUESTIONS

11–1. Name and locate the general somatic sensory losses anticipated as a result of the following:

    a. Rupture of disc into left intervertebral foramen between LV5 and SV1
    b. Left hemisection of spinal cord at T10
    c. Ventral white commissure from T2–T4
    d. Left lateral third of medulla at the obex
    e. Right medial third of medulla near the pontomedullary junction
    f. Left ventral posterior nucleus
    g. Right paracentral lobule

THE VISUAL SYSTEM: ANOPSIA

■ **A hypertensive patient, admitted because of stroke, is found to have paralysis of the left upper and lower limbs, left hemianesthesia, and blindness of the left half of the field of vision in both eyes.**

We receive most of the information about our surroundings through the visual system. The medical importance of this system includes the fact that blindness is the most devastating of all sensory deficits and that clinical examination of the visual system provides precise localization of lesions.

We "see" when light rays are focused on the retina; these rays are transduced by photoreceptor cells into retinal potentials, and nerve impulses are transmitted to the thalamus and thence to the cerebral cortex. Three anatomical features of the visual pathways are of medical significance:

1. These pathways extend from the front to the back of the head.

2. They are entirely supratentorial.

3. Visual information travels in both crossed and uncrossed paths.

THE RETINA

The retina contains seven types of cells: the receptors for vision, the first two neurons in the visual pathway, two types of interneurons, supporting cells, and pigment epithelial cells. The cells and their processes are arranged in 10 layers. The light rays pass from internal to external through the retina, but the layers are numbered from external to internal (Fig. 12–1).

The outermost layer is the pigment epithelial layer, a single layer of cells that contain melanin. The pigment cells absorb the light that has passed through the retina.

Two clinical conditions related to the pigment epithelial layer are retinitis pigmentosa and retinal detachment. In retinitis pigmentosa, debris from photoreceptor cells accumulates between the photoreceptor cell layer and the pigment epithelial cell layer. Normally the pigment epithelial cells phagocytose this debris.

Retinal detachment occurs between the pigment epithelial cell layer and the photoreceptors. The photoreceptor cells at the site of detachment cease to function, resulting in blurred vision in the affected part of the visual field.

Layer 2 contains the photoreceptors, the rods and cones. The human retina contains 110 to 125 million rods and 6 to 7 million cones. The cones are responsible for visual acuity and color vision (**photopic vision**); the rods are responsible for vision in light of low intensity (**scotopic vision**). The rods are uniformly slender, whereas the cones have wide bases and tapered, narrow ends. Each rod and cone cell consists of four parts: outer segment, inner segment, cell body, and synaptic terminal (Fig. 12–1). Actually, the photoreceptor layer contains only the outer and inner segments of the photoreceptors.

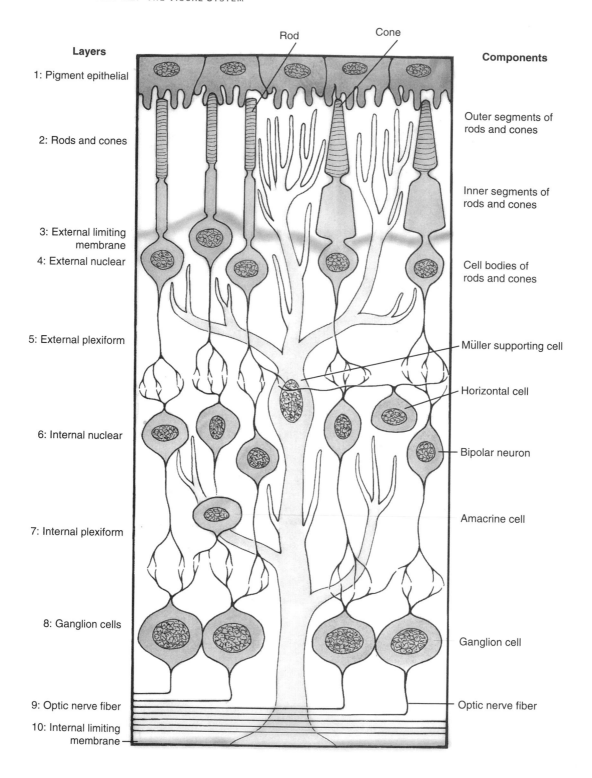

Layers

1: Pigment epithelial

2: Rods and cones

3: External limiting membrane

4: External nuclear

5: External plexiform

6: Internal nuclear

7: Internal plexiform

8: Ganglion cells

9: Optic nerve fiber

10: Internal limiting membrane

Components

Rod

Cone

Outer segments of rods and cones

Inner segments of rods and cones

Cell bodies of rods and cones

Müller supporting cell

Horizontal cell

Bipolar neuron

Amacrine cell

Ganglion cell

Optic nerve fiber

FIGURE 12-1.   The retina: Layers, cells and their connections.

The outer segments contain the visual photopigments, **rhodopsin** in the rods and **iodopsin** in the cones. On absorbing light, rhodopsin is broken down into retinal, the light-absorbing molecule, and opsin. After absorbing light, rhodopsin is then restored by a series of chemical reactions, some of which depend on vitamin A.

The rods, which are much more sensitive to light than the cones, are chiefly used in dim or nocturnal vision. Because of its vital role in the restoration of rhodopsin, vitamin A deficiency reduces nocturnal vision, a condition called night blindness. Although only one type of rod exists in the human eye, there are three types of cones: red-, green-, and blue-sensitive cones. The light-absorbing molecule in each cone type appears to be similar to the retinal found in rods. Different wavelength sensitivities are determined by the specific type of opsin to which the retinal is bound. The absence of either the red-, green-, or blue-sensitive cones results in blindness to that color. Thus, cones respond to colors, but only when the illumination is great enough.

Whereas the outer segments of the photoreceptor cells transduce light rays into electrical energy, the inner segments supply the energy necessary for the restoration of the visual pigments. This is accomplished by the numerous mitochondria located in the inner segments.

With the exception of the pigment epithelial cells in layer 1, all the other cell bodies are in retinal layers 4, 6, and 8 (Fig. 12–1). Layer 4, the external nuclear layer, contains the cell bodies and nuclei of the rods and cones. Layer 6, the internal nuclear layer, contains chiefly the cell bodies of the bipolar neurons, the first neurons in the visual pathway. Local circuit neurons, the **horizontal cells** and **amacrine cells,** are interspersed among the bipolar neurons. The horizontal cells, located in the outer part of layer 6, modulate the synaptic activity between the photoreceptors and bipolar cells, whereas the amacrine cells, located in the inner part of layer 6, modulate such activity between the bipolar and the second neurons in the visual path, ganglion cells. Most of the cell bodies of the supporting cells of the retina, the **Müller cells,** are located in the internal nuclear layer also.

Layer 8 is the ganglion cell layer, formed by the cell bodies of the second neurons in the visual pathway. The axons of these second order neurons form layer 9, the optic nerve fiber layer. Until they emerge from the eye, these axons are unmyelinated, an optical advantage because myelin is highly refractile.

The remaining layers of the retina are the external and internal plexiform layers, layers 5 and 7, respectively, and the external and internal limiting membrane layers, layers 3 and 10, respectively. The plexiform layers are the synaptic layers and consist of the axons and dendrites of the cells in the adjacent layers. The limiting membranes are formed by the external and internal ends of the Müller supporting cells, the modified glial cells of the retina.

Two parts of the retina that are structurally and functionally different from the rest of the retina are the central area and the **optic disc.** The central area contains the **macula lutea** and the **fovea centralis.** At the fovea, the inner layers of the retina are displaced, forming a pit or **foveola.** Only cones are present in the floor of the foveola. The fovea is the area for acute vision, and, therefore, the line connecting it with the viewed object is the visual axis.

Acuity occurs at the fovea not only because of displacement of the inner retinal layers, which allows the light rays to reach the cones without having to traverse the other layers, but also because cones are densest in the fovea, where they number about 200,000 per square millimeter.

The rest of the retina participates in nonacute paramacular and peripheral vision. Most of the photoreceptors in the paramacular and peripheral parts of the retina are the rods. Because of their longer outer segments, the rods can detect very small amounts of light, and because the impulses from many rods converge on the same bipolar neuron, the rods have low acuity.

The optic disc or papilla is the area at which the unmyelinated optic nerve fibers exit from

At the point of attachment of the optic nerve to the back of the eye, the external layer of the eye, the sclera, becomes continuous with the dura mater that completely encloses the nerve. The optic nerve, therefore, is surrounded by the dura as well as the arachnoid and pia mater. Hence, increased intracranial pressure can exert pressure via the cerebrospinal fluid-filled subarachnoid space onto the optic nerve especially at its emergence from the eyeball. When this occurs, the axoplasmic flow in the individual optic nerve axons is obstructed and they become swollen at the optic disc. This condition is known as **disc edema, papilledema,** or choked disc and can be observed with an ophthalmoscope.

the retina. At this point the outer eight layers of the retina are interrupted; hence, because of the absence of photoreceptors, it is the **blind spot.** As the fibers emerge to form the optic nerve they become myelinated.

Embryologically, the retina develops from the diencephalon; hence, it is a central nervous system (CNS) derivative. As a result, the optic nerve, unlike all other cranial nerves, is a CNS structure. Like other CNS structures, the optic nerve fibers do not regenerate when damaged.

VISUAL PATHWAY

Light rays striking the retina travel from the internal layers to the external layers where the rods and cones are stimulated. The visual impulses then pass from the external to the internal layers. Thus, within the retina the light rays and visual impulses travel in opposite directions.

The visual impulses from the rods and cones are transmitted to the bipolar cells, the primary or first order neurons in the visual system. Axons from the bipolar neurons synapse with the dendrites of the retinal ganglion cells, the second neurons in the pathway. The optic nerve axons coming from the ganglion cells radiate toward the optic disc, where they become myelinated and emerge to form the optic nerve. The optic nerves from each eye proceed posteriorly and medially, enter the cranial cavity through the optic foramina, and unite to form the optic chiasm (Fig. 12–2).

The optic chiasm rests on the diaphragma sellae in close relation to the stalk of the pituitary gland. Laterally, it is related to the internal carotid arteries. A pituitary tumor may damage the median portion of the chiasm, whereas an **aneurysm** on one of the internal carotid arteries may damage the lateral part of the chiasm.

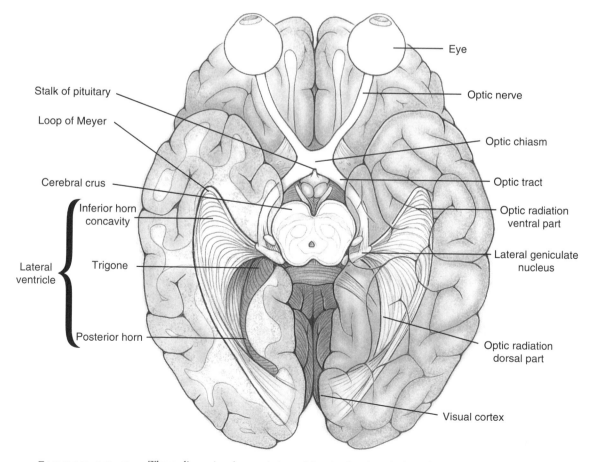

FIGURE 12–2.   Three-dimensional ventral view of the visual path with the right temporal lobe dissected.

Leaving the optic chiasm is the optic tract, which passes posterolaterally along the surfaces of the hypothalamus and cerebral crus and enters the ventral surface of the lateral geniculate nucleus. Here, axons from the retinal ganglion cells finally reach the tertiary visual path neurons.

The lateral geniculate nucleus has a triangular shape, somewhat similar to a Napoleonic hat. It consists of six layers. The two ventral layers are composed of large neurons, whereas the four dorsal layers consist of small neurons. Both types are the tertiary neurons that send axons to the cerebral cortex. The magnocellular layers are the part of the visual pathway concerned with the location and movement of an object in the visual field, whereas the parvicellular layers are concerned with the color and form of the object. Hence, the magnocellular is part of the "where" pathway and the parvicellular is part of the "what" pathway.

The tertiary lateral geniculate neurons give rise to the geniculocalcarine tract or optic radiation, which initially enters the retrolenticular part of the posterior limb of the internal capsule. As it enters the internal capsule, the optic radiation forms a conspicuous triangular area referred to as **Wernicke zone** (Fig. 12–3).

From the internal capsule, the fibers of the optic radiation sweep to the lateral surface of the lateral ventricle (Fig. 12–2). The more dorsal fibers proceed directly posteriorly, initially within the parietal lobe and then the occipital lobe. The more ventral fibers pass anteriorly

> The location of the optic radiation in the triangular zone of Wernicke is of clinical importance. Because of its close anatomical relation to the pyramidal tract and somatosensory thalamocortical radiations that are immediately adjacent in the posterior limb of the internal capsule, a small lesion (approximately 1.5 cm) in this area, gives rise to a contralateral paralysis and hemianesthesia and blindness in the opposite half of the field of vision in each eye (as given in the case at the introduction of this chapter). These abnormalities result from anterior choroidal artery disease.

and loop over the inferior horn of the lateral ventricle. Those fibers that proceed most anteriorly form the **loop of Meyer.** Therefore, after emerging from the internal capsule, the ventral part of the optic radiation is located initially in the temporal lobe and then in the occipital lobe.

> Parts of the optic radiation can be damaged by a lesion in the parietal, temporal, or occipital lobe.

The optic radiation sweeps posteriorly near the lateral wall of the posterior horn of the lateral ventricle and terminates in the primary visual cortex located in the walls of the calcarine sulcus (Fig. 12–4). The more dorsal fibers terminate in the cuneus; the more ventral fibers pass to the lingual gyrus. The visual cortex is also referred to as the striate cortex because, unlike other parts of the cerebral cortex, it con-

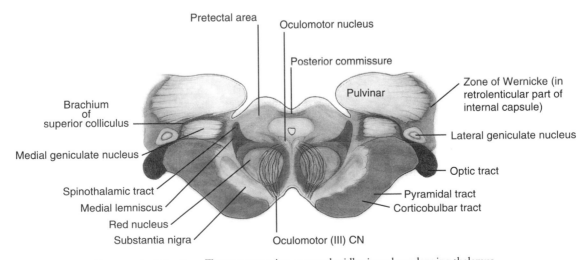

FIGURE 12-3.   Transverse section at rostral midbrain and overlapping thalamus.

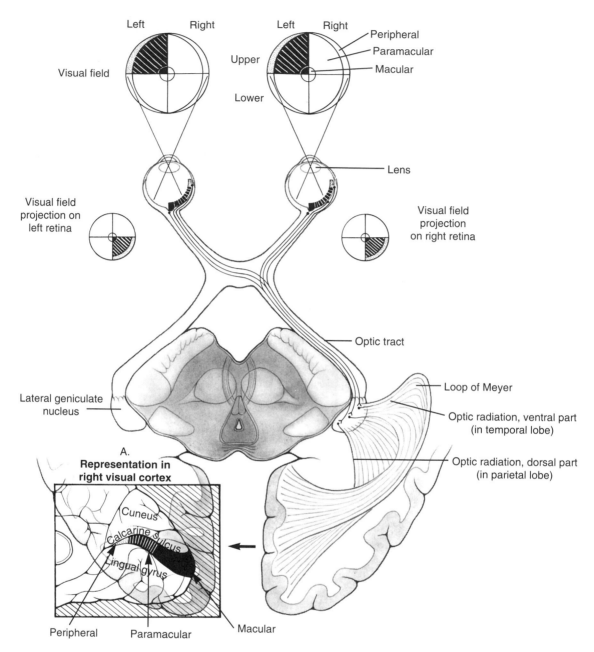

FIGURE 12–4. Visual field representation in visual paths. **A.** Visual field and retinal representation in primary visual cortex.

tains a very conspicuous horizontal stripe, called the line of Gennari. Within the visual cortex, the macula of the retina is represented in the posterior half and the paramacular and peripheral parts of the retina are represented successively more anteriorly (Fig. 12–4A).

VISUAL FIELDS AND VISUAL PATHS

Lesions in various parts of the visual path are described according to the visual field deficits that result. Knowledge of the representation of the fields of vision in the visual paths is of medical importance.

The field of vision is divided into four quadrants: upper right, upper left, lower right, and lower left. The quadrants are demarcated by imaginary horizontal and vertical lines through the **fixation point,** that is, the point on which vision is focused.

These visual field quadrants are projected onto each retina in a reversed and inverted pattern through the action of the lens (Fig. 12–4). Within the optic chiasm, the optic nerve fibers from the nasal or medial halves of the retinae cross, but those from the temporal or lateral halves of the retinae do not cross. This partial decussation serves to bring all of the optic nerve fibers transmitting impulses from either the right or the left half of the field of vision into the contralateral optic tract. Thus, the right and left visual pathways distal to the chiasm are carrying all of the impulses from the contralateral halves of the visual field.

Moreover, due to the point-to-point relations that exist between the retina, lateral geniculate nucleus, and primary visual cortex, impulses from the upper and lower halves of the visual field are located in different parts of the optic radiation. Impulses from the contralateral upper field take a ventral course and sweep into the temporal lobe before proceeding posteriorly to the occipital lobe where they end in the lower wall of the calcarine sulcus, the lingual gyrus (Fig. 12–4A). Impulses from the contralateral lower field, however, take a dorsal course and sweep posteriorly through the parietal lobe to the occipital cortex, where they end in the upper wall of the calcarine sulcus, the cuneus.

Damage to the visual pathways results in the loss of vision, anopsia, that is described according to the field of vision that is lost. Visual defects are **homonymous** when confined to the same part of the visual field in each eye. They are **heteronymous** when the part of the visual field lost in each eye is different. A homonymous defect results from lesions in the visual pathway distal to the optic chiasm. Thus, total destruction of the optic tract, lateral geniculate nucleus, geniculocalcarine tract, or visual cortex results in loss of the entire opposite field of vision in each eye, a phenomenon referred to as contralateral homonymous hemianopsia.

Lesions of the optic chiasm cause several types of heteronymous defects. Most commonly, the crossing fibers are involved and this results in an interruption of the nasal retinal fibers, which are carrying impulses from the temporal fields of vision. The defect in this case is referred to as **bitemporal hemianopsia.** Examples of lesions in various parts of the visual pathway, the visual field defects, and the principal causes of the lesions that result are given in Figure 12–5.

VISUAL REFLEXES

The size of the pupil and the curvature of the lens are governed by three groups of visual reflexes whose afferent components include parts of the visual system and whose efferent components involve, with only one exception, the autonomic system. These reflexes are the light or pupillary constriction reflex, the pupillary dilation reflex, and the accommodation reflexes.

THE LIGHT REFLEX

When light entering the eye becomes brighter, the pupil constricts. The reflex pupillary constriction of this eye is referred to as the **direct light reflex.** In addition to the pupillary constriction of the stimulated eye, constriction in the opposite eye also occurs; this reflex is referred to as the **consensual light reflex.**

The afferent components of the light reflex involve the receptor and neuronal elements of the retina, the optic nerve, the optic chiasm, and the optic tract (Fig. 12–6). From the optic tract, the impulses enter the brachium of the superior colliculus (superior brachium) (Fig. 12–3), which carries them to the light reflex center in the pretectal region. Neurons in the pretectal region have axons that terminate on visceromotor neurons of the oculomotor nuclear complex, commonly referred to as the Edinger-Westphal nucleus. For the consensual phenomenon, crossing occurs in the optic chiasm or in the posterior commissure, thus involving the contralateral Edinger-Westphal nucleus.

The efferent limb of the light reflex involves preganglionic parasympathetic axons from the

Visual field defects

A. **Right optic nerve:** Blindness of right eye (trauma, optic neuritis).

B. **Optic chiasm:** Complete midline transection causes bitemporal hemianopsia (pituitary tumors, craniopharyngiomas).

C. **Right angle of chiasm:** Right nasal hemianopsia (pressure by aneurysm of internal carotid artery).

D. **Right optic tract:** Left homonymous hemianopsia (abscess or tumor of temporal lobe that compresses optic tract against the crus cerebri).

E. **Complete capsular destruction of right optic radiation:** Left homonymous hemianopsia (anterior choroidal artery dysfunctions, tumors).

F. **Right Meyer loop or lower part of geniculocalcarine tract:** Left homonymous superior quadrantic anopsia (temporal or occipital lobe tumor).

G. **Upper part of right geniculocalcarine tract:** Left homonymous inferior quadrantic anopsia (parietal or occipital lobe tumor).

H. **Right striate area (visual cortex):** Left homonymous hemianopsia. Macular vision may be preserved if posterior part of the visual cortex is not involved (posterior cerebral artery dysfunctions, tumors, trauma).

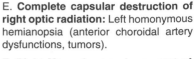
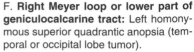
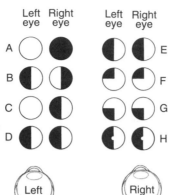
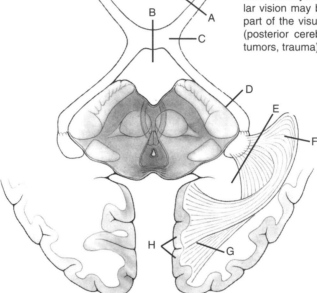

FIGURE 12-5. Visual field defects resulting from lesions in various parts of the visual pathway, and chief causes of the lesions.

The light reflex may be used to distinguish an optic tract lesion from lesions more distal in the visual pathway, all of which result in hemianopsia. With lesions distal to the optic tract, a small beam of light directed into only the blind halves of each retina results in pupillary constriction because the visual pathway is interrupted beyond the optic tract and superior brachium. In other words, the afferent components of the light reflexes in the optic tract are intact. Conversely, when the optic tract is damaged, shining light into the blind halves of each retina does not elicit the light reflexes because the afferent limb from the blind hemifield is interrupted.

Edinger-Westphal nucleus that travel in the oculomotor nerve and its branches to the ciliary ganglion. Postganglionic fibers from this ganglion course to the eye through the short ciliary nerves and terminate on the constrictor muscle of the iris.

The preganglionic pupilloconstrictor fibers in the oculomotor nerve are usually the first components affected when the nerve is compressed. Thus, an early sign of oculomotor nerve compression, such as occurs in herniation of the brain into the tentorial notch, is ipsilateral pupillary dilation.

A. Enlarged anterior part of eye

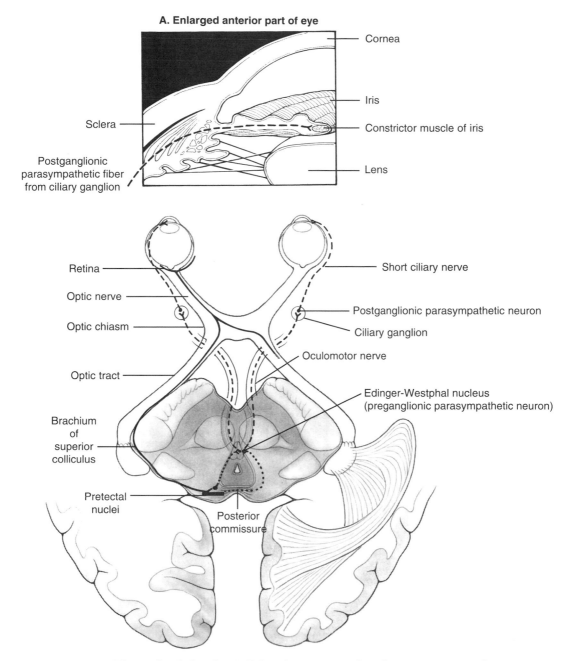

FIGURE 12-6. The pupillary light reflex. **A.** Enlarged anterior part of eye showing innervation of constrictor muscle of iris.

An optic nerve lesion interrupts the afferent limb of the light reflex and abolishes both the direct and the consensual responses from the blind eye. However, both pupils react when the good eye is stimulated by increased light. An oculomotor nerve lesion interrupts the efferent limb of the reflex, resulting in pupillary dilation (mydriasis) and a loss of both the direct and consensual responses in the ipsilateral eye.

THE PUPILLARY DILATION REFLEX

Pupillary dilation occurs passively when the parasympathetic tone is decreased, and actively when sympathetic tone is increased. The latter is usually a result of emotional expressions (fear, rage, etc.) or pain. Impulses from sympathetic centers in the posterior hypothalamus travel via the brainstem reticular formation to the **ciliospinal center,** which is composed of preganglionic sympathetic neurons located at the C8 and T1 spinal cord segments (Fig. 12–7). These preganglionic sympathetic neurons have axons that emerge with the ventral roots of spinal nerves T1 and T2, traverse the white communicating rami to enter and ascend in the sympathetic trunk, and terminate in the superior cervical ganglion. Postganglionic sympathetic fibers then travel in the **carotid plexuses** and via the nasociliary and long ciliary nerves to the dilator muscle of the iris. Interruption of this pathway, centrally as it descends from the hypothalamus to the ciliospinal center in the spinal cord, in the spinal cord at C8–T1, or in the periphery, leads to constriction of the pupil (miosis) due to the unopposed action of the parasympathetically innervated pupillary constrictor. In spite of the miosis the pupil still reacts to light and accommodation.

The miosis resulting from interruption of the pupillary dilation path is included in a triad of symptoms referred to as **Horner syndrome.** In addition to the miosis, the syndrome includes a mild ptosis and an **anhidrosis.** The mild ptosis occurs because of the denervation of smooth muscle in the upper eyelid (Müller muscle). The anhidrosis occurs because of the sympathetic denervation of facial sweat glands.

Horner syndrome commonly results from tumors or vascular lesions involving the lateral medulla; cervical spinal cord injuries, tumors, or syringomyelia; trauma to T1 and T2 ventral roots; cervical sympathetic trunk involvement by pulmonary carcinoma; and diseases of the internal carotid artery.

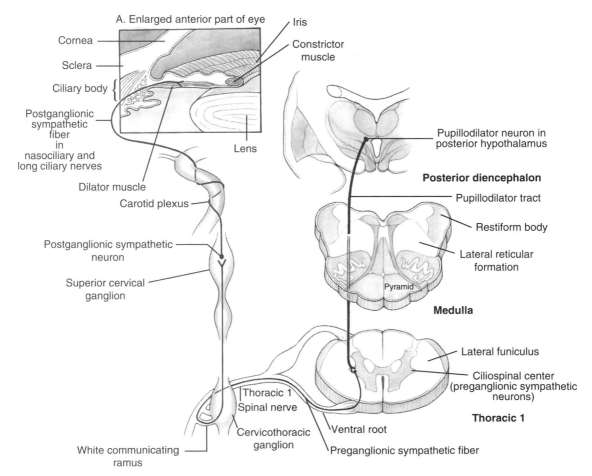

FIGURE 12-7.   The pupillodilator reflex. **A.** Enlarged anterior part of eye showing innervation of dilator muscle of iris.

THE ACCOMMODATION REFLEXES

Accommodation is the process in which a clear visual image is maintained as gaze is shifted from a distant to a near point. There are three components of the accommodation reaction: convergence of the eyes, pupillary constriction, and thickening of the lens.

When vision is changed from a distant ob-ject to a near one the light rays become more divergent on passing through the lens. In order for the image to remain focused on the retina, the curvature of the lens increases. The mechanism for this accommodation of the lens is based on an inherently elastic lens that is suspended by ligaments from the ciliary body. On contraction of its muscles the ciliary body moves closer to the lens, thereby decreasing the

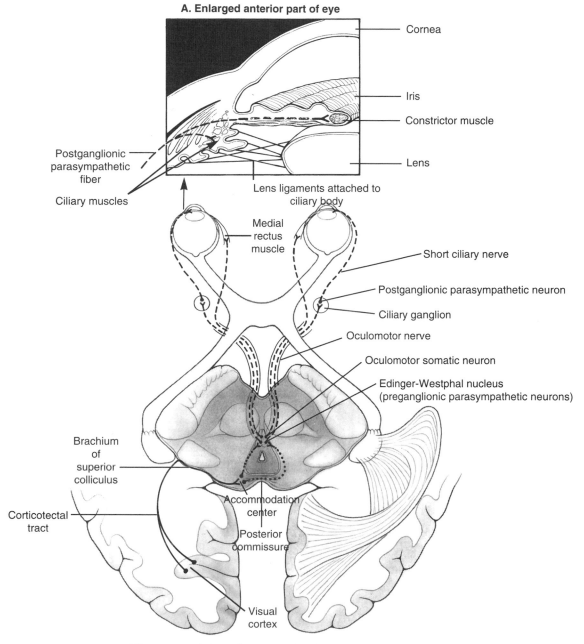

FIGURE 12–8. The accommodation reflexes. **A.** Enlarged anterior part of eye showing innervation of ciliary muscles and constrictor muscle of iris.

tension on the suspensory ligaments. This allows the lens to increase its anteroposterior diameter by bulging. To facilitate visual acuity further, convergence of the eyes and constriction of the pupils are combined with the accommodation of the lens. The accompanying constriction of the pupil enhances visual acuity by keeping light rays from the more peripheral part of the lens where chromatic and spherical aberrations are more likely to result.

The stimulus for accommodation is the perception of an object. The accommodation reflexes are initiated by the occipital cortex (Fig. 12–8). The afferent limbs in the reflexes are represented by corticotectal projections from the occipital lobe that pass to the **accommodation center** in the region of the superior colliculus and pretectal area.

From the accommodation center impulses go to appropriate nuclei of the oculomotor complex: the parasympathetic Edinger-West-

phal nucleus for changes in the lens and pupil and the somatic nuclei for convergence of the eyes. The efferent limb is the oculomotor nerve with a synapse in the ciliary ganglion for the parasympathetic impulses responsible for the involuntary accommodation and constriction. Short ciliary nerves carry the postganglionic parasympathetic fibers to the eye. The somatic impulses for convergence pass uninterruptedly from lower motor neurons of the oculomotor complex to the medial rectus muscles.

In certain pathologic conditions, such as tabes dorsalis resulting from neurosyphilis or tumors near the posterior part of the third ventricle, an Argyll Robertson pupil sign occurs. This sign is characterized by a small pupil that does not react to increased light, but does react well on accommodation. The underlying mechanism is not understood, nor has the lesion that causes the symptoms been located.

CHAPTER REVIEW QUESTIONS

12–1. Between what layers does detachment of the retina occur?

12–2. What morphologic features are common to retinal layers 4, 6, and 8?

12–3. Night blindness is associated with functional deficits in what structures? What vitamin may be involved?

12–4. Color blindness is associated with functional deficits in what structures?

12–5. Compare the fovea centralis and optic disc as to morphology and function.

12–6. What is the medical significance of the morphologic features unique to the optic nerve?

12–7. What visual field deficits result from destructive lesions of the following:

  a. Left optic nerve
  b. Median part of optic chiasm
  c. Retrolenticular part of right internal capsule
  d. Left Meyer loop
  e. Right striate cortex

12–8. What cranial nerves and which parts of the brain are essential for the integrity of the direct and consensual light reflexes?

12–9. Name three CNS and three PNS structures that when damaged interrupt the pupillodilator path unilaterally.

12–10. Describe the phenomenon associated with accommodation and give its neural substrate.

THE AUDITORY SYSTEM: DEAFNESS

■ **A middle-aged woman complains of dizziness, loss of hearing in the left ear, and a sagging of the left side of the face, all of which have gradually become more severe during the past 6 months.**

The paths conveying auditory impulses are organized in such a manner that nerve impulses must pass through at least four neurons in order to reach the cerebral cortex: number 1 in a ganglion of VIII CN, number 2 in the caudal brainstem, number 3 in the rostral brainstem, and number 4 in the thalamus. Unlike other sensory systems, the central auditory paths have bilateral representation of sounds, i.e., input from both ears reaches the auditory cortex in both hemispheres.

THE EAR

The ear, a vestibulocochlear organ concerned with hearing and equilibrium, consists of three parts: external, middle, and internal (Fig. 13–1). The external ear includes the auricle or pinna, the external acoustic meatus, and the tympanic membrane (ear drum). The auricle gathers the sound waves and the external acoustic meatus amplifies and directs the waves to the tympanic membrane. The tympanic membrane, the partition between the external and middle parts of the ear, is set into vibration by the sound waves.

The middle ear, or tympanic cavity, is an air-filled space in the temporal bone. The middle ear contains three **auditory ossicles** and two small muscles. The malleus, incus, and stapes

are the auditory ossicles. The malleus is attached to the internal surface of the tympanic membrane and to the incus. The incus articulates with the stapes. The vibrations of the tympanic membrane are transferred to the malleus and then conducted through the incus and stapes to the internal ear. Sound vibrations can also be conducted to the internal ear by the temporal bone. This phenomenon, **bone conduction,** is far less efficient than the conduction via the ossicles in the middle ear.

Movements of the ossicles may be dampened reflexly by the two small muscles in the middle ear. The tensor tympani muscle, innervated by the trigeminal nerve, is attached to the malleus. This tensor muscle dampens low tones by pulling the malleus internally, thereby increasing the tension on the tympanic membrane. The stapedius muscle, innervated by the facial nerve, is attached to the stapes. This muscle decreases sound intensity by pulling the stapes away from the opening into the internal ear.

> A lesion of the facial nerve proximal to its branches to the stapedius muscle results in hyperacusis, abnormally loud sounds in the affected ear.

The internal ear is located in the temporal bone and consists of fluid-filled spaces that form the bony and membranous labyrinths. The bony labyrinth contains perilymph and consists of vestibular parts, the semicircular canals and vestibule, and an auditory part, the **cochlea.** The membranous labyrinth is located within the bony labyrinth and is composed of a series of

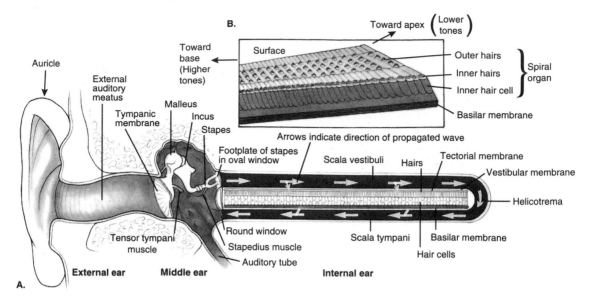

FIGURE 13–1. Principal parts of the auditory apparatus. **A.** The external, middle, and internal parts of the ear. **B.** Surface and side view of the basilar membrane and spiral organ, which increases in width from base to apex.

connecting ducts filled with endolymph. The vestibular receptors within the membranous labyrinth are described in Chapters 7 and 10.

The cochlea, so named because it is shaped like the shell of a snail, consists of three fluid-filled spaces: scala vestibuli, scala tympani, and cochlear duct (Fig. 13–2). The scalae vestibuli and tympani, partially enclosed in bone, are parts of the bony labyrinth, contain perilymph, and are continuous with each other at the helicotrema (Fig. 13–1). The cochlear duct is part of the membranous labyrinth and contains endolymph. The **vestibular,** or **Reissner membrane,** separates the scala vestibuli and cochlear duct, whereas the **basilar membrane** separates the scala tympani and cochlear duct.

Two openings or windows are located between the cochlea and the middle ear: the **oval window** into the scala vestibuli and **round window** into the scala tympani (Fig. 13–1). The footplate of the stapes occupies the oval window; the round window is occupied by a flexible membrane. When the stapes moves inward, the round window moves outward, and vice versa. The inward and outward movements of the stapes produce perilymphatic pressure waves between the scala vestibuli and the scala tympani and set the cochlear duct into motion.

Because the cochlear duct rests on the basilar membrane, it, too, is set into motion. Movement of the basilar membrane stimulates the auditory receptors located on this membrane.

Tonotopic localization occurs in the basilar membrane, which increases in width from its base, the part nearest the oval window, to its apex at the end of the two and one-half coils (Fig. 13–1). In addition, the structure of the basilar membrane is such that its narrow end is taut but its wide end is more flexible. Consequently, the highest frequencies set the base in motion, whereas the lowest frequencies set the apex in motion.

AUDITORY RECEPTORS

The **spiral organ** consists of neuroepithelial receptor and supporting cells (Fig. 13–3). The neuroepithelial receptor cells are classified as inner and outer hair cells. The inner hair cells are arranged in a single row, whereas the outer hair cells increase from three rows at the base of the cochlea to five rows at the apex (Fig. 13–1B). Projecting from the free surface of the hair cells are stereocilia whose tips are embedded in the overlying tectorial membrane. Therefore, when the basilar membrane is in motion, the stereocilia bend, resulting in changes in the membrane potentials of their hair cells. The inner hair cells have 1:1 synaptic relations with the primary auditory neurons and play a big role in auditory discrimination. Each outer hair cell receives synapses from large numbers of primary auditory neurons; the function of the outer hair cells is unknown.

AUDITORY PATHWAY

The primary or first order auditory neurons are located in the spiral ganglion (Figs. 13–2, 13–3). The dendrites of these bipolar neurons synapse on the hair cells of the spiral organ. Their central processes form the cochlear nerve, which passes toward the cranial cavity in the internal acoustic meatus and enters the brainstem in the cerebellar angle.

> The relation of the cochlear nerve to the vestibular and facial nerves in the internal acoustic meatus is of medical importance, especially in the case of an **acoustic neurinoma.** This benign Schwann cell tumor almost always arises from part of the vestibular nerve in the internal acoustic meatus. After its initial growth within the meatus, the tumor spreads into the cerebellar angle. This phenomenon results in a sequence of signs and symptoms that are caused by pressure damage to the structures in the internal acoustic meatus: cochlear nerve = progressive deafness, vestibular nerve = dysequilibrium, and facial nerve = facial weakness (as given in the clinical illustration starting this chapter). Later, in the posterior cranial fossa near the cerebellar angle, there is loss of the corneal reflex and, occasionally, somatosensations in the face, and ipsilateral limb ataxia, due to trigeminal nerve and cerebellar pathways, respectively.

The cochlear nerve terminates on second order neurons in the dorsal and ventral cochlear nuclei, which hang on the inferior cerebellar peduncle like saddlebags (Fig. 13–4). The dorsal cochlear nucleus is posterolateral to the inferior cerebellar peduncle and forms the acoustic tubercle in the floor of the lateral recess of the fourth ventricle. The ventral cochlear nucleus is slightly more rostral and is located anterolateral to the inferior cerebellar peduncle.

As axons from the dorsal and ventral cochlear nuclei pass toward the midline prior to decussating, they travel rostrally into the pons and form three groups of acoustic striae

named for their locations in the caudal pontine tegmentum: dorsal, intermediate, and ventral. Of the three acoustic striae, the ventral is most prominent and as it decussates it forms the trapezoid body (Fig. 13–2, 13–3, 13–4). After decussating, fibers from all three acoustic striae join the **lateral lemniscus,** which ascends through the pons to the midbrain. On reaching the midbrain, all auditory fibers in the lateral lemniscus enter the inferior colliculus and synapse. Most of the fibers from the inferior colliculus emerge laterally and ascend along the lateral surface of the midbrain as the brachium of the inferior colliculus (inferior brachium).

> This bundle of the inferior colliculus forms a conspicuous eminence on the lateral surface of the rostral half of the midbrain and has been used as a landmark for the surgical interruption of pain fibers traveling in the spinothalamic tract, which is located several millimeters medial to the brachium.

The brachium of the inferior colliculus terminates in the medial geniculate nucleus (Figs. 13–2, 13–3, 13–4). This thalamic auditory center then gives rise to the **auditory radiation,** which passes laterally to join the posterior limb of the internal capsule beneath the posterior part of the lentiform nucleus. Hence, the auditory radiation lies in the sublenticular part of the posterior limb. From here it travels to the primary auditory cortex, located in the transverse temporal gyri (of Heschl). These gyri are on the dorsal surface of the superior temporal gyrus and are buried in the lateral fissure (Fig. 13–3). Tonotopic localization is thought to exist in the primary auditory cortex; high tones are represented posteromedially and low tones anterolaterally.

BILATERALISM IN THE AUDITORY PATHWAYS

The central auditory pathways are unlike other ascending sensory paths due to (1) the presence of accessory nuclei that are intimately related to the ascending paths and (2) the bilateral representation of auditory impulses on each side.

Three groups of nuclei are found along the

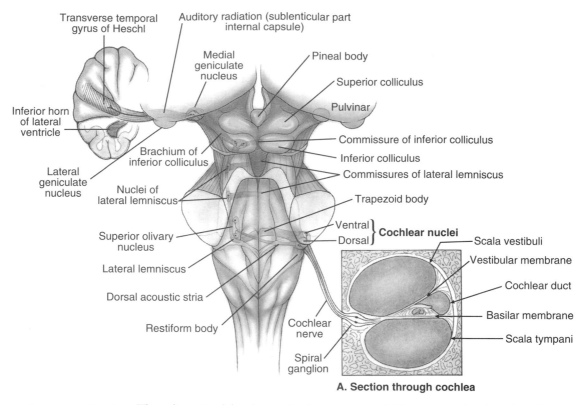

Transverse temporal gyrus of Heschl

Auditory radiation (sublenticular part internal capsule)

Medial geniculate nucleus

Pineal body

Superior colliculus

Pulvinar

Inferior horn of lateral ventricle

Brachium of inferior colliculus

Commissure of inferior colliculus

Inferior colliculus

Commissures of lateral lemniscus

Lateral geniculate nucleus

Nuclei of lateral lemniscus

Trapezoid body

Ventral ⎱ **Cochlear nuclei**
Dorsal ⎰

Superior olivary nucleus

Dorsal

Scala vestibuli

Vestibular membrane

Lateral lemniscus

Cochlear duct

Dorsal acoustic stria

Basilar membrane

Cochlear nerve

Scala tympani

Restiform body

Spiral ganglion

A. Section through cochlea

FIGURE 13–2.   Three-dimensional dorsal view of auditory pathways. **A.** Transverse section through cochlea.

A unilateral lesion of the auditory cortex or of the ascending paths distal to the cochlear nuclei, results in virtually no loss of hearing. The abnormality most often accompanying such a lesion is impairment of the ability to localize the direction and distance of sounds reaching the contralateral ear.

auditory pathways between the cochlear nuclei and the inferior colliculus. These are the superior olivary nucleus, the nuclei of the trapezoid body, and the nuclei of the lateral lemniscus.

The superior olivary nucleus is located in the caudal pons near the lateral border of the trapezoid body (Figs. 13–2, 13–3, 13–4). It receives input from the ipsilateral and contralateral cochlear nuclei, and it gives rise to fibers that join the ipsilateral and contralateral lateral lemnisci. The superior olivary nucleus plays a key role in the localization of sounds in space. The nuclei of the trapezoid body are scattered among the trapezoid bundles, and its afferent and efferent connections are similar to those of the superior olive.

The nuclei of the lateral lemniscus are lo-cated in and adjacent to the lateral lemniscus at middle and rostral pontine levels. They receive lemniscal fibers and their collaterals, and these nuclei send axons to both the ipsilateral and the contralateral lateral lemnisci. The nuclei of the inferior colliculi also aid in the bilateralism of the auditory paths by sending axons to the contralateral side via the commissure of the inferior colliculus (Figs. 13–2, 13–3, 13–4).

Conduction deafness results from any interference with the passage of sound waves through the external or middle ear (air-ossicular route). Bone conduction (transmission of sound waves through the cranial bones) can still occur. Therefore, conduction deafness is never complete or total.

Nerve deafness (perception deafness) results from damage to the receptor cells of the spiral organ or to the cochlear nerve. The defect or damage is in the portion of the auditory mechanism common to both air and bone conduction and, therefore, hearing failure or loss in both routes occurs. The degree of hearing loss is, of course, related to the amount of damage to the spiral organ or nerve.

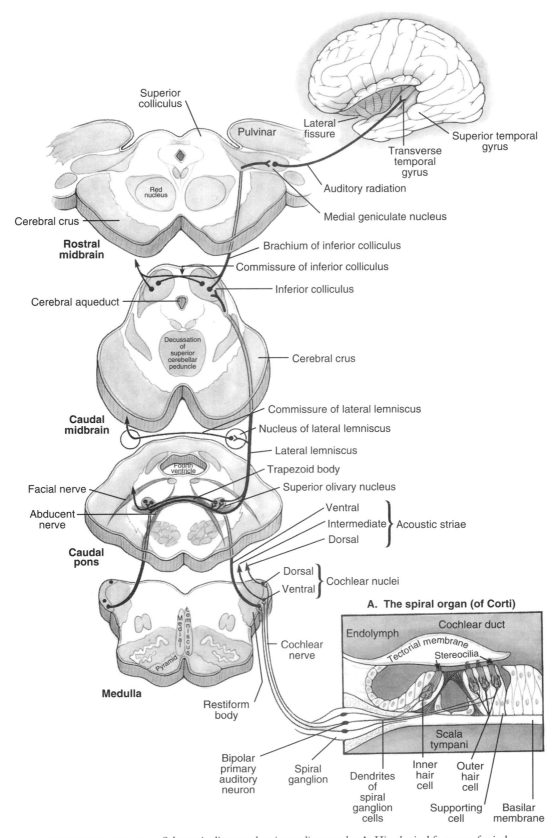

Superior colliculus

Pulvinar

Lateral fissure

Transverse temporal gyrus

Superior temporal gyrus

Auditory radiation

Medial geniculate nucleus

Red nucleus

Cerebral crus

Rostral midbrain

Brachium of inferior colliculus

Commissure of inferior colliculus

Cerebral aqueduct

Inferior colliculus

Decussation of superior cerebellar peduncle

Cerebral crus

Caudal midbrain

Commissure of lateral lemniscus

Nucleus of lateral lemniscus

Lateral lemniscus

Fourth ventricle

Trapezoid body

Facial nerve

Superior olivary nucleus

Abducent nerve

Ventral
Intermediate } Acoustic striae
Dorsal

Caudal pons

Dorsal } Cochlear nuclei
Ventral

A. The spiral organ (of Corti)

Medial Lemniscus

Pyramid

Cochlear duct

Endolymph

Tectorial membrane

Stereocilia

Medulla

Cochlear nerve

Restiform body

Scala tympani

Bipolar primary auditory neuron

Spiral ganglion

Dendrites of spiral ganglion cells

Inner hair cell

Outer hair cell

Supporting cell

Basilar membrane

FIGURE 13-3. Schematic diagram showing auditory paths. **A.** Histological features of spiral organ.

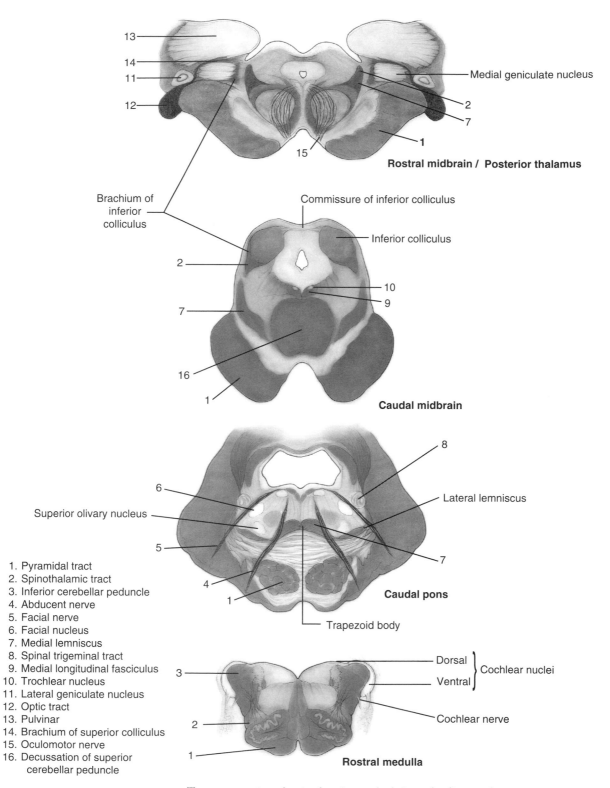

1. Pyramidal tract
2. Spinothalamic tract
3. Inferior cerebellar peduncle
4. Abducent nerve
5. Facial nerve
6. Facial nucleus
7. Medial lemniscus
8. Spinal trigeminal tract
9. Medial longitudinal fasciculus
10. Trochlear nucleus
11. Lateral geniculate nucleus
12. Optic tract
13. Pulvinar
14. Brachium of superior colliculus
15. Oculomotor nerve
16. Decussation of superior
    cerebellar peduncle

FIGURE 13-4.   Transverse sections showing locations and relations of auditory pathways.

Unilateral lesions in the spiral organ, spiral ganglion, cochlear nerve, or cochlear nuclei produce deafness on the ipsilateral side. Due to the bilateralism of auditory impulses as they ascend in the brainstem, unilateral lesions in the pathway beyond the cochlear nuclei result in deficits not nearly as serious as those resulting from unilateral lesions of the other sensory pathways.

AUDITORY MODULATION

Reciprocal connections between the various auditory central nuclei permit descending modulation of ascending auditory activity. Thus, the auditory cortex sends axons back to the medial geniculate nucleus and inferior colliculus. The inferior colliculus, along with the lateral lemniscus and superior olivary nuclei, send fibers to the cochlear nuclei. Moreover, the efferent olivocochlear bundle, which arises from neurons in the superior olivary and trapezoid nuclei, as well as the adjacent reticular for-

mation, terminates on the hair cells of the spiral organ and on the afferent terminals innervating them. This auditory feedback system provides a mechanism for regulating selective attention to certain sounds.

Two tuning fork tests may be used to determine types of deafness. The **Weber tuning fork test** is performed by placing the stem of a vibrating tuning fork at the middle of the forehead and asking the patient in which ear the tone is heard. A patient with unilateral nerve deafness hears the tone in the unaffected ear because that ear is more sensitive. The patient with a unilateral conduction deafness hears the tone louder in the affected ear.

The **Rinne tuning fork test** compares hearing via air conduction and bone conduction. A vibrating tuning fork is held near the patient's auricle (air conduction) until it can no longer be heard. Then the stem of the vibrating tuning fork is placed in contact with the mastoid process (bone conduction). Normally the sound is heard louder and longer by air conduction.

CHAPTER REVIEW QUESTIONS

13–1. Account for the bilateral representation of sound in the auditory system.

13–2. Where in the auditory system does a unilateral lesion produce total deafness in the ipsilateral ear?

13–3. As an acoustic neurinoma on the vestibular nerve in the internal acoustic meatus expands, what other nerves become impaired

    a. In the internal acoustic meatus?
    b. In or near the cerebellar angle?

13–4. Contrast conduction deafness and neural deafness.

THE GUSTATORY AND OLFACTORY SYSTEMS: AGEUSIA AND ANOSMIA

■ A 50-year-old patient has right facial paralysis, right hyperacusis, and the loss of taste on the anterior two thirds of the right side of the tongue, as well as a headache in the right frontal area and loss of smell in the right nasal cavity.

Taste and smell are chemical senses that provide information about a wide range of stimuli, from the pleasant taste of certain foods and drinks to the unpleasant or noxious odors of decay and danger. Both senses arise from specific chemical receptors, which when activated transmit neural impulses to the cerebral cortex, where perception occurs.

GUSTATORY SYSTEM

Taste arises chiefly from receptors embedded in the mucosa of the tongue. A few receptors may also exist on the epiglottis and adjacent part of the pharynx. The gustatory pathways consists of three neurons: number 1 in the ganglia of the VII, IX, and X cranial nerves; number 2 in the medulla; and number 3 in the thalamus.

GUSTATORY RECEPTORS

Taste receptors, or gustatory receptors, are activated by sweet, salty, bitter, and sour. The tip of the tongue responds to all four tastes, but is most sensitive to sweet and salty. The lateral parts of the tongue are more sensitive to sour, but also respond to sweet. The root of the tongue responds to bitter substances.

The taste buds are composed of three types of cells: receptor, supporting, and basal. Gustatory receptors are the neuroepithelial cells in the taste buds (Fig. 14–1). At the apex of each gustatory cell, microvilli form the gustatory hairs, which project into a small cavity beneath the gustatory pore. The base of each taste bud is penetrated by nerve fibers that branch and spiral around the receptor cells. Individual receptor cells have a life span of approximately 2 weeks. They are replaced by the supporting cells, the daughter cells of the basal cells.

GUSTATORY PATHWAY

Taste buds in different parts of the tongue are innervated by different cranial nerves (Fig. 14–1). Taste buds in the anterior two thirds of the tongue are innervated by the facial nerve; taste buds in the posterior third of the tongue are innervated by the glossopharyngeal nerve; and taste buds in the epiglottic and palatal portions of the oral cavity are innervated by the vagus nerve. The primary or first order neurons in the gustatory pathway are unipolar cells in the geniculate ganglion of the facial nerve (VII CN), inferior or petrosal ganglion of the glossopharyngeal nerve (IX CN), and inferior or nodose ganglion of the vagus nerve (X CN).

The axons of these ganglia cells enter the brainstem, pass to the solitary tract, and synapse in the rostral part of the solitary nucleus, commonly referred to as the **gustatory nucleus** (Figs. 14–1–14–3).

Secondary connections of the gustatory nucleus ascend near either the medial lemniscus

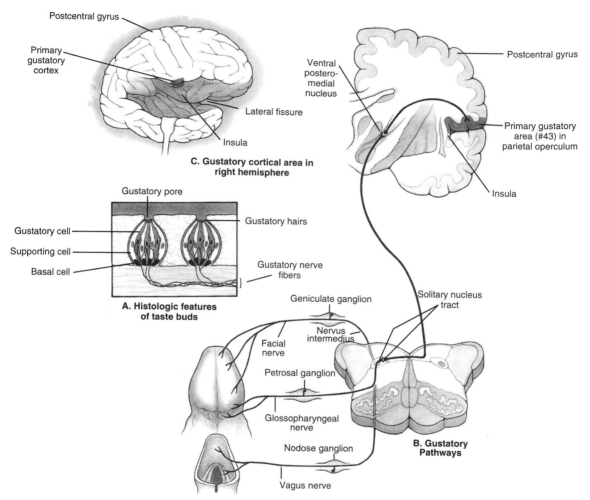

FIGURE 14–1. Schematic diagram of gustatory pathways. **A.** Histologic features of taste buds. **B.** Gustatory pathways. **C.** Gustatory cortical area in right hemisphere.

or central tegmental tract to reach the ventral posteromedial (VPM) nucleus of the thalamus. The most medial part of the VPM nucleus, the small cell parvicellular part, receives projections from the gustatory nucleus. From this parvicellular part, fibers travel in the gustatory radiation through the posterior limb of the internal capsule to the cortical gustatory area.

According to clinical reports, damage to the VPM nucleus or to the parietal operculum results in a loss of taste. The clinical evidence, however, is controversial as to whether the loss is ipsilateral or contralateral.

The primary gustatory cortex, is located in the parietal **operculum** and the adjacent part of the **insula.**

In experimental animals, a pontine gustatory center in the parabrachial area, consisting of nuclei near the brachium conjunctivum (superior cerebellar peduncle) as it enters the tegmentum of the rostral pons, receives input from the gustatory nucleus. The parabrachial area projects, at least partially, to the hypothalamus and amygdaloid nuclei, components of the limbic system that may be important in the affect related to the perception of taste.

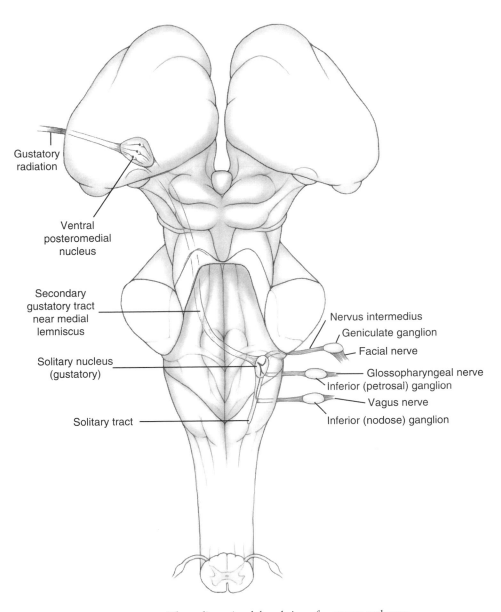

Gustatory
radiation

Ventral
posteromedial
nucleus

Secondary
gustatory tract
near medial
lemniscus

Solitary nucleus
(gustatory)

Solitary tract

Nervus intermedius

Geniculate ganglion

Facial nerve

Glossopharyngeal nerve

Inferior (petrosal) ganglion

Vagus nerve

Inferior (nodose) ganglion

FIGURE 14–2.   Three-dimensional dorsal view of gustatory pathways.

OLFACTORY SYSTEM

Humans are **microsmatic,** i.e., their sense of smell is poorly developed; hence, the sense of smell and its pathways are considerably less important clinically than the visual, auditory, and somatosensory senses and their pathways. The central nervous system (CNS) structures associated with olfaction form the rhinencephalon "nose-brain," which chiefly includes the olfactory structures on the base of the brain and the medial parts of the temporal lobe in the vicinity of the **uncus.**

OLFACTORY RECEPTORS

The primary olfactory neurons are located in the yellowish olfactory mucosa, which con-

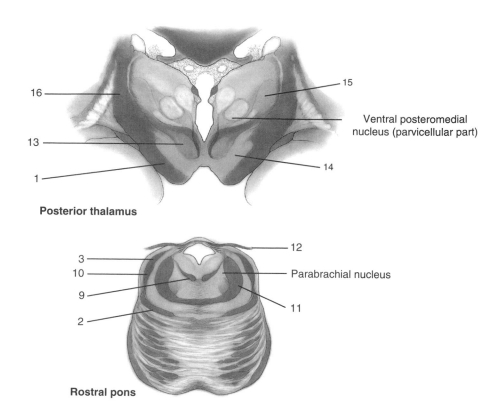

Posterior thalamus

Ventral posteromedial
nucleus (parvicellular part)

Rostral pons

Parabrachial nucleus

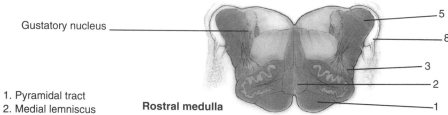

Gustatory nucleus

Rostral medulla

1. Pyramidal tract
2. Medial lemniscus
3. Spinothalamic tract
4. Spinal trigeminal tract
5. Inferior cerebellar peduncle
6. Vestibular nuclei
7. Hypoglossal nucleus
8. Ventral cochlear nucleus
9. Medial longitudinal fasciculus
10. Lateral lemniscus
11. Superior cerebellar peduncle
12. Trochlear nerve
13. Red nucleus
14. Substantia nigra
15. Ventral posterolateral nucleus
16. Posterior limb, internal capsule

Solitary tract

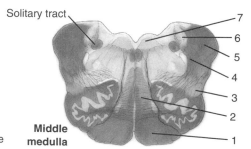

**Middle
medulla**

FIGURE 14-3. Transverse sections showing the relations of gustatory central pathways.

sists of about 1 in² of epithelium on the superior nasal concha and the upper part of the nasal septum. The olfactory neurons are bipolar and number several million on each side. Each neuron possesses a dendrite that extends to the surface where it expands to form a bulbous olfactory vesicle. Each of these vesicles, in turn, gives rise to a number of olfactory cilia (Fig. 14–4). These cilia spread over the surface of the olfactory mucosa and are bathed in mucus secreted mainly by specialized glands and by cells in the olfactory epithelium and the neighboring nasal mucosa. In order for odors to be smelled, they must dissolve in the mucus and stimulate the chemosensitive cilia.

A unique feature of the primary olfactory neurons is that they are constantly replaced throughout a person's lifetime. It is estimated that the life span of these neurons is only 4 to 6 weeks, and, on degenerating, new neurons are formed from undifferentiated basal cells in the deeper part of the olfactory epithelium.

OLFACTORY PATHWAY

The central branches of the bipolar olfactory neurons form the axons of the olfactory nerves (Fig. 14–4). These nonmyelinated fibers are collected into about 20 bundles, which traverse the foramina in the cribriform plate of the ethmoid bone. Collectively these bundles form the olfactory nerve and they terminate in the olfactory bulb located on the floor of the anterior cranial

fossa above the cribriform plate. How the axons of olfactory neurons newly formed throughout life reach synaptic sites on the secondary neurons in the olfactory bulb is not known.

> The sudden loss of smell (**anosmia**) is not uncommon after sudden blows to the head. Anosmia occurs most frequently as the result of head injuries that injure the olfactory nerves or nasal infections that damage the olfactory receptors. However, the gradual loss of smell may be related to the growth of a tumor at the base of the anterior cranial fossa; hence, this type of loss should be investigated.

The olfactory bulb is the flattened oval structure on the orbital surface of the frontal lobe near the anterior end of the olfactory sulcus (Fig. 14–5). It is composed of several types of cells, the most prominent of which are the mitral cells (Fig. 14–4). The synaptic contacts between the olfactory nerve fibers and the mitral cells are made via dense arborizations that form the olfactory glomeruli. In these structures, thousands of olfactory nerve fibers may synapse on the dendrites of one mitral cell. The axons of the mitral cells enter the olfactory tract.

The olfactory tract is the narrow band that continues posteriorly from the olfactory bulb along the olfactory sulcus. It is mainly composed of the efferent fibers of the bulb, although it does contain clumps of neurons that form the anterior olfactory nucleus as well as

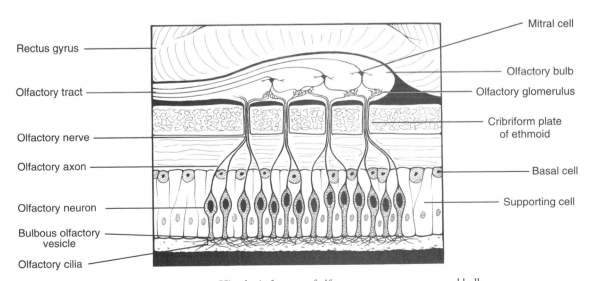

Rectus gyrus

Olfactory tract

Olfactory nerve

Olfactory axon

Olfactory neuron

Bulbous olfactory vesicle

Olfactory cilia

Mitral cell

Olfactory bulb

Olfactory glomerulus

Cribriform plate of ethmoid

Basal cell

Supporting cell

FIGURE 14–4. Histologic features of olfactory receptors, nerves, and bulb.

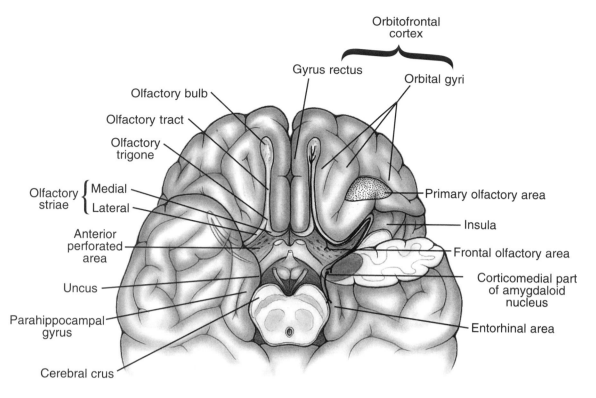

FIGURE 14–5.   Ventral view of frontal and temporal lobes showing the olfactory pathway from the olfactory bulb to the primary olfactory cortex. Left temporal lobe removed from temporal pole to uncus to expose pathway.

centrifugal fibers from the contralateral anterior olfactory nucleus and from neurons in the basal forebrain whose axons modulate the olfactory bulb neurons.

At the posterior end of the olfactory tract is the olfactory trigone (Fig. 14–5) where the fibers of the tract diverge to form two bundles, the lateral and medial olfactory striae, which border the anterior perforated substance. The fibers of the medial olfactory stria arise chiefly in the anterior olfactory nucleus and project via the anterior or olfactory part of the **anterior commissure** to the contralateral olfactory bulb. The medial olfactory stria becomes buried in the **anterior perforated substance** shortly after emerging from the olfactory trigone.

The lateral olfactory stria carries the efferent projections of the olfactory bulb toward the insula where they bend medially to enter the temporal lobe. On entering the temporal lobe, the fibers of the lateral olfactory stria terminate in the region of the uncus. The uncus is the enlargement in the anterior part of the parahip-

pocampal gyrus and is located on the medial surface of the temporal lobe (Fig. 14–5). The uncus is actually the medial part of the amygdaloid nucleus, which sends axons to the medial dorsal nucleus of the thalamus. The medial dorsal nucleus, in turn, sends axons to the posterolateral part of the orbitofrontal cortex, the primary olfactory area.

Unlike all the other senses, olfactory sensations reach the cerebral cortex without passing through the thalamus. This nonthalamic pathway passes from the uncus to more posterior parts of the parahippocampal gyrus, which, in turn, sends axons via the **uncinate fasciculus** directly to the primary olfactory cortex.

Lesions in the olfactory area of the orbitofrontal cortex result in the loss of ability to discriminate different odors.

Irritative lesions in the region of the uncus result in olfactory hallucinations usually disagreeable in character. These olfactory hallucinations commonly occur in temporal lobe epilepsy and frequently constitute the aura that precedes the phenomenon referred to as "uncinate fits."

CHAPTER REVIEW QUESTIONS

14–1. Which cranial nerves contain taste fibers and what are their peripheral distributions and central connections?

14–2. Locate the primary gustatory area in the cerebral cortex.

14–3. Give the location and morphologic features of the olfactory membrane.

14–4. Locate the primary olfactory area.

THE CEREBRAL CORTEX:
APHASIA, AGNOSIA, AND APRAXIA

■ *A 62-year-old patient experiences sudden loss of speech, accompanied by weakness of the right lower facial muscles and the right hand. The episode lasts about 5 minutes and is immediately followed by the return of normal speech and muscle strength in the face and hand.*

The cerebral cortex is the "highest center" in the brain, and, as such, it perceives sensations, commands skilled movements, provides awareness of emotions and is necessary for memory, thinking, language abilities, and all other higher mental functions.

SUBDIVISIONS OF THE CEREBRAL CORTEX

There are three types of cortex in the human brain: neocortex, paleocortex, and archicortex. The neocortex appeared last in evolution and constitutes about 90% of the total cerebral cortex. The paleocortex is restricted to the base of the cerebral hemispheres and is associated with the olfactory system, whereas the archicortex, the phylogenetically oldest cortex, makes up the **hippocampal formation.** Both the paleocortex and archicortex are parts of the limbic system, which is described in Chapter 16.

The cerebral cortex reaches its greatest development in the human. It contributes about half the total brain weight and consists of a sheet of neurons 2.5 ft^2 in area that is folded or convoluted with only about one third of the neocortex found on the surface and the remainder buried in the grooves between the convolutions. A fold or convolution is called a gyrus (pl.

gyri) and the groove between adjacent gyri is called a sulcus (pl. sulci).

HISTOLOGIC FEATURES

The young adult cortex contains billions of neurons. The two main neuronal cell types are the **pyramidal** and **granule cells** (Fig. 15–1). The pyramidal cells have a pyramid-shaped cell body with a large apical dendrite directed toward the surface of the cortex and several large basal dendrites that pass horizontally from the base of the cell. The axon proceeds from the base of the cell and in most cases leaves the cortex to reach other cortical areas or subcortical nuclei. The pyramidal cells are the chief cortical efferent or output neurons.

> The surfaces of the dendrites of mature pyramidal cells contain numerous synaptic sites, called spines (Fig. 15–1). During postnatal maturation of the cortex, the pyramidal cell dendritic trees expand and the number of spines increases. The finding that the faulty development of these dendritic trees and their spines is seen in cases of mental retardation such as **Down syndrome** suggests that these phenomena may be related to learning.

The granule or stellate cells are the main interneurons of the cortex and greatly outnumber the pyramidal cells. These small cells have numerous short dendrites that extend in all directions and a short axon that arborizes on other neurons in the vicinity. Granule cells occur in large numbers in all cortical areas and are especially numerous in the sensory and association areas.

Layers

Cells

I: Molecular

II: External
granular

III: External
pyramidal

IV: Internal
granular

V: Internal
pyramidal

VI: Multiform

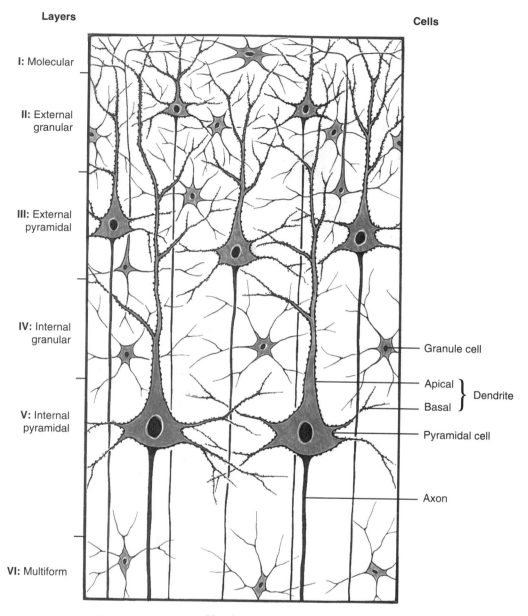

Granule cell

Apical
Basal } Dendrite

Pyramidal cell

Axon

FIGURE 15–1.   Histology of cerebral cortex: Layers and cells.

FUNCTIONAL HISTOLOGY

The neurons of the neocortex are arranged in six horizontal layers. The most superficial is the cell-poor molecular layer (I) and the deepest is the multiform layer (VI). In between these layers are alternating external and internal granular layers (II and IV) and pyramidal layers (III and V), each of which is named according to its predominant cell type (Fig. 15–1).

Although the neurons of the cortex are arranged in six layers oriented parallel to the surface, the functional units of cortical activity are organized in groups of neurons oriented perpendicular to the surface. These vertically oriented functional units are called **cortical columns,** and they contain thousands of neurons that are interconnected in the vertical direction.

Within each cortical column the internal granular layer (IV) is the chief input layer (Fig. 15–2)

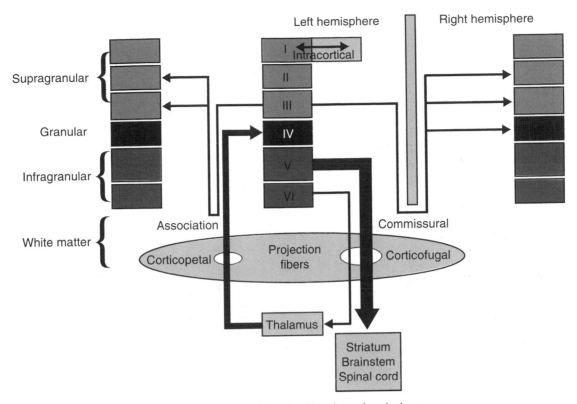

FIGURE 15-2.   Functional histology of cerebral cortex.

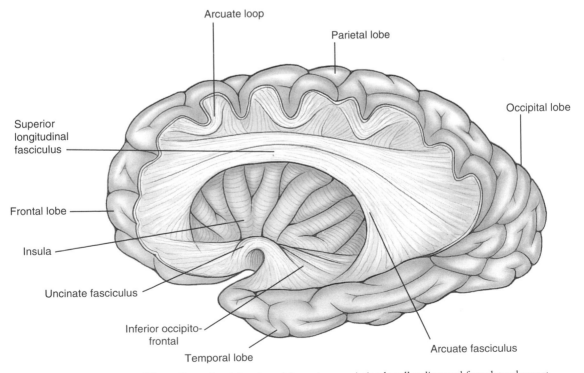

FIGURE 15-3.   Three-dimensional drawing of the major association bundles dissected from lateral aspect.

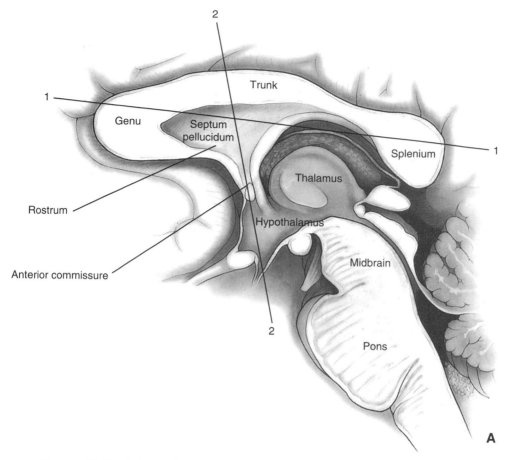

FIGURE 15–4. Median brainstem showing locations of hemispheric commissural fibers: The corpus callosum and anterior commissure. **A.** Plane of horizontal section (*line 1-1*); plane of coronal section (*line 2-2*). **B.** Horizontal section through genu and splenium of corpus callosum. **C.** Coronal section through corpus callosum and anterior commissure.

and receives afferent fibers from the thalamic nuclei. The infragranular layers (V and VI) are for output, layer V giving rise to fibers destined for the corpus striatum, brainstem, and spinal cord. Layer VI projects fibers to the thalamus. The supragranular layers (I, II, and III) are associative and connect with other parts of the cerebral cortex.

CORTICAL CONNECTIONS

The connections of each cortical column are of four types: intracortical, association, commissural, and subcortical (Fig. 15–2).

INTRACORTICAL FIBERS

Intracortical connections are quite short and occur chiefly through horizontally oriented

neurons in layer I and the horizontally coursing branches of pyramidal cell axons.

ASSOCIATION FIBERS

Association connections occur from gyrus to gyrus and from lobe to lobe in the same hemisphere. The short association fibers, called arcuate fibers or loops, connect adjacent gyri, and the long association fibers form bundles connecting more distant gyri (Fig. 15–3). The long association bundles give fibers to and receive fibers from the overlying gyri along their routes. The main long association bundles are the **superior longitudinal fasciculus** and its temporal component, the **arcuate fasciculus**, the inferior occipitofrontal and uncinate fasciculi, and the **cingulum.** The superior longitudinal fasciculus is located above the insula and

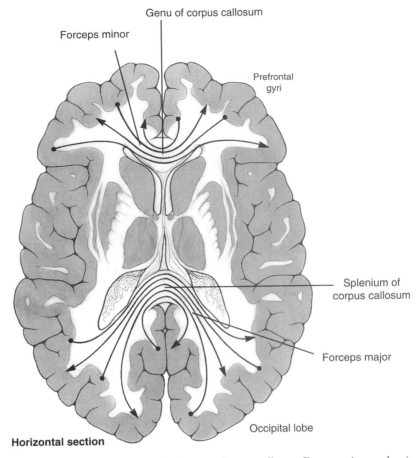

Horizontal section

FIGURE 15–4B. Connections of genu and splenium of corpus callosum: Forceps minor and major (*line 1-1*).

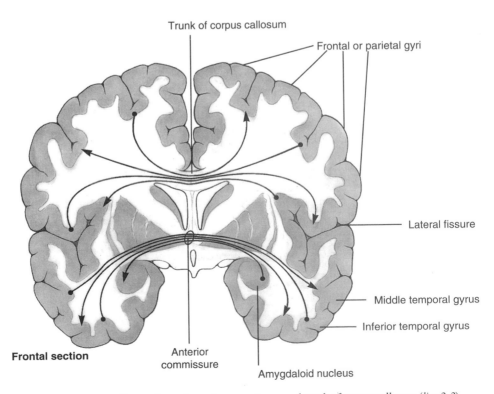

Frontal section

FIGURE 15–4C. Connections of anterior commissure and trunk of corpus callosum (*line 2-2*).

connects the frontal, parietal, and occipital lobes. Posterior to the insula is the arcuate fasciculus, which arches from the superior longitudinal fasciculus into the temporal lobe, thereby connecting the frontal and temporal lobes. The inferior occipitofrontal fasciculus passes below the insula as it interconnects the frontal, temporal, and occipital lobes. The uncinate fasciculus joins the orbital (inferior) part of the frontal lobe with the temporal lobe. The cingulum is located beneath the cingulate and parahippocampal gyri, components of the limbic lobe. The association fibers arise from pyramidal neurons chiefly in layers II and III.

COMMISSURAL FIBERS

Commissural connections occur between homologous areas of the two hemispheres. Two major bundles exist: the corpus callosum and the anterior commissure (Fig. 15–4A). The corpus callosum is divided, from anterior to posterior, into rostrum, genu, trunk, and **splenium.** The rostrum and genu interconnect the anterior part of the frontal lobe (Fig. 15–4B). The trunk interconnects the posterior part of the frontal lobe, the entire parietal lobe, and the superior part of the temporal lobe. The splenium interconnects the occipital lobes. The fibers arching anteriorly from the genu and rostrum form the forceps minor, and those arching posteriorly from the splenium form the forceps major. Cortical connections of the anterior commissure include the inferior and middle temporal gyri (Fig. 15–4C). The commissural fibers arise from pyramidal cells chiefly in layers II and III (Fig. 15–2).

> Surgical transection of the corpus callosum is sometimes performed for the relief of epilepsy. Such **split brain** patients have served to elucidate the importance of the corpus callosum, especially for language functions.

PROJECTION FIBERS

Projection fibers connect the cerebral cortex with subcortical nuclei and are classified as **corticofugal** or efferent if they carry impulses away from the cortex, or **corticopetal** or afferent if they carry them toward the cortex (Fig. 15–2). The corticofugal projection fibers are distributed to the corpus striatum and nuclei at all levels of the brainstem and spinal cord. The major corticofugal projections are described with the motor system (Chapters 6–9). Corticopetal projection fibers arise predominantly in the thalamus and are called thalamic radiations. These radiations can be distributed to specific or to widespread cortical areas. In most cases the connections between the thalamic nuclei and the cerebral cortex are reciprocal.

As projection fibers course between the thalamus and the corpus striatum, they are gathered together in a conspicuous band called the internal capsule. In the horizontal plane, the internal capsule is V-shaped (Fig. 15–5) and is divided into an anterior limb located between the head of the caudate and lentiform nuclei, a posterior limb located between the thalamus and lentiform nucleus, and a genu where the two limbs meet. The anterior limb of the internal capsule is for frontal lobe connections exclusively, e.g., corticofugal projections to the striatum and pontine nuclei and corticopetal projection fibers from the anterior and medial thalamic nuclei. The genu and adjacent part of the posterior limb contain corticopetal projection fibers from the motor thalamus (i.e., the ventral anterior and ventral lateral nuclei), which project to the premotor and motor areas, respectively. Posteriorly, the posterior limb contains the corticonuclear (corticobulbar) and corticospinal (pyramidal) tracts as well as the somatosensory thalamic radiations from the ventral posterior nucleus. The precise location of the corticonuclear and corticospinal tracts in the posterior limb varies according to the superior-inferior level of the capsule. Superiorly, the pyramidal tract is in the anterior half of the posterior limb, whereas inferiorly it is in the posterior half (Fig. 15–5). The corticobulbar tract is slightly anterior to the pyramidal tract. The part of the internal capsule lateral to the thalamus and posterior to the lentiform nucleus is the retrolenticular part and contains the optic radiations as they emerge from the lateral geniculate nucleus (Fig. 15–5B). The auditory radiations from the medial geniculate nucleus are located in that part of the internal capsule lateral to the thalamus and ventral to the lentiform nucleus, the sublenticular part of the internal capsule.

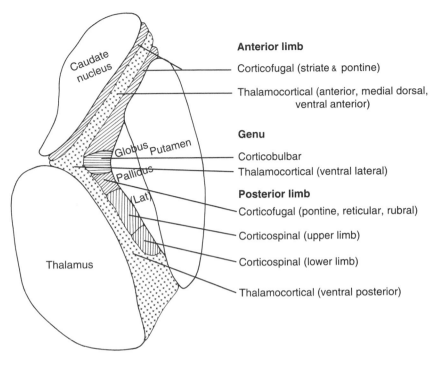

Anterior limb

Corticofugal (striate & pontine)

Thalamocortical (anterior, medial dorsal,
ventral anterior)

Genu

Corticobulbar
Thalamocortical (ventral lateral)

Posterior limb

Corticofugal (pontine, reticular, rubral)

Corticospinal (upper limb)

Corticospinal (lower limb)

Thalamocortical (ventral posterior)

A

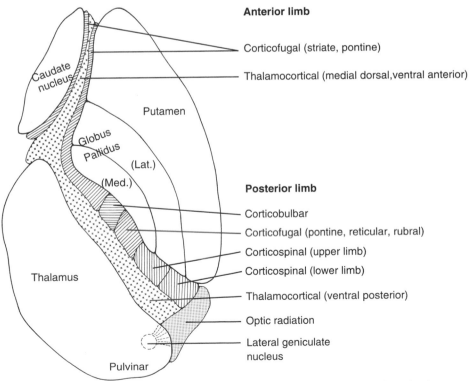

Anterior limb

Corticofugal (striate, pontine)

Thalamocortical (medial dorsal,ventral anterior)

Posterior limb

Corticobulbar
Corticofugal (pontine, reticular, rubral)
Corticospinal (upper limb)
Corticospinal (lower limb)
Thalamocortical (ventral posterior)
Optic radiation
Lateral geniculate
nucleus

B

FIGURE 15-5.   Components of internal capsule. **A.** Superior level. **B.** Inferior level.

The posterior limb of the internal capsule is of great clinical importance because it is the most frequent site of cerebral hemorrhage or "stroke." Moreover, when this area is damaged the signs and symptoms are more widespread than those associated with a lesion of comparable size anywhere in the nervous system. Following a capsular stroke, the patient has contralateral spastic hemiplegia, resulting from damage to the corticospinal tract and contralateral hemianesthesia, resulting from damage to the somatosensory thalamic radiation. In addition, contralateral lower facial paralysis results from damage to the corticobulbar tract. If the damaged capsular area includes the retrolenticular part, contralateral homonymous hemianopsia results from interruption of the optic radiation.

FUNCTIONAL AREAS

Anatomically, the cerebral cortex is described according to lobes (frontal, parietal, temporal, occipital, limbic, and insular) that are subdivided into gyri (Figs. 15–6**A**, 15–7**A**). Functionally, the cortex is described according to the numbered areas (Figs. 15–6**B**, 15–7**B**) that were originally demarcated by Brodmann. Interestingly, Brodmann designated these areas not on the basis of function but of cytoarchitecture. A summary of the cortical areas, the localization of cortical functions, and the effects of destructive lesions is given in Table 15–1.

Because the density of the pyramidal and granule cells and the thickness of the various cortical layers are not uniform, the various parts of the cortex have different patterns or cytoarchitecture. On the basis of its different cytoarchitecture the cerebral cortex was divided into numbered areas by Brodmann in 1909. With the advent of functional studies by electrical stimulation of the human cortex, it became apparent that Brodmann numbered map corresponded well with functions of the various cortical areas. Hence, **Brodmann numbered areas** have become functional areas in addition to cytoarchitectonic areas.

FRONTAL LOBE

The frontal cortex constitutes about one third of the entire cerebral cortex and its size and connections are far more differentiated in humans than in any other animal, including the highest subhuman primates. It contains the following six main functional areas: (1) primary motor, (2) premotor, (3) frontal eye field, (4) supplementary motor, (5) prefrontal, and (6) Broca speech.

The primary motor area corresponds to Brodmann area 4 and occupies the posterior part of the precentral gyrus and the adjoining part of the paracentral lobule (Figs. 15–6**B**, 15–7**B**). Within the motor cortex somatotopic localization of contralateral movements is represented in an upside-down fashion with the lower limb in the paracentral lobule, the upper limb in the dorsal part of the precentral gyrus, and the face most ventral (Figs. 15–6**C**, 15–7**C**). The size of the area representing various movements is directly proportional to the degree of skill or finesse associated with the particular movement. Lesions of the primary motor area result in a weakness in the body part contralateral to the specific area damaged (Figs. 15–6**D**, 15–7**D**).

The premotor cortex, area 6, is located in the anterior part of the precentral gyrus, although dorsally it enlarges and includes the more posterior part of the superior frontal gyrus as well. Electrical stimulation of this area also produces contralateral movements, but they are slower in nature and include larger groups of muscles as compared to area 4 stimulation. The premotor area contains the programming necessary for movements. Focal lesions of the premotor area often result in **apraxia,** the inability to perform purposive movement even though no paralysis exists. For example, an apraxic patient who is unable to protrude the tongue when asked, spontaneously does so a few minutes later to lick the lips.

The frontal eye field, area 8, is located immediately in front of area 6, chiefly in the middle frontal gyrus, although it extends into the superior frontal gyrus as well (Fig. 15–6**B**). Stimulation of this area produces conjugate deviation of the eyes to the contralateral side; a unilateral destructive lesion here results in a transient deviation of the eyes to the same side and paralysis of contralateral gaze (Fig. 15–6**D**).

The supplementary motor area consists of the extensions of areas 6 and 8 into the medial aspect of the frontal lobe (Fig. 15–7**B**). Thus, it lies in the medial part of the superior frontal gyrus just in front of the paracentral lobule. Stimulation of this area results in posturing re-

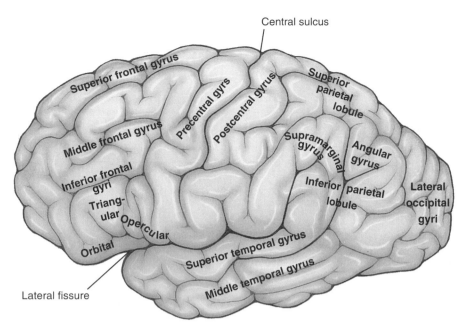

A. Principal gyri and sulci

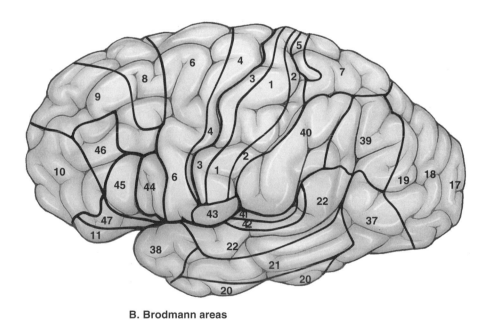

B. Brodmann areas

FIGURE 15–6.   Lateral views of left hemisphere. **A.** Gyri and sulci. **B.** Brodmann areas.

sponses such as turning the head and eyes toward the elevated contralateral arm. This area contains the programming necessary for complex movements involving several parts of the body.

The prefrontal cortex includes almost one fourth of the entire cerebral cortex and is located on the lateral, medial, and inferior surfaces of the frontal lobe in front of areas 6, 8, and 45 (Figs. 15–6**B**, 15–7**B**). It is referred to as

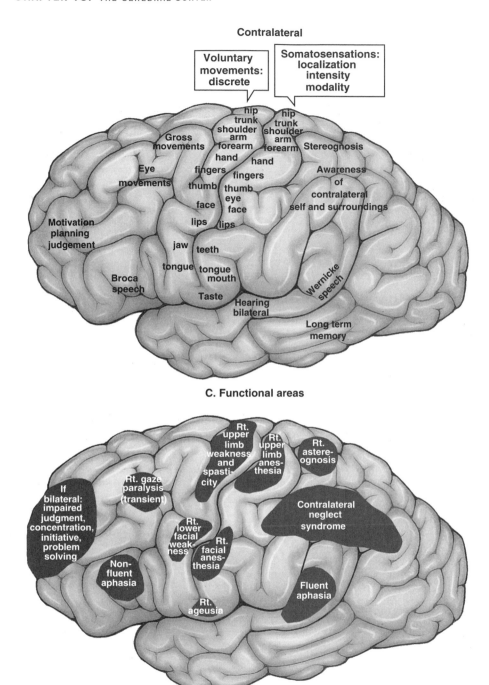

C. Functional areas

D. Results of lesions

FIGURE 15–6 (CONTINUED).   **C.** Functional areas. **D.** Results of lesions.

the frontal association cortex and is divided into two main regions: orbital and lateral. The orbital region, sometimes called the orbitofrontal region, is located on the inferior surface of the frontal lobe and includes the orbital gyri; the lateral area, frequently called the dorsolateral prefrontal region, includes the gyri on the convexity of the frontal lobe in front of areas 8 and 45. The orbitofrontal area appears to be associated with visceral and emo-

TABLE 15–1. LOCALIZATION OF CORTICAL FUNCTIONS

LOBE	STRUCTURE	FUNCTION	DESTRUCTIVE LESION
Frontal	Area 4	Discrete volitional movements	Contralateral paralysis and paresis (most pronounced in distal parts of limbs and lower part of face)
	Area 8	Conjugate eye movements	Transitory paralysis of conjugate eye movements to opposite side
	Broca Speech (areas 44 and 45)	Language production	Nonfluent aphasia
	Prefrontal Cortex Dorsolateral	Motivation, problem solving, judgment	Bilateral lesions: Impaired ability to concentrate, easily distracted, loss of initiative, apathy, cannot make decisions
	Orbitofrontal	Emotions, behavior	Unstable emotions; unpredictable and frequent unacceptable behavior
	Orbital Gyri (posterolateral part)	Olfaction	Inability to discriminate odors
Parietal	Areas 3, 1, 2	Somesthetic sensations	Loss of contralateral stimulus location and intensity; severe impairment of two-point and limb position senses
	Area 43	Taste	Impairment of taste in contralateral side of tongue
	Superior and Inferior Parietal Lobules	Processing of somatic and visual information especially related to use of hands	Tactile and visual agnosia, visual disorientation, neglect of contralateral self and surroundings
Temporal	Area 41	Hearing	Subtle decrease in hearing and ability to localize sounds, both contralaterally
	Wernicke Speech (area 22)	Language understanding and formulation	Fluent aphasia
	Middle Inferior, and Occipitotemporal Gyri (dominant side)	Storage of auditorially presented information	Impairment of learning and memory
	Temporal Cortex (nondominant side)	Storage of visually presented information	Impairment of learning and memory
	Parahippocampal Region	Recent memory	Bilateral lesions: Profound memory loss of recent events and no new learning
Occipital	Area 17	Vision	Contralateral homonymous hemianopsia
	Parastriate and Peristriate (areas 18 and 19)	Visual association	Bilateral lesions: Color agnosia and loss of spatial relationships (cannot draw floor plan of home, map of route to work or church, etc.)

tional activities, whereas the dorsolateral area is concerned with such intellectual abilities as conceptualizing, planning, judgment, and problem solving. Lesions of the prefrontal cortex may result in loss of initiative and judgment. The patient becomes careless of appearance and dress and loses the sense of acceptable social behavior. Prefrontal leucotomy, isolation of the prefrontal cortex by cutting its connections with the rest of the brain, or prefrontal lobotomy, removal of the prefrontal cortex, were once fairly common surgical procedures used to treat patients with severe behavioral disorders.

> Insight into the functions of the prefrontal cortex was first reported in the middle of the 19th century when a railroad construction worker, Phineas Gage, suffered prefrontal lobotomy when a dynamite tamping rod was accidentally blown through the front of his head. Prior to the accident, Gage was a model employee—punctual, hardworking, gentlemanly, and highly respectable. Following recovery from the accident, Gage lost all sense of responsibility, became impulsive, irascible and profane, and drifted aimlessly the rest of his life.

Even though many functions are attributed to the prefrontal cortex, massive bilateral lesions often result in changes so subtle they are difficult to detect. As a result, it has been suggested that instead of having specific functions, the prefrontal cortex may be the orchestrator for other cortical areas and may elicit the behavior appropriate to the situation at hand.

The **Broca area,** located in areas 44 and 45 of the inferior frontal gyrus, is associated with speech and is described later.

PARIETAL LOBE

The parietal cortex constitutes slightly over one fifth of the entire cerebral cortex and contains the following four functional areas: (1) primary somatosensory, (2) secondary somatosensory, (3) gustatory, and (4) association.

The primary somatosensory area (SI) occupies the postcentral gyrus and the adjoining part of the paracentral lobule (Figs. 15–6A, 15–7A). It consists of three longitudinal zones: area 3 that includes the cortical tissue in the floor and posterior wall of the central sulcus, area 1 in the anterior two thirds of the convex surface of the postcentral gyrus, and area 2 in the remaining one third of the convex surface and the adjoining anterior wall of the postcentral sulcus. The somatotopic representation is contralateral with parts of the head located ventrally and the upper limb located dorsally in the postcentral gyrus (Fig. 15–6C), and the lower limb medially, in the posterior part of the paracentral lobule (Fig. 15–7C). The total area associated with a particular region of the body is directly related to the sensitivity of the particular region and not to its size. Stimulation of the primary sensory cortex in humans produces sharply localized contralateral sensations described as tingling or numbness. Lesions of this area result in the loss of tactile discrimination and position sense on the contralateral side (Figs. 15–6D, 15–7D). Pain cannot be elicited from this area nor is it abolished or relieved following its ablation.

The secondary somatosensory area (SII) is composed of a strip of cortex that extends from the parietal operculum into the posterior part of the insula. The parietal operculum (operculum means lid) is the cortical tissue continuous with the postcentral gyrus that forms the upper wall of the lateral fissure. Hence, it overlies and covers the insula. Somatotopic localization in

the SII area is poorly defined and bilateral. There is evidence that the sensation of pain is perceived here.

The primary gustatory cortex appears to be in area 43 of the postcentral gyrus and includes the more anterior part of the parietal operculum (Fig. 15–6B). It extends along the wall of the lateral fissure toward the insula and is adjacent to the tongue regions of the primary sensory and motor areas. A lesion in this area results in contralateral ageusia, i.e., loss of taste (Fig. 15–6D).

The parietal association area consists of the superior and inferior parietal lobules. The superior parietal lobule contains areas 5 and 7 (Figs. 15–6B, 15–7B). Area 5 receives input primarily from the SI cortex, whereas area 7 has widespread connections with the visual and motor areas of the cortex. The inferior parietal lobule includes two gyri: the supramarginal (area 40) and the angular (area 39) gyri. These receive input from the other parts of the parietal lobe as well as from association areas in the frontal, occipital, temporal, and limbic lobes. The parietal association areas process tactile and visual information and are intimately concerned with the cognition of the body itself and the objects surrounding it. These areas are also important in the orderly or sequential performance of tasks, especially those involving the hands. Lesions in the parietal association areas are associated with **astereognosis** and the **neglect syndrome,** a perceptual disorder related to recognition of the opposite side of the body and its surroundings (Fig. 15–6D).

> In the neglect syndrome, the patient fails to recognize the opposite side of the body and its surroundings. For example, when the damage is in the right hemisphere the patient does not bathe the left side of the body and may actually deny that the left limbs belong to him. Moreover, objects located in the left side of the visual field, e.g., cup of coffee on the left side of a food tray, do not exist in the mind of the patient.

TEMPORAL LOBE

The temporal cortex forms almost one fourth of the entire cortex and contains the primary auditory area as well as areas associated with emotions and higher mental functions such as memory and speech. The primary auditory cortex (areas 41 and 42) is situated in the transverse temporal gyri of Heschl, which are buried in the floor of the lateral fissure (Fig. 15–6, Fig. 13–3). Area 41 is mostly in the anterior gyrus but extends slightly into the adjacent part of the posterior gyrus. Immediately adjacent to area 41 is area 42, and adjacent to this area is the auditory association part of area 22, located in the superior temporal gyrus. Electrical stimulation of the auditory area results in noises described as humming, buzzing, clicking, or ringing, and stimulation of the adjacent part of area 22 produces sounds perceived as a whistle, a bell, etc. A unilateral lesion in the primary auditory area results in no significant hearing loss because of the bilateralism of the central auditory pathways. Such a lesion does, however, cause difficulty in recognizing the distance and direction from which sounds are coming, especially in the ear contralateral to the lesion.

The anterior and inferomedial parts of the temporal lobe are strongly connected with the limbic system and are concerned with mechanisms related to visceral activity, emotions, behavior, and some forms of memory. The posterior parts of the temporal lobe appear to record and store experiences. Electrical stimulation here produces illusions of past events that include not only the scenes and sounds but also the emotions associated with them. Lesions of the left posterior temporal cortex may impair the learning or remembering of verbally based information, whereas lesions of the right posterior temporal cortex (areas 20, 21, and 37) may impair the learning and remembering of visually based information. Bilateral lesions of areas 20 and 21 may result in prosopagnosia, the inability to recognize faces.

OCCIPITAL LOBE

The occipital cortex makes up only about one eighth of the entire cortex and contains the primary visual and visual association areas. The primary visual cortex (area 17), also called the striate area, receives the optic radiation and is located in the gyri forming the walls of the calcarine fissure (Fig. 15–7**A,B**). The cuneus

forms the upper wall of the calcarine fissure and herein is represented the lower half of the contralateral field of vision. The upper half of the contralateral visual field is represented in the lingual gyrus that forms the lower wall of the calcarine fissure. Macular vision is represented in the entire posterior half of area 17 (Fig. 12–4**A**). Unilateral lesions of the primary visual cortex result in contralateral homonymous hemianopsia (Fig. 15–7**D**).

The rest of the occipital lobe consists of area 18, which borders area 17 and is called the parastriate cortex, and area 19, the peristriate cortex, which is larger and forms most of the lateral surface of the occipital lobe. These areas receive visual information from the striate areas bilaterally and are important in the complex visual perceptions related to color, movement, direction of objects, etc. Lesions in the visual association areas and the adjoining parts of the temporal lobe result in visual agnosia, the inability to recognize objects and their colors.

HEMISPHERIC LATERALIZATION OF FUNCTION

In terms of motor and sensory functions (other than olfaction), each cerebral hemisphere contains contralateral representation of the body and its surroundings. Thus, lesions in the primary motor, primary somatosensory, or primary visual areas in one hemisphere result in contralateral hemiparesis, contralateral hemianesthesia, or contralateral hemianopsia. Higher functions such as analytical thinking, language comprehension and production of emotional and intuitive thinking, spatial orientation, and artistic and music abilities—to cite only a few—are functions of only one hemisphere. The hemisphere that contains the centers for language comprehension and production is called the **dominant hemisphere.**

As the result of numerous tests to determine the language-dominant hemisphere in patients in need of neurosurgical removal of cerebral cortical tissue, it has been found that language is represented in the left hemisphere in a high percentage of people: more than 95% of right-handed persons and almost 75% of left-handed persons.

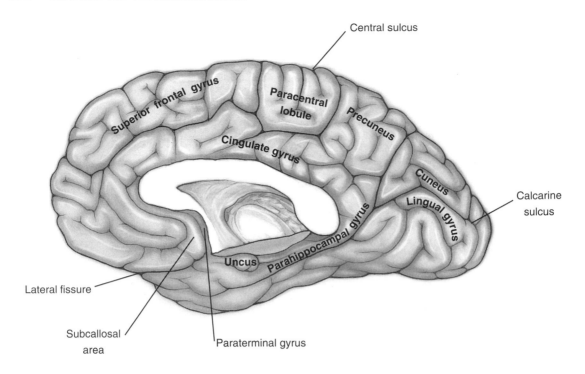

A. Principal gyri and sulci

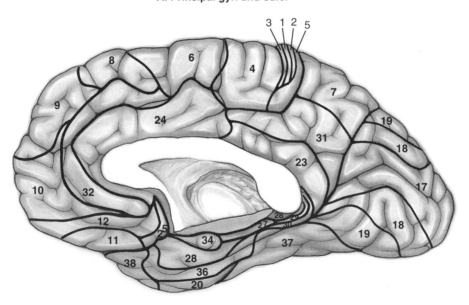

B. Brodmann areas

FIGURE 15-7.   Medial views of right hemisphere. **A.** Gyri and sulci. **B.** Brodmann areas.

Handedness and language dominance develop before a child has learned to speak. A unilateral lesion in the left hemisphere of a child does not hinder the development of speech because the right hemisphere assumes dominance. Furthermore, lesions occurring in children even toward the end of the first decade of life usually result in language difficulties only until the other hemisphere assumes the language function.

In addition to language dominance, the left hemisphere excels in intellectual processes such

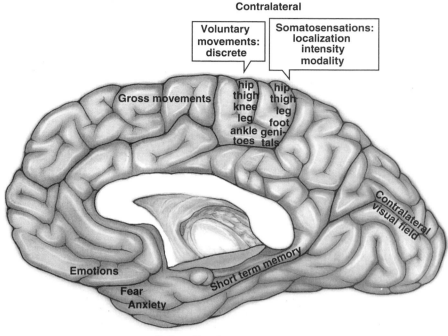

C. Functional areas

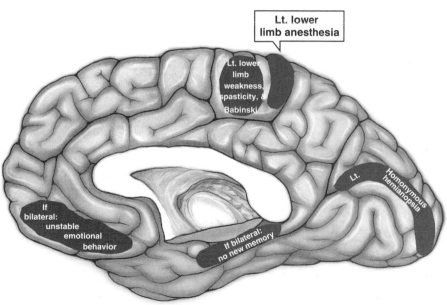

D. Results of lesions

FIGURE 15-7 (CONTINUED).   **C.** Functional areas. **D.** Results of lesions.

as analytical thinking or rationalizing, calculating, and verbalization (Fig. 15–8). In contrast, the nondominant hemisphere, usually the right, excels in sensory discrimination, in emotional, nonverbal thinking, and in artistic skills such as drawing and composing music, spatial perception, and, perhaps, recognition of faces.

LANGUAGE AREAS

Language is represented in cortical areas bordering the lateral fissure of the dominant hemisphere. Two areas exist: **Broca** and **Wernicke** (Fig. 15–9). Broca area, the motor speech center, comprises the opercular and triangular

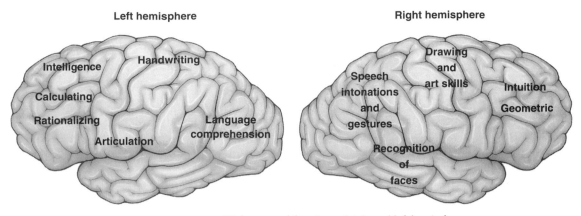

FIGURE 15-8.   Higher mental functions of right and left hemispheres.

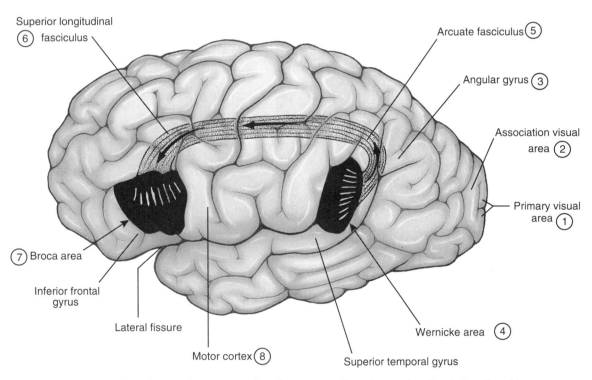

FIGURE 15-9.   Speech areas. Structures numbered represent pathway for a spoken description of an object or scene.

parts of the inferior frontal gyrus (Fig. 15–6**A**). This area contains the motor programs for the production of words and it projects fibers to the parts of the motor cortex that control the muscles used in articulation, i.e., the muscles in the vocal cords, tongue, and lips. A lesion in the Broca area is associated with an **expressive** or **motor aphasia,** characterized as **nonfluent** (Fig. 15–6**D**) because of the slow and prolonged out-put of words, poor articulation, and short sentences containing only the necessary verbs, nouns, and pronouns.

The Wernicke area, the sensory or receptive speech area, is in the posterior part of area 22 in the superior temporal gyrus. This area contains the mechanisms for the comprehension and formulation of language. A lesion in the Wernicke area, is associated with **receptive** or **sen-**

sory aphasia, characterized as **fluent** (Fig. 15–6**D**) because production of words is normal but the use of words is defective. The patient substitutes one word for another, inserts meaningless words, or strings together words or phrases of great length but no meaning. The patient with receptive aphasia is fluent but cannot comprehend language in any form—heard, read, or spoken.

The Wernicke area projects into the Broca area via association fibers in the arcuate and superior longitudinal fasciculi (Figs. 15–3, 15–9). A lesion interrupting these fibers produces a **conduction aphasia** in which speech deficiency is similar to a receptive aphasia. But, because comprehension remains intact, the patient makes repeated attempts to say the right words.

Other forms of aphasia also exist and may result from lesions not only in the cortical tissue bordering the lateral fissure (the perisylvian language areas) but also in cortical areas some distance from these and even in some subcortical structures, such as the thalamus.

The simplified pathway for a spoken description of an object or a scene is as follows:

1. Visual input to area 17 bilaterally with further processing in areas 18 and 19 (Fig. 15–9);
2. Input from the visual association areas to the left angular gyrus where the objects are recognized and named;
3. Input to the Wernicke area, where words are assembled into sentences and the appropriate impulses are sent via the arcuate and superior longitudinal fasciculi to the Broca area;
4. Motor programs in the Broca area are projected to the motor cortex, which then elicits speech via the appropriate brainstem centers and the muscles under their control.

CHAPTER REVIEW QUESTIONS

15–1. How many layers are present in the neocortex and what are the connections of each?

15–2. Locate the cortical area whose damage results in the following:

    a. Nonfluent aphasia
    b. Left lower limb anesthesia, weakness, and a Babinski response
    c. Paralysis of gaze to the right
    d. Left homonymous hemianopsia
    e. Weakness of right upper limb
    f. Fluent aphasia
    g. Left neglect syndrome
    h. Weakness of right lower facial muscles

16

THE LIMBIC SYSTEM: ANTEROGRADE AMNESIA AND INAPPROPRIATE BEHAVIOR

■ During the past 18 months a 60-year-old patient has become increasingly forgetful and disoriented and now requires assistance with daily activities.

The term limbic system is the arbitrary name of a functional system of cortical and subcortical neurons. The interconnections between these neurons form complex circuits that play an important role in memory and behavior.

LIMBIC LOBE

The term limbic means border. Limbic was first used by Broca in 1878 to describe a lobe on the medial surface of the cerebral hemisphere bordering the corpus callosum and rostral brainstem. The limbic lobe (Fig. 16–1) comprises the cingulate gyrus and its anterior extension and **septal region,** both of which border the corpus callosum, and the parahippocampal gyrus of the temporal lobe bordering the rostral brainstem.

The limbic lobe is anatomically and functionally connected with other structures. The entire complex is called the limbic system. The two centers most closely related to the limbic lobe are the hippocampal formation, deep to the posterior part of the parahippocampal gyrus, and the **amygdala** or amygdaloid nucleus, deep to the anterior part of the parahippocampal gyrus (Fig. 16–1). These two structures are the key functional centers of the limbic system. Also closely associated with the limbic system is the hypothalamus, which has abundant connections with the hippocampal formation and amygdaloid nucleus.

HIPPOCAMPAL FORMATION

The hippocampal formation plays a key role in memory and learning. It is composed of three parts: dentate gyrus, hippocampus proper, and subiculum (Fig. 16–2). The dentate gyrus and hippocampus proper are the archicortex, the phylogenetically oldest part of the cerebral cortex. The subiculum is a transitional zone of cortex between the hippocampus proper and **entorhinal area,** part of the parahippocampal gyrus. The parahippocampal gyrus is neocortex, the phylogenetically newest part of the cortex.

CONNECTIONS

The hippocampal formation resembles a sea horse about 2 in long in the floor of the temporal horn of the lateral ventricle (Fig. 16–3). The major input to the hippocampal formation comes from the entorhinal part of the parahippocampal gyrus. The entorhinal area receives its input from the cingulum, a large bundle of fibers deep to the cingulate and parahippocampal gyri. The cingulum receives input from widespread areas of the neocortex, especially the cingulate gyrus and the prefrontal cortex. The hippocampal formations in the right and left hemispheres are connected via the hippocampal commissure.

The hippocampal formation is the initial center in a reverberating pathway called the **Papez circuit** (Fig. 16–4). A major part of the Papez circuit is the fornix, which connects the hippocampal formation to the hypothalamus. The fornix originates from the alveus of the

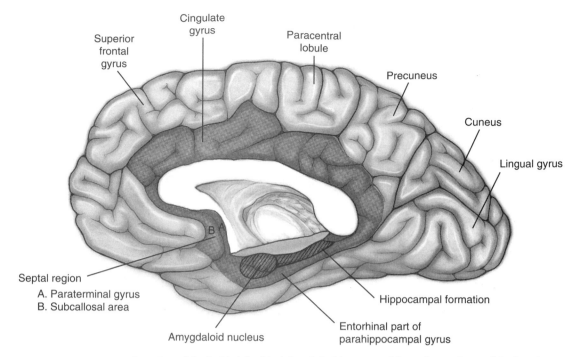

FIGURE 16-1. Location of the limbic lobe (*shaded*) and the hippocampal formation, and amygdaloid nucleus.

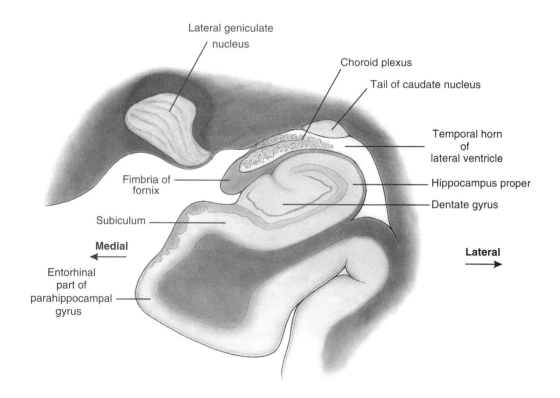

FIGURE 16-2. Coronal section of the hippocampal formation showing its relations.

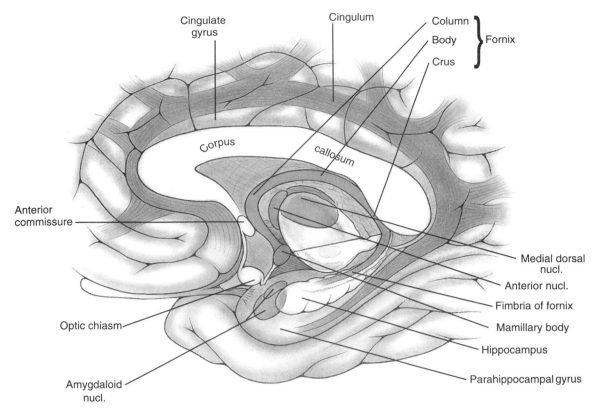

Cingulate gyrus

Cingulum

Column
Body } Fornix
Crus

Corpus
callosum

Anterior
commissure

Medial dorsal
nucl.

Anterior nucl.

Fimbria of fornix

Mamillary body

Optic chiasm

Hippocampus

Parahippocampal gyrus

Amygdaloid
nucl.

FIGURE 16-3. Three-dimensional view of cerebral hemisphere showing relations of hippocampal formation, fornix, and cingulum.

1. Hippocampus
2. Fimbria of fornix
3. Body of fornix
4. Column of fornix
5. Mamillary body
6. Mamillothalamic
   tract
7. Anterior nucl.
8. Thalamocingulate
   radiation
9. Cingulate gyrus
10. Cingulum
11. Entorhinal area
12. Medial dorsal
    nucl.

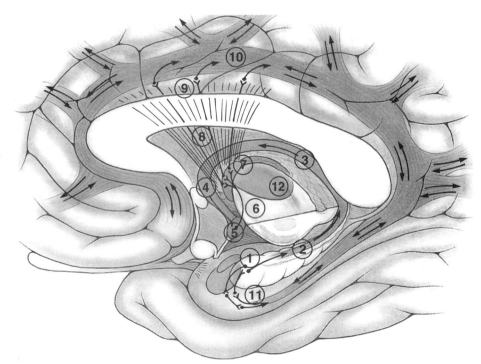

FIGURE 16-4. Papez circuit and other connections of the hippocampal formation.

hippocampus as the **fimbria** of the fornix (Figs. 16–2–16–4). Beneath the splenium of the corpus callosum, the fibers of the fimbria leave the hippocampal formation and become the crus of the fornix. As the two crura converge toward the midline they exchange fibers, forming the hippocampal commissure. Each crus then continues forward as the body of the fornix. The body passes forward beneath the corpus callosum suspended in the free margin of the septum pellucidum and arches downward toward the anterior commissure as the column of the fornix. At the anterior commissure, the fornix separates into two parts: a precommissural part, located in front of the anterior commissure, and a postcommissural part, located behind it. The precommissural fibers arise from the hippocampus proper and terminate in the septal area and basal forebrain structures. The postcommissural fibers arise from the subiculum and are distributed primarily to nuclei in the mamillary body.

The mamillary body gives rise to the mamillothalamic tract, which passes dorsally between the medial and lateral thalamic nuclei and terminates in the anterior thalamic nucleus (Fig. 16–4). This nucleus then projects axons via the thalamocingulate radiation to the cingulate gyrus, which projects to the prefrontal, posterior parietal, and temporal association areas chiefly through the cingulum. From the cingulum, impulses also reach the entorhinal area of the parahippocampal gyrus and then pass to the hippocampal formation, thus completing the Papez circuit.

Besides the fornix, another important output of the hippocampal formation is from both the hippocampus proper and the subiculum directly to the entorhinal area from which impulses enter the cingulum and reach the association areas in all lobes of the cerebral hemisphere.

FUNCTION

The hippocampal formation is essential for the formation of new memories and learning. Bilateral removal of the hippocampal formations, a rare surgical procedure used for the treatment of epilepsy, results in a profound loss of recent or short-term memory and the ability to learn. Persons who have undergone such surgery cannot remember anything that has occurred longer than a few minutes beforehand (anterograde amnesia). Memories of the distant past and intelligence remain intact.

Through the cingulum and its connections with all parts of the cerebral cortex, the hippocampal formation receives all types of information. When particular items of information are important to remember or one desires to remember them, the hippocampal formation emits signals that enable these items to be rehearsed over and over until they are stored permanently in the areas of the cerebral cortex for long-term memory.

Alzheimer disease is characterized by progressive dementia in patients under 65 years of age. In patients over 65 years of age, progressive dementia is referred to as senile dementia. In both cases, the individuals become increasingly forgetful and develop progressive abnormalities of memory, cognition, orientation, and behavior. These types of dementia are associated with (a) a loss of neurons in the hippocampal formation and adjacent parahippocampal cortex (Fig. 16–5) and (b) a reduction in the cholinergic innervation of the cerebral cortex. The neurons lost in the parahippocampal cortex are those providing input to the hippocampus from the association and limbic cortices. The neurons lost in the hippocampal formation are those providing output from the hippocampus to the association cortices and diencephalon. Thus, the loss of these hippocampal connections with the neocortex undoubtedly accounts for the characteristic loss of recent memory in persons with these dementias. The reduction in the cholinergic innervation of the cerebral cortex is the result of the degeneration of the large cholinergic neurons in the **basal nucleus of Meynert** located in the anterior perforated substance, more commonly referred to as the **substantia innominata.** The anterior perforated substance extends from the olfactory striae anteriorly to the optic tracts posteriorly. Normally, the axons of these cholinergic neurons in the basal nucleus provide acetylcholine to the neocortex. The absence of neocortical acetylcholine may account for the cognitive deficits that occur in more advanced stages of dementia.

Korsakoff syndrome or psychosis is characterized by the loss of recent memory and a tendency to fabricate false accounts of recent events. This syndrome most often results from chronic alcoholism and associated nutritional deficiency. Although morphologic changes have been described in the hippocampus and the mamillary bodies, the most frequent alterations occur in the medial parts of the medial dorsal thalamic nuclei (Fig. 16–5).

Limbic system syndromes

++++
++++ Alzheimer: loss of recent memory

vvvv
vvvv Klüver-Bucy: behavioral changes

▒▒ Korsakoff: loss of recent memory & confabulation

Structures

1. Hippocampal formation
2. Amygdaloid nucleus
3. Medial dorsal nucleus
4. Parahippocampal gyrus
5. Uncus
6. Mamillary body
7. Mamillothalamic tract

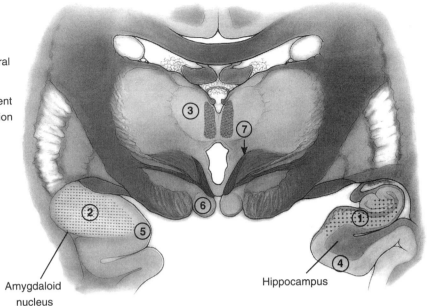

Amygdaloid nucleus

Hippocampus

FIGURE 16−5. Coronal section at mamillary bodies showing sites associated with limbic system syndromes.

AMYGDALOID NUCLEUS

The amygdaloid nucleus or amygdala plays an important role in behavior and emotions. It resembles an almond and is located beneath the uncus near the dorsomedial tip of the temporal lobe. It consists of a number of subnuclei that are divided into a large basolateral group and small corticomedial and central groups.

CONNECTIONS

The basolateral nuclear group is especially well developed in humans and receives strong connections from the sensory areas of the cerebral cortex and thalamus. The corticomedial nucleus is poorly developed in humans and receives input directly from the olfactory bulb via the lateral olfactory stria. From the basolateral and corticomedial nuclei, information passes to the central nucleus.

The major output of the amygdala (Fig. 16–6) is the ventral amygdaloid path. This output courses within the anterior perforated substance (Fig. 16–7), and provides input to the basal nucleus, hypothalamus, and the medial

dorsal thalamic nucleus. The medial dorsal nucleus has strong reciprocal connections with the prefrontal cortex via the thalamoprefrontal radiation. Strong connections between the basolateral amygdala and the prefrontal cortex are also made directly via the uncinate fasciculus (Fig. 16–6), an association bundle connecting the anterior part of the temporal lobe and the orbitofrontal part of the frontal lobe. Connections from the central nucleus to the anterior hypothalamus and septal region occur through the terminal stria, a small bundle of fibers located medial to the caudate nucleus. The right and left amygdalae are interconnected by the anterior commissure (Fig. 16–7).

FUNCTIONS

The amygdaloid nucleus programs appropriate behavioral responses. In animals that largely depend on the sense of smell to seek food, search for a mate to reproduce, and sense danger, olfactory sensations are the primary inputs to the amygdaloid nuclei. On receiving the aforementioned types of information, the amygdaloid nuclei program the appropriate behavioral responses by emitting signals to the vari-

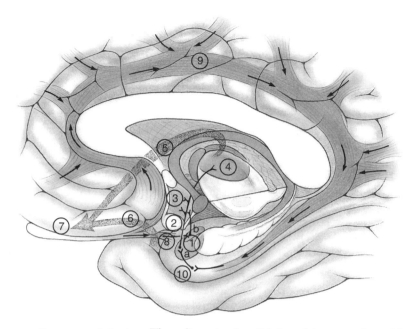

1. Amygdaloid nucl.
   a) basolateral
   b) corticomedial
2. Ventral amygdaloid path
3. Hypothalamus
4. Medial dorsal nucl.
5. Thalamo-prefrontal radiation
6. Uncinate fasciculus
7. Orbitofrontal cortex
8. Lateral olfactory stria
9. Cingulum
10. Parahippocampal gyrus

FIGURE 16-6. Three-dimensional medial view of the connections of the amygdaloid nucleus.

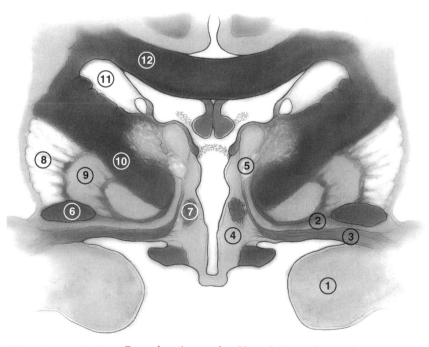

1. Amygdaloid nucl.
2. Anterior perforated substance
3. Ventral amygdaloid path
4. Hypothalamus
5. Medial dorsal nucl.
6. Anterior commissure
7. Column of fornix
8. Putamen
9. Globus pallidus (lat. seg.)
10. Internal capsule
11. Caudate nucleus
12. Corpus callosum

FIGURE 16-7. Coronal section at tuberal hypothalamus showing hypothalamic and thalamic connections of the amygdala.

ous centers that control appropriate activities. In these types of animals the amygdalae consist primarily of the corticomedial nuclei. Human behavior, however, is based chiefly on non-olfactory experiences that are projected from all parts of the cerebral cortex via the cingulum to the large basolateral nuclei of the amygdalae. After assessing the nature of the input, i.e., pleasant, unpleasant, frightening, dangerous, etc., the basolateral nucleus sends signals to centers mainly in the hypothalamus but also in the thalamus, other limbic centers, and the cerebral cortex that elicit the appropriate visceral and motor responses. The orbitofrontal cortex and cingulate gyrus provide the perception of emotions, whereas the hypothalamus provides the expression of emotions.

Bilateral lesions of the amygdaloid nuclei result in profound behavioral alterations. For example, surgical lesions of the amygdalae in patients with socially unacceptable aggressive behavior result in placid behavior and decreased emotional excitability.

The **Klüver-Bucy syndrome** is characterized by
1. An absence of emotional responses so that fear, rage, and aggression cease to exist;
2. A compulsion to be overly attentive to all sensory stimuli, to examine all objects visually, tactilely, and orally;
3. Hypersexuality;
4. Psychic blindness or visual agnosia, in which objects are not recognized visually.

These disturbances are seen experimentally and clinically after bilateral removal of the temporal lobes as far posteriorly as the auditory areas. The docility, compulsive attentiveness, oral tendencies, and hypersexuality result from the bilateral destruction of the amygdaloid nuclei (Fig. 16–5); the visual agnosia results from damage to the neocortical parts of the temporal lobe.

SEPTAL REGION

A third limbic system center, the septal region, is poorly developed in humans. This region includes the paraterminal gyrus and subcallosal area anterior to the lamina terminalis (Fig. 16–1) and the septal nuclei above the median part of the anterior commissure. The septal region receives input from the hippocampus and has reciprocal connections with the hypothalamus, amygdalae, and cingulate gyrus. The septal region and adjacent parts of the anterior hypothalamus project to the midbrain reticular formation via the **medial forebrain bundle,** a diffuse hypothalamic fiber system, and the stria medullaris of the thalamus. The latter passes along the dorsomedial surface of the thalamus and terminates in the habenular nuclei. The habenulointerpeduncular tract (**fasciculus retroflexus**) then carries impulses to the interpeduncular nuclei, considered part of the midbrain reticular formation. This connection of the septal region provides reticular formation input to respiratory, cardiovascular, salivatory, and other centers, which respond to emotional events. In experimental animals, electrical stimulation of the septal region, areas in the hypothalamus along the medial forebrain bundle as well as parts of the thalamus and midbrain, suggest that this path may be associated with reward or pleasure phenomena.

Studies in humans suggest that brainstem connections with the septal region may be modified by antipsychotic drugs and that the septal region and areas with which it connects may be involved in the euphoria associated with the use of narcotics. In addition, recent clinical evidence of marked increased sexual activity in elderly male patients following septal damage has been reported.

CHAPTER REVIEW QUESTIONS

16–1. What are the parts of the limbic lobe and the limbic system?

16–2. What are the two key functional centers of the limbic system and where are they located?

16–3. Describe the Papez circuit.

16–4. Based on clinical evidence, what are the functions of the hippocampal formation and amygdaloid nuclei?

16–5. Alterations in what limbic system structures are associated with Alzheimer disease, the Klüver-Bucy syndrome, and Korsakoff psychosis?

THE HYPOTHALAMUS: VEGETATIVE AND ENDOCRINE IMBALANCE

■ **During the past year, a 15-year-old girl became obese and listless, had episodes of high fever without apparent cause, ceased menstruating, drank copious amounts of water due to severe thirst, passed excessive amounts of urine, frequently fell asleep during the day, often had reversed sleep-wake cycles, and on occasion erupted into a violent state of rage without provocation.**

The hypothalamus controls visceral activity and, as the chief effector of the limbic system, elicits the phenomenon associated with emotions. Because it has both neural and endocrine components, the hypothalamus exerts its influence through the nervous system and the circulatory system. It plays an important role in self-preservation and in preservation of the species. Through its neural and vascular connections it influences water balance, food intake, the endocrine system, reproduction, sleep, behavior, and the entire autonomic nervous system.

HYPOTHALAMIC SUBDIVISIONS AND NUCLEI

Despite its enormous number of connections and functions, the hypothalamus is extremely small, weighing about 4 g and making up less than 1% of the total human brain mass. In the median plane, the hypothalamus extends from the lamina terminalis anteriorly through the mamillary bodies posteriorly. The hypothalamus is divided into anterior or supraoptic, middle or tuberal, and posterior or mamillary regions (Fig. 17–1). Lateral to the lamina terminalis, the preoptic area extends anteriorly to the septal region and is considered part of the anterior hypothalamus.

The hypothalamus is also divided into three sagittal zones: lateral and medial, which are on either side of the fornix, and periventricular, which is deep to the ependyma of the third ventricle (Fig. 17–2). Although numerous hypothalamic nuclei are described, it is difficult to define the precise boundaries of most of them.

The lateral zone, interspersed with longitudinally arranged fibers, contains diffuse neurons and influences widespread areas of the cerebral cortex. The longitudinal fibers in the lateral zone belong to the medial forebrain bundle, a diffuse system of axons interconnecting the septal region, hypothalamus, and brainstem. The medial forebrain bundle is associated with reward mechanisms and behavior. The lateral zone also influences the autonomic nervous system.

The medial zone and its periventricular part are divided into many nuclei (Fig. 17–3). The anterior region contains the preoptic, supraoptic, paraventricular, anterior, and suprachiasmatic nuclei (Fig. 17–2); the middle region has the dorsomedial, ventromedial, and arcuate nuclei; and, the posterior region contains the mamillary and posterior nuclei.

CONNECTIONS

INPUT

Input to the hypothalamus is both neural and humoral. The neural input is primarily from the

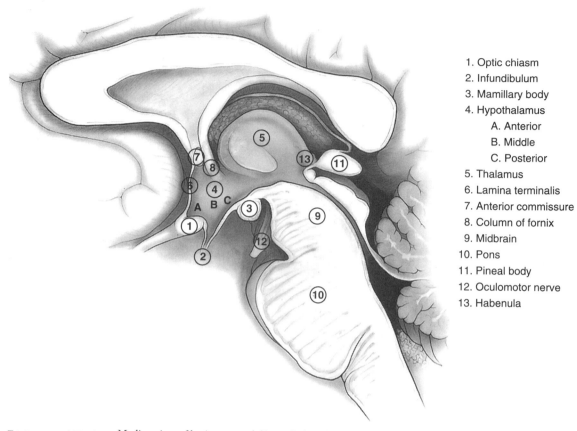

1. Optic chiasm
2. Infundibulum
3. Mamillary body
4. Hypothalamus
    A. Anterior
    B. Middle
    C. Posterior
5. Thalamus
6. Lamina terminalis
7. Anterior commissure
8. Column of fornix
9. Midbrain
10. Pons
11. Pineal body
12. Oculomotor nerve
13. Habenula

FIGURE 17–1.   Median view of brainstem and diencephalon. **A.** Anterior part of the hypothalamus. **B.** Middle part of the hypothalamus. **C.** Posterior part of the hypothalamus.

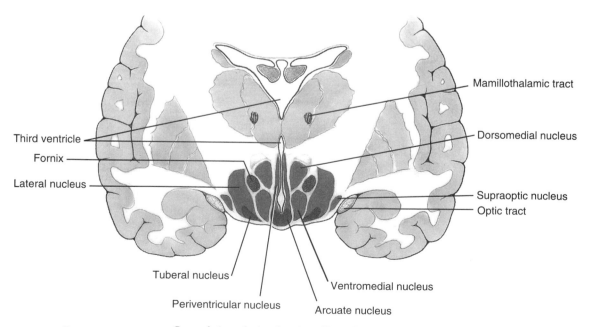

FIGURE 17–2.   Coronal view of tuberal region of hypothalamus showing the principal nuclei.

Hypothalamic nuclei:
1. Preoptic
2. Suprachiasmatic
3. Paraventricular
4. Supraoptic
5. Anterior
6. Dorsomedial
7. Ventromedial
8. Arcuate
9. Posterior
10. Mamillary

Tracts:
11. Hypothalamo-
    hypophysial
12. Tubero-
    hypophysial
13. Column of fornix
14. Mamillothalamic

Other structures:
15. Mamillo-
    tegmental
16. Anterior pituitary
17. Posterior pituitary
18. Hypophysial portal system
19. Hypophysial arteries
20. Hypophysial veins
21. Optic chiasm
22. Lamina terminalis
23. Anterior commissure
24. Oculomotor nerve
25. Infundibulum

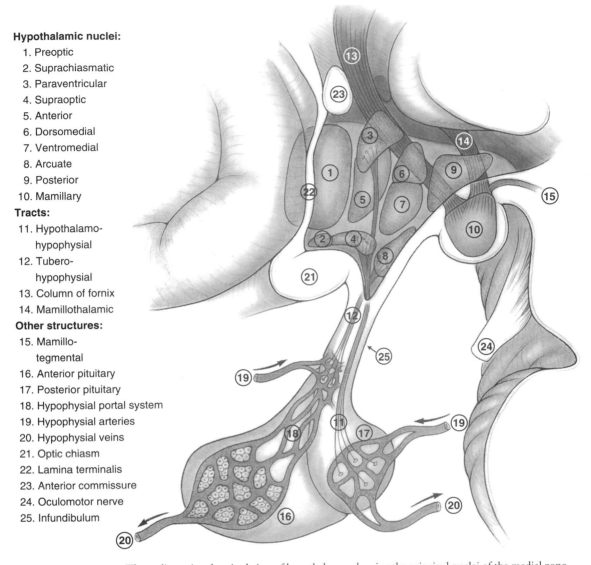

FIGURE 17-3. Three-dimensional sagittal view of hypothalamus showing the principal nuclei of the medial zone and their connections with the pituitary gland, thalamus, and midbrain tegmentum.

limbic system. As previously described, hypothalamic afferent projections from the hippocampal formation travel via the fornix (Figs. 16–4, 17–3) and from the amygdaloid nucleus via the ventral amygdaloid path (Figs. 16–6, 16–7). Projections also reach the hypothalamus from the orbitofrontal cortex, the midline thalamic nuclei, and the retina. The medial forebrain bundle interconnects the basal forebrain and septal region with the lateral hypothalamic area. Afferent fibers from the brainstem reach the hypothalamus chiefly through the reticular formation.

The humoral input is vascular, and through it various hypothalamic neurons are stimulated chemically by substances such as glucose and hormones, and physically by factors such as temperature changes and osmolality. In addition to chemically sensitive or physically sensitive hypothalamic neurons, **circumventricular organs** located in the wall of the third ventricle also detect chemical changes in the cerebrospinal fluid and blood and relay this information to the nearby hypothalamus.

OUTPUT

The output of the hypothalamus is also neural and humoral. The four major targets of neural output are:

1. The anterior thalamic nucleus, which receives the mamillothalamic tract relaying impulses from the hippocampal formation (Figs. 16–4, 17–3);

2. The midbrain reticular formation, which receives hypothalamic impulses from the medial forebrain bundle and the mamillotegmental tract (Fig. 17–3)

3. The amygdaloid nucleus via the ventral amygdaloid path (Figs. 16–6, 16–7);

4. Brainstem and spinal cord autonomic centers, which receive direct input from the hypothalamic nuclei and indirect input via the reticular formation.

Pathways from hypothalamic nuclei to autonomic centers in the brainstem and spinal cord are not clearly demarcated. In the midbrain and rostral pons, descending hypothalamic paths are located dorsomedially, i.e., near the periaqueductal gray and floor of the fourth ventricle, respectively. From here the paths sweep laterally and descend through the caudal pons and the medulla in the lateral part of the reticular formation.

The hypothalamic humoral output influences the endocrine system and occurs directly by secretion into the general circulation and indirectly by secretion into the **hypophysial portal system** (Fig. 17–3). The direct humoral route involves large neurons in the supraoptic and paraventricular nuclei whose axons pass via the hypothalamo-hypophysial tract to the posterior pituitary where they release **vasopressin** and **oxytocin** into the general circulation. Vasopressin, or **antidiuretic hormone (ADH),** controls water balance, and oxytocin causes constriction of smooth muscle in the uterus and myoepithelial cells in the mammary glands. The indirect humoral route involves small neurons chiefly in the tuberal region that produce **hypothalamic regulatory hormones,** which enter the hypophysial portal system and are transported to the anterior pituitary. The hypophysial portal system is a vascular connection between the hypothalamus and anterior pituitary. Capillaries, derived from the superior hypophysial artery and located in the **median eminence** and infundibulum, form portal vessels that pass down the pituitary stalk to a second capillary bed in the anterior pituitary. It is through this route that the hypothalamus regulatory hormones reach the anterior pituitary.

HYPOTHALAMIC FUNCTIONS

The functions of the tiny hypothalamus are Herculean (Table 17–1). Perhaps they can be best described by considering the manifestations of hypothalamic lesions. The **hypothalamic syndrome** is manifested by (a) **diabetes insipidus,** (b) endocrine imbalance, (c) impairment of temperature regulation, (d) abnormalities of sleep patterns, and (e) behavioral changes.

Diabetes insipidus occurs as a result of the absence of vasopressin, the ADH that is produced in the large neurons of the supraoptic and paraventricular nuclei and released into the bloodstream in the posterior pituitary or neurohypophysis. ADH increases the permeability of the distal convoluted tubules and collecting ducts of the kidney. In the absence of ADH, water is not reabsorbed by the kidney, and urine production is extremely high.

Endocrine imbalance is the result of the absence of hypothalamic regulatory hormones that influence the anterior pituitary or adenohypophysis. These hormones are produced by small neurons mainly in the tuberal region (particularly in the arcuate nucleus), although similar neurons in the supraoptic region are also involved. The regulatory hormones are transported via the axons of the tuberoinfundibular tract to capillaries in the infundibulum where these hormones are released and carried to the anterior pituitary via the hypophysial portal system (Fig. 17–3). Within the pituitary gland these hormones regulate the production and release of the adrenocorticotropic, growth, thyrotropic, follicle-stimulating, and luteinizing hormones. Damage to the hypothalamus or to the hypophysial portal system results in decreased secretion of all the anterior pituitary hormones except prolactin. As a result the patient exhibits hypoadrenalism, hypothyroidism, and abnormalities in the reproductive system cycles.

TABLE 17-1. HYPOTHALAMIC FUNCTIONS AND NUCLEI

ANTERIOR	MIDDLE	POSTERIOR
Heat loss (preoptic)	Endocrine activity (tuberal and arcuate)	Heat conservation (posterolateral)
Drinking (preoptic)	Satiety (ventromedial ?)	Cortical activation waking (posterior)
Sleep (preoptic?)	Feeding (lateral?)	Recent memory (mamillary)
Water balance	Emotions	
Milk ejection and uterine contraction (supraoptic and paraventricular)	(dorsomedial?) (lateral?)	
Circadian rhythm (suprachiasmatic)		
Parasympathomimetic		Sympathomimetic

Body temperature is regulated in the hypothalamus by a **heat loss center** located anteriorly and a **heat gain center** located posteriorly. Temperature-sensitive neurons located near capillary beds in the hypothalamus respond to very small changes in temperature. Neurons in the preoptic area are sensitive to a small increase in blood temperature and these neurons initiate heat loss responses. Neurons in the posterior hypothalamic nucleus are sensitive to decreased blood temperature and initiate heat gain mechanisms. Lesions in the anterior hypothalamus result in **hyperthermia** because the neurons that initiate sweating and cutaneous vasodilation when the body temperature increases are not functional. Lesions in the posterior hypothalamus may result in a decrease in body temperature because of the absence of shivering and vasoconstriction mechanisms. But, most frequently, posterior hypothalamic lesions result in **poikilothermy,** the condition in which body temperature varies with the environment. Poikilothermy occurs because the posterior hypothalamic heat gain center that normally elicits cutaneous vasoconstriction, piloerection, and shivering is no longer functional and the impulses from the anterior hypothalamic heat loss center, which normally elicit sweating and vasodilation, are interrupted enroute to the brainstem reticular formation.

Food intake is influenced by several hypothalamic areas such as the ventromedial and paraventricular nuclei and the lateral hypothalamic zone. Glucose-sensitive neurons in these areas influence the endocrine glands associated with metabolism. Lesions of the ventromedial and paraventricular nuclei result in increased appetite and, eventually, obesity. Lesions of the lateral hypothalamus result in decreased food and drink intake.

Reproduction and sexual functions are influenced by the preoptic and ventromedial nuclei. Estrogen-sensitive and androgen-sensitive neurons in these areas elicit the production of appropriate hormones that regulate the production and release of the anterior pituitary gonadotropins. Hypothalamic lesions may result in menstrual cycle disturbances or precocious puberty.

Sleep and the sleep-wake cycle are influenced by several areas of the hypothalamus. The suprachiasmatic nucleus, which receives input from the retina, is the biologic clock that plays a role in the **circadian rhythm** of approximately 24 hours. The preoptic area can induce sleep and the lateral hypothalamic area is involved in cortical arousal.

Although a specific hypothalamic sleep center has not been identified, it is well known that hypothalamic lesions result in abnormalities of sleep patterns. The most frequent alteration is an impairment of wakefulness that varies from drowsiness to permanent coma. The posterior hypothalamus appears to be associated with this abnormality; lesions here often result in hypersomnia. Perhaps some of the influence the hippocampus exerts on the electrical activity of the cerebral cortex is exerted through the posterior hypothalamus into the midbrain tegmentum where it complements the **ascending reticular activating system.**

The expression of emotions such as anger, fear, embarrassment, etc. occurs through hypothalamic connections with appropriate brainstem and spinal cord centers. The hypothalamus has reciprocal connections with nuclei associated with behavior such as the amygdaloid nuclei (via the ventral amygdaloid path) and the medial dorsal thalamic nucleus (via the periventricular fibers). Bilateral hypothalamic lesions, especially in or near the ventromedial nuclei, result in extreme viciousness. Animals with such lesions fly into a rage and attack repeatedly without provocation. A similar phe-

nomenon occurs in humans with such hypothalamic lesions. Patients with these lesions exhibit violent, aggressive behavior toward anyone present, including loved ones. It seems probable, therefore, that the ventromedial area of the hypothalamus normally exerts a regulatory effect on more posterior parts of the hypothalamus where the mechanisms associated with aggressive behavior are centered. Such mechanisms include increased heart rate, elevated blood pressure, increased respiration, pupillary dilation, piloerection, etc., phenomena that are associated with activity of the sympathetic nervous system. It is generally accepted that the posterior hypothalamus controls sympathetic activity. In contrast, the anterior hypothalamus controls parasympathetic events (Table 17–1).

CHAPTER REVIEW QUESTIONS

17–1. What are the anteroposterior subdivisions of the hypothalamus?

17–2. What is the chief neural output of the hypothalamus?

17–3. What is the hypophysial portal system?

17–4. Which parts of the hypothalamus are associated with:

    a. Temperature regulation
    b. Parasympathomimetic activity
    c. Sympathomimetic activity
    d. Hypothalamic regulatory hormones
    e. Water balance
    f. Sleep-wake cycle
    g. Sleep
    h. Emotions

THE AUTONOMIC SYSTEM: VISCERAL ABNORMALITIES

■ A 28-year-old man involved in an automobile accident several months ago had recovered from all the abnormalities resulting from brainstem damage except for a right-sided mild ptosis, miosis, and facial anhidrosis.

The autonomic or involuntary system regulates visceral activity throughout the body. The autonomic system may be described as divided into efferent and afferent parts, both of which innervate the involuntary musculature (smooth and cardiac) and glandular tissue. The autonomic efferent system is composed of two divisions, sympathetic and parasympathetic. The autonomic afferent system consists of visceral afferent fibers that travel in the nerves making up the sympathetic and parasympathetic divisions. Because all viscera are supplied by both sympathetic and parasympathetic nerves, all visceral organs are innervated by four types of fibers: sympathetic efferents and afferents and parasympathetic efferents and afferents.

AUTONOMIC EFFERENTS

BASIC PRINCIPLES

The anatomical features of the autonomic and somatic efferent systems differ considerably: two efferent neurons exist in the autonomic path, whereas only a single neuron exists in the somatic path (Fig. 18–1).

The autonomic efferent system is divided into two parts: sympathetic and parasympathetic. The basic anatomical features of the two parts significantly differ. First, sympathetic ac-

tivity enters the peripheral nervous system only via the thoracolumbar spinal nerves, whereas parasympathetic activity enters the peripheral nervous system only via cranial nerves and sacral spinal nerves (Table 18–1). Second, due to its short postganglionic fibers and the small ratio of preganglionic fibers:postganglionic neurons (1:2) (Fig. 18–2), the parasympathetic division has a localized influence. The parasympathetic division, with its very localized influence, is associated with the protection, rest, and recuperation of individual organs and bodily functions, i.e., pupillary constriction, decreased heart rate, salivation and digestion, elimination of waste products from bowel and bladder, etc.

Conversely, the sympathetic division, with its long postganglionic fibers and large ratio of postganglionic neurons to preganglionic fibers, has a widespread influence. Because of these anatomical features, sympathetic system activity results in diffuse phenomena associated with emergency situations such as "fight or flight," i.e., increased heart rate and respiration, dilated pupils, increased blood supply to voluntary muscles, etc.

PARASYMPATHETIC DIVISION

All activity in parasympathetic nerve fibers originates in the brainstem or spinal cord (Fig. 18–3). The brainstem preganglionic parasympathetic neurons are found in four locations:

1. The Edinger-Westphal nucleus, the visceromotor component of the oculomotor nuclear complex;

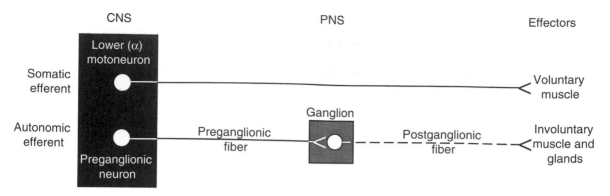

FIGURE 18–1.   Comparison of somatic and autonomic efferent systems.

TABLE 18–1.   PRINCIPAL FEATURES OF AUTONOMIC EFFERENT DIVISIONS

	SYMPATHETIC	PARASYMPATHETIC
Preganglionic location	Thoracolumbar	Craniosacral
Postganglionic location	Paravertebral and prevertebral ganglia	Terminal ganglia
Postganglionic fibers	Relatively long, thus a more diffuse action	Relatively short, thus a more discrete action
Preganglionic to postganglionic ratio	Larger (e.g., 1:17)	Smaller (e.g., 1:2)
Function	Prepares organism for emergencies: "Fight or flight"	Prepares organism for "rest and recuperation"

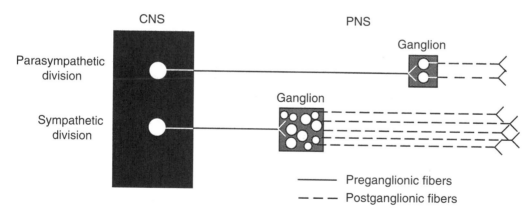

FIGURE 18–2.   Comparison of parasympathetic and sympathetic divisions of autonomic efferent system. Preganglionic fibers (*solid line*); postganglionic fibers (*broken line*).

2. The superior salivatory nucleus, the viscerosecretory component of the facial nuclear complex;

3. The inferior salivatory nucleus, found near the rostral part of the nucleus ambiguus and contributing viscerosecretory fibers to the glossopharyngeal nerve;

4. The dorsal nucleus of the vagus as well as neurons scattered near the caudal part of the nucleus ambiguus; the visceromotor and viscerosecretory axons of these neurons emerge in the vagus nerve.

The cranial ganglia that give rise to the postganglionic parasympathetic fibers are the ciliary ganglion, which receives preganglionic fibers from the oculomotor nerve; the pterygopalatine and submandibular ganglia, which receive preganglionic fibers from the facial nerve; and the otic ganglion, which receives preganglionic fibers from the glossopharyngeal nerve. The preganglionic fibers in the vagus nerve synapse in terminal ganglia both extrinsic and intrinsic to the thoracic, abdominal, and pelvic viscera that are vagally innervated (Fig. 18–3).

The sacral preganglionic parasympathetic neurons are in and near the intermediolateral nucleus in spinal cord segments S2,S3,S4. The preganglionic fibers emerge from the spinal cord and pass to the terminal ganglia of the colon and rectum, urinary bladder, prostate and vaginal glands, and erectile tissues of the penis and clitoris. The sacral parasympathica control defecation, urination, and erection.

SYMPATHETIC DIVISION

All activity in sympathetic nerve fibers originates in the spinal cord (Fig. 18–3). The preganglionic sympathetic neurons are found in several columns extending from about C8 to L2 or L3. These sympathetic columns are an intermediolateral nucleus in the lateral horn, an intermediomedial nucleus in the medial part of the intermediate zone (lamina VII), and an intercalated nucleus bridging the previous two. Some sympathetic preganglionic neurons are also scattered in the lateral funiculus near the lateral horn.

The sympathetic neurons that give rise to postganglionic fibers are in the paravertebral (sympathetic trunk) ganglia and in the prevertebral (collateral or autonomic plexus) ganglia. The sympathetic trunk ganglia comprise 20 to 25 pair along the vertebral column, whereas the

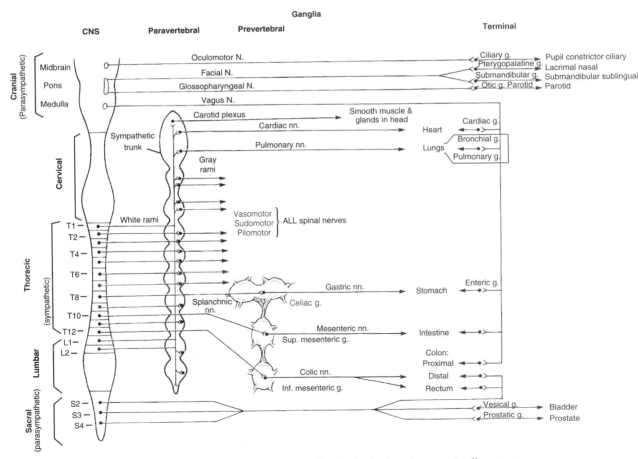

FIGURE 18–3.   Schematic diagram showing basic plan of autonomic efferent system.

1. Preganglionic neurons
   Preganglionic axons:
2. In ventral root
3. In spinal nerve
4. In white communicating ramus
5. Synapsing in same level ganglion
6. Ascending to more cranial ganglion
7. Synapsing in superior cervical ganglion
8. Descending to more caudal ganglion
9. Coursing in splanchnic nerves
10. Synapsing in autonomic plexus ganglia
    Postganglionic axons:
11. In carotid plexus
12. In gray communicating rami to
    All spinal nerves
13. In visceral nerves to thoracic organs
14. In perivascular plexuses

Ganglia:
15. Sympathetic trunk
16. Superior cervical
17. Celiac
18. Superior mesenteric
19. Inferior mesenteric

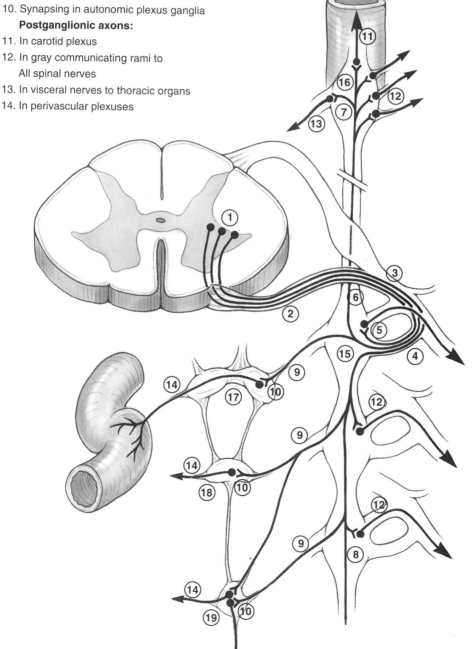

FIGURE 18-4.   Basic circuitry of sympathetic system.

autonomic plexus ganglia are found along the abdominal aorta, especially around the origins of the celiac and superior mesenteric and inferior mesenteric arteries.

The basic circuitry of the sympathetic system (Fig. 18–4) is as follows:

1. All preganglionic sympathetic fibers emerge from the spinal cord in spinal nerves T1–L2.

2. The preganglionic sympathetic fibers reach the sympathetic trunk by passing through the ventral roots, the spinal nerves, and the white communicating rami.

3. Within the sympathetic trunk, the preganglionic sympathetic fibers may

    a. Synapse at the same level;

    b. Ascend and synapse in a higher or more cranial sympathetic trunk ganglion;

    c. Descend and synapse in a lower or more caudal sympathetic trunk ganglion, or

    d. Emerge via thoracic splanchnic nerves and lumbar splanchnic nerves without synapsing.

4. The sympathetic trunk neurons give rise to three types of postganglionic fibers:

    a. Perivascular, which travel along the walls of blood vessels, e.g., carotid plexus, to their destinations;

    b. Spinal, which pass via the gray communicating rami to each spinal nerve, through which they are distributed to blood vessels, sweat glands, and piloarrector muscles;

    c. Visceral, which pass directly to the viscera, e.g., cardiac nerves.

5. The autonomic plexus ganglia receive their preganglionic fibers from the splanchnic nerves and send their postganglionic fibers to the viscera via perivascular plexuses around the arteries supplying the abdominal and pelvic viscera, e.g., gastric, mesenteric, colic, etc.

GENERAL FUNCTIONS OF AUTONOMIC EFFERENTS

The autonomic efferent system plays an indispensable role in the maintenance of the internal environment. At times the sympathetic and parasympathetic divisions exert antagonistic effects. However, in most instances, the two divisions collaborate, both of them regulating and adjusting visceral functions. Most visceral organs are innervated by both divisions. One division usually produces effects opposite those of the other division (Table 18–2). The primary postganglionic neurotransmitters are acetylcholine for the parasympathetic system and norepinephrine for the sympathetic system.

TABLE 18–2. EXAMPLES OF VISCERAL INNERVATION

ORGAN	SYMPATHETIC			PARASYMPATHETIC		
	PREGANGLIONIC	POSTGANGLIONIC	FUNCTION	PREGANGLIONIC	POSTGANGLIONIC	FUNCTION
Iris	C8–T3	Superior cervical ganglion	Dilation of pupil	Edinger-Westphal nucleus	Ciliary ganglion	Constriction of pupil
Parotid gland	T1–T3	Superior cervical ganglion	Secretion reduced and viscid	Inferior salivatory nucleus	Otic ganglion	Secretion increased and watery
Heart	T1–T5	Cervical and upper thoracic ganglia	Increased rate	Dorsal vagal nucleus	Intracardiac ganglia	Decreased rate
Coronary vessels	T1–T5	Cervical and upper thoracic ganglia	Dilation or constriction	Dorsal vagal nucleus	Intracardiac ganglia	Constriction
Bronchi	T2–T5	Upper thoracic ganglia	Dilation	Dorsal vagal nucleus	Pulmonary ganglia	Constriction
Stomach	T6–T10	Celiac ganglion	Inhibition of peristalsis and secretion	Dorsal vagal nucleus	Myenteric and submucosal ganglia	Increased peristalsis and secretion
Sex organs	T10–L2	Inferior hypogastric ganglia	Ejaculation	S2–S4	Cavernous ganglia	Erection
Urinary bladder	T12–L2	Hypogastric ganglia	Contraction of trigone muscle	S2–S4	Vesical ganglion	Contraction of detrusor muscle

However, sweat glands are an exception because they are innervated by cholinergic (acetylcholine) sympathetic fibers.

AUTONOMIC AFFERENTS

The importance of impulses arising from visceral organs and blood vessels is mainly the initiation of visceral reflexes; most visceral impulses do not reach the level of consciousness. Those autonomic afferent impulses that do reach levels of awareness result in sensations that are vague and poorly localized, e.g., hunger, nausea, fullness of urinary bladder and rectum, etc. In certain conditions visceral sensations may become painful.

PRIMARY VISCERAL AFFERENTS

Peripheral nerves carrying autonomic preganglionic and postganglionic fibers to the viscera and blood vessels also contain nerve fibers carrying visceral impulses in the opposite direction, i.e., toward the brain and spinal cord. These are the autonomic afferents responsible for visceral input. Such afferent fibers come from unipolar neurons located in the spinal and some cranial nerve ganglia.

Various forms of free and encapsulated nerve endings in viscera and in the walls of blood vessels are the receptors for visceral input. The glossopharyngeal nerves; vagus nerves; and second, third, and fourth sacral nerves distribute visceral afferent fibers along parasympathetic paths, whereas the thoracic and upper lumbar spinal nerves distribute visceral afferent fibers through communicating rami to sympathetic nerves and peripheral blood vessels. In general, those fibers associated with reflex control of visceral activity accompany the parasympathetic nerves; those fibers that convey visceral sensations accompany the sympathetic nerves. An exception to this general rule is visceral pain fibers from certain pelvic viscera (sigmoid colon, rectum, neck of the bladder, prostate gland, and cervix of the uterus) that accompany the sacral parasympathetic nerves.

In addition to a vagal route to the brainstem, the thoracic and abdominal viscera send afferent fibers to the spinal cord via the sympathetic trunks (Fig. 18–5). From the heart, coronary vessels, bronchial tree, and lungs, visceral afferent fibers travel in the cardiac and pulmonary nerves to the sympathetic trunk. From the abdominal viscera, afferent fibers travel through the mesenteric and celiac plexuses and the thoracic and lumbar splanchnic nerves to the sympathetic trunk. After following an uninterrupted course, these afferent fibers enter the thoracic and upper lumbar spinal nerves through the white communicating rami. Their cell bodies are located in the dorsal root ganglia of T1–L2, and their first synapse is in the spinal cord at these segments.

The phrenic nerve contains visceral afferent fibers coming from the pericardium, diaphragm, hepatic ligaments and capsule, pancreas, and suprarenal glands. Visceral afferent fibers from peripheral blood vessels travel centrally in all spinal nerves. The cell bodies of these autonomic afferent components are also unipolar neurons in appropriate dorsal root ganglia.

Receptors in the sigmoid colon, rectum, urinary bladder, proximal part of the urethra, and cervix of the uterus initiate visceral afferent impulses for reflexes and sensations. The visceral afferent impulses from these pelvic viscera also travel centrally by two routes. One route is taken by the fibers that course in the pelvic splanchnic nerves and have their cell bodies located in the dorsal root ganglia of the second, third, and fourth sacral spinal nerves. The other route is through the various hypogastric plexuses, lumbar splanchnic nerves, and sympathetic trunk and its white communicating rami to the cells of origin in the dorsal root ganglia of the lower thoracic and upper lumbar spinal nerves.

BRAINSTEM CENTRAL CONNECTIONS

The solitary tract and solitary nucleus are the only conspicuous brainstem structures that can be identified with the visceral afferent system. The solitary tract extends from the lower part of the pons to the obex of the medulla and is closely related throughout its course to the

1. Visceral afferent receptors in abdominal organ
2. Perivascular nerves
3. Celiac ganglion
4. Superior mesenteric ganglion
5. Inferior mesenteric ganglion
6. Splanchnic nerves
7. Sympathetic trunk
8. White communicating rami
9. Spinal nerves
10. Cell bodies in spinal (dorsal root) ganglia
11. Dorsal root
12. Synapse in spinal gray
13. Visceral afferent from thoracic organ
14. Superior cervical ganglion

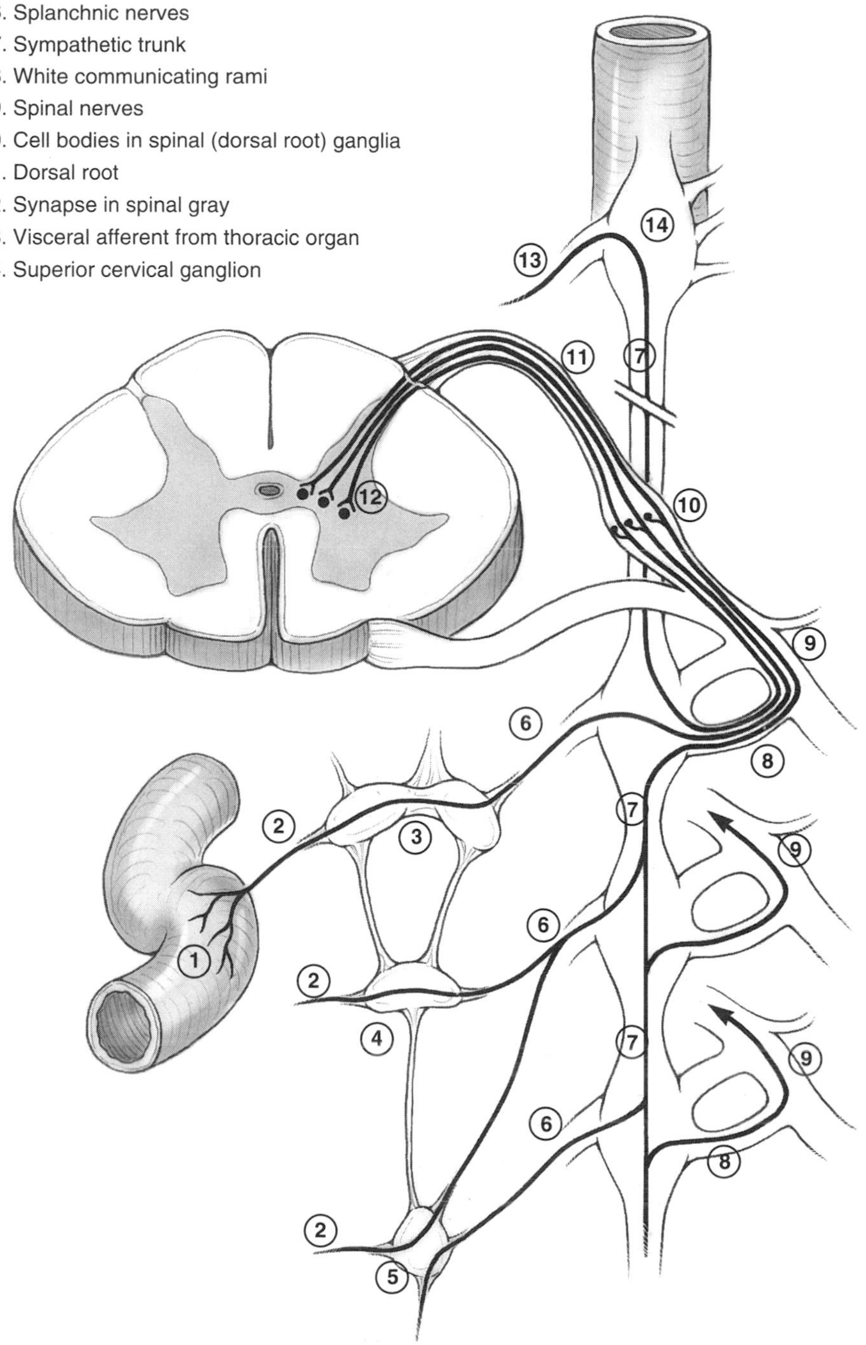

FIGURE 18-5.   Routes of autonomic afferents travelling with sympathetic nerves.

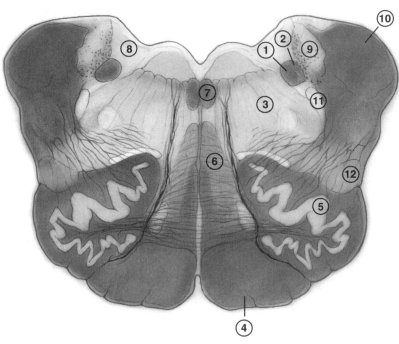

1. Solitary tract
2. Solitary nucleus
3. Medullary reticular formation
4. Pyramid
5. Inferior olivary nucleus
6. Medial lemniscus
7. Medial longitudinal fasciculus
8. Medial vestibular nucleus
9. Spinal (inf.) vestibular nucleus
10. Restiform body
11. Spinal trigeminal nucleus
12. Spinothalamic tract

FIGURE 18–6. Transverse section of medulla showing central components of autonomic afferents from vagus nerve.

solitary nucleus (Fig. 18–6). The primary autonomic afferent fibers in the solitary tract come from the glossopharyngeal nerves and vagus nerves and synapse in the solitary nucleus. Fibers from the solitary nucleus synapse in the reticular formation. From the reticular formation, connections are made with the respiratory center and cardiovascular center, visceral and somatic motor nuclei, and higher centers.

SPINAL CENTRAL CONNECTIONS

Visceral afferent fibers destined for the spinal cord enter through the lateral division of the dorsal root and synapse on cells located in the dorsal horn and intermediate zone. Impulses associated with the initiation of reflexes make secondary connections with visceral or somatic motor neurons of the spinal gray. Visceral impulses destined to reach conscious levels ascend bilaterally in the lateral and posterior parts of the anterolateral quadrants, and, on reaching the brainstem, continue through multisynaptic pathways in the reticular formation to higher centers. One exception to this route is

the path subserving the sensation that urination is imminent. This sensation arises from the urethra and ascends in the dorsal column–medial lemniscus system.

VISCERAL SENSATIONS

True visceral sensations, e.g., heartburn, nausea, hunger, fullness of bladder or bowels, tend to be vague and poorly localized. This vagueness is due to the multisynaptic nature of the central pathways and the meager representation of viscera in the cerebral cortex.

Visceral organs, including the brain and spinal cord, are insensitive to ordinary mechanical and thermal stimuli. Even though handling, cutting, crushing, or burning of viscera occurs during surgical procedures, sensations are not felt. Painful sensations do result from excessive stretch, violent or spasmodic contractions, or decreased blood supply (ischemia). In such conditions the pain may be felt in the region of the organ itself (true visceral pain) or in a cutaneous or even other somatic tissue region (**referred pain**).

Pain of visceral origin is not necessarily confined to visceral pathways in its conduction to the spinal cord, because the abdominal wall or the diaphragm may be involved by the disease process. Thus, pain of inoperable carcinoma of the stomach may not be favorably affected by sympathectomy (removal of the sympathetic trunks) because the body wall may be involved. Sympathectomy is, therefore, not a cure-all for visceral pain.

REFERRED PAIN

In pathologic conditions, visceral pain radiates to cutaneous areas and is therefore as-

sumed by the patient to arise mainly or exclusively in surface areas of the body (Fig. 18–7). This kind of pain is called referred pain. It is important to recall that most visceral pain fibers travel with sympathetic nerves and reach the thoracic and upper lumbar spinal nerves through the 14 or 15 pair of white rami communicating with the sympathetic trunks. Although the region to which the pain is referred may seem unrelated to the pathologic visceral organ, the two loci are part of the same segmental level.

The commonly accepted explanation for re-

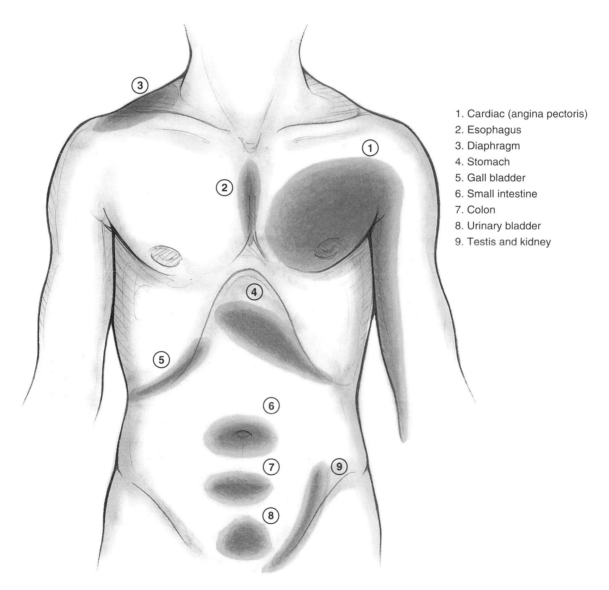

1. Cardiac (angina pectoris)
2. Esophagus
3. Diaphragm
4. Stomach
5. Gall bladder
6. Small intestine
7. Colon
8. Urinary bladder
9. Testis and kidney

FIGURE 18-7.   Common cutaneous areas of referred pain.

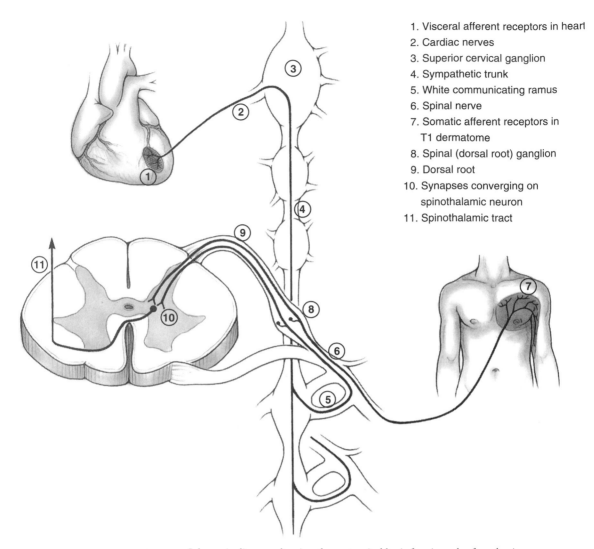

1. Visceral afferent receptors in heart
2. Cardiac nerves
3. Superior cervical ganglion
4. Sympathetic trunk
5. White communicating ramus
6. Spinal nerve
7. Somatic afferent receptors in
   T1 dermatome
8. Spinal (dorsal root) ganglion
9. Dorsal root
10. Synapses converging on
    spinothalamic neuron
11. Spinothalamic tract

FIGURE 18–8.   Schematic diagram showing the anatomical basis for visceral referred pain.

ferred pain is that within the spinal gray matter the visceral afferent impulses converge on secondary somatic afferent neurons (Fig. 18–8) and lower their threshold of excitation. Thus, an abnormally large volley of visceral afferent impulses causes spinothalamic neurons to fire, resulting in deception of the cerebral cortex.

AUTONOMIC CONTROL CENTERS

Many types of autonomic phenomena have been elicited from various parts of the cerebral hemispheres, e.g., frontal lobe, cingulate gyrus,

orbitoinsulotemporal cortex, hippocampus, amygdala, caudate nucleus, etc. Most of the visceral responses are diffuse and tend to overlap somatic reactions. The autonomic or visceral responses elicited by stimulation in the cerebral hemispheres are funneled through the hypothalamus, the highest center for the regulation of autonomic responses.

In addition to hypothalamic nuclei, other groups of neurons at various levels also strongly influence autonomic activities. At the level of the midbrain, pupillary constriction and lens accommodation centers are located in the pretectal area and superior colliculus. In the pons,

TABLE 18–3.	PRINCIPAL AUTONOMIC CENTERS AND THEIR OUTPUT	
FUNCTION	**LOCATION**	**OUTPUT**
Vasomotor cardioaccelerator and pressor	Medullary reticular formation	Sympathetic nucleus in spinal cord
Depressor and cardiodecelerator	Medullary reticular formation	Neurons in dorsal vagal nucleus and reticular formation
Respiratory[a]: Inspiration and expiration	Medullary reticular formation	Phrenic, intercostal and abdominal motoneurons
Apneusis and pneumotaxis	Pontine reticular formation	Medullary respiratory centers
Vomiting	Medullary centers	Emetic center, vagal and parasympathetic preganglionic neurons
Micturition: Initiation	Pontine reticular formation	Sacral parasympathetic neurons for detrusor contraction and inhibition of Onuf neurons supplying sphincter
Micturition: cessation[a] or prevention[a]	Frontal lobe	Onuf nucleus for contraction of sphincter

[a]*Not autonomic.*

a micturition center rostrally governs the initiation of urination, and pneumotaxic and apneustic centers more caudally influence respiration. Within the medulla are the cardiovascular and the expiratory and inspiratory respiratory centers.

Although these various centers receive input from many sources (hypothalamus, cranial nerves, ascending pathways, etc.), their output is funneled to autonomic efferent and, in many cases, associated somatic neurons (Table 18–3). Examples of such connections are those that control the heart, the urinary bladder, and the sex organs.

CONTROL OF THE HEART

The heart is abundantly supplied by parasympathetic, sympathetic, and afferent nerves (Fig. 18–9).

Visceral afferent impulses arising from the heart travel centrally via the vagus and sympathetic nerves. Those in the vagus have cell bodies located in the nodose ganglion. The cardiac vagal afferent fibers enter the solitary tract and synapse in the solitary nucleus. The cardiac afferent fibers traveling via the sympathetic nerves do so on the left side. Their cell bodies are located in the upper four or five thoracic dorsal root ganglia and they synapse in the upper thoracic spinal cord segments.

Cardiac control centers are located in the medullary reticular formation. These control centers are influenced mainly by impulses de-

scending from the hypothalamus and by visceral afferent impulses from mechanoreceptors and chemoreceptors located in the walls of the heart, aorta, and carotid arteries. The mechanoreceptors or baroreceptors respond to blood pressure; the chemoreceptors respond to oxygen–carbon dioxide levels in the circulating blood. From these receptors, impulses are carried in the glossopharyngeal and vagus nerves to the solitary tract. After a synapse in the solitary nucleus, these visceral afferent impulses pass to cardiovascular centers in the adjacent reticular formation. Increases in blood pressure elicit vagal responses, and decreases in blood pressure cause sympathetic responses.

Cardiac parasympathetic neurons are located in the medulla in the vicinity of the dorsal vagal nucleus and nucleus ambiguus. The preganglionic fibers travel in the vagus nerves and synapse on ganglion cells in the cardiac plexus and epicardium and along the conducting system of the heart. Postganglionic fibers pass to the sinus and atrioventricular nodes and, to a lesser extent, the atria. The cardiac vagal innervation decreases heart rate and results in bradycardia.

Cardiac sympathetic neurons are located in and near the intermediolateral nucleus of the upper six to eight thoracic spinal cord segments. The preganglionic fibers emerge in spinal sympathetic ganglia. Postganglionic fibers travel via the cardiac nerves to the cardiac plexus and are distributed to the sinus and atrioventricular nodes, the atria and ventricles, and

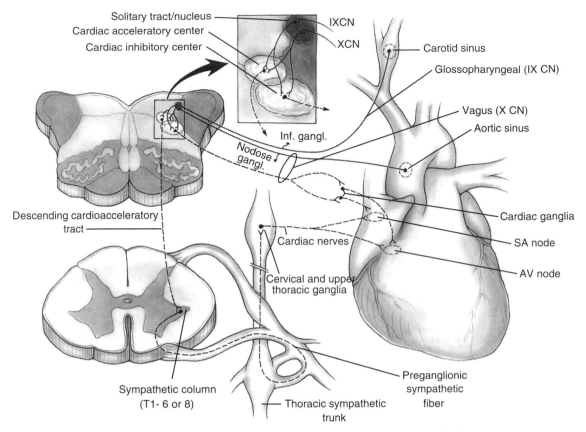

FIGURE 18-9. Schematic diagram showing the nervous control of the heart.

the coronary arteries. The cardiac sympathetic innervation increases heart rate and results in **tachycardia.**

The coronary arteries are chiefly controlled by local metabolic factors. Increased metabolism accompanying increased heart rate results in dilation of the coronary arteries and increased blood flow to the heart muscle. Conversely, decreased heart rate results in decreased metabolic rate and constriction of the coronary arteries.

CONTROL OF THE URINARY BLADDER

The urinary bladder and its sphincters are supplied by parasympathetic, sympathetic, somatic motor, and visceral afferent fibers (Fig. 18–10).

Several groups of visceral afferent fibers supply the urinary bladder. Pain and temperature impulses from the mucosa of the fundus travel with the sympathetic nerves and reach the spinal cord via the dorsal roots of T12 and L1. From the mucosa at the neck of the bladder, pain and temperature impulses travel with the sacral parasympathetic nerves to S2,S3,S4. The spinothalamic tract then transmits impulses of both groups of pain and temperature fibers to higher centers.

Fullness of the bladder is detected by mechanoreceptors in the bladder wall that send impulses to the spinal cord via the sacral parasympathetic route. The spinothalamic tracts carry "fullness" impulses to higher centers in the thalamus and cerebral cortex. The sensation that micturition is imminent arises from mechanoreceptors in the trigone of the bladder; these visceral afferent impulses travel with the sacral parasympathetic nerves to S2,S3,S4 and ascend in the dorsal column–medial lemniscus system.

Parasympathetic visceromotor neurons located in S2,S3,S4 give rise to preganglionic fibers that travel in the pelvic nerve to the hy-

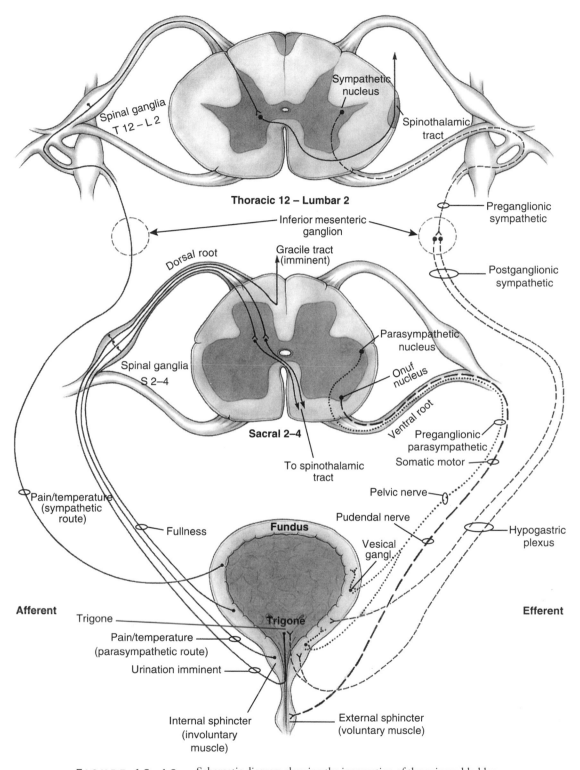

Thoracic 12 – Lumbar 2

Sacral 2–4

Fundus

Trigone

Afferent

Efferent

FIGURE 18–10. Schematic diagram showing the innervation of the urinary bladder.

pogastric and then to the vesical plexuses. Vesical ganglion cells give postganglionic parasympathetic fibers that supply the **detrusor muscle** that, on contraction, empties the bladder.

Sympathetic visceromotor neurons in spinal cord segments T11–L2 give preganglionic fibers that travel in the lumbar splanchnic nerves to the inferior mesenteric ganglion. Postganglionic sympathetic fibers from the inferior mesenteric ganglion reach the bladder via the hypogastric and vesicle plexuses and supply the internal urethral sphincter. During bladder filling, the sympathetic fibers relax the detrusor muscle directly and also indirectly by inhibiting the parasympathetic cells in the vesical ganglia. The sympathetic fibers elicit contraction of the internal urethral sphincter.

Lower motor neurons that make up the Onuf nucleus in S2,S3,S4 send axons via the internal pudendal nerve and its perineal branch to the skeletal muscle that forms the external urethral sphincter.

Micturition centers are located in the brainstem and cerebral cortex. A cortical center for voluntary control of the initiation and cessation of micturition is located in the superior frontal gyrus on the medial surface of the hemisphere. Two micturition centers are located in the pons. One pontine micturition center sends excitatory impulses to the sacral parasympathetic neurons that elicit contraction of the detrusor muscle. A second pontine micturition center sends excitatory impulses to the lower motoneurons of the Onuf nucleus that supply the external urethral sphincter. During micturition the pontine parasympathetic excitatory center inhibits the other pontine center. Thus, the external urethral sphincter relaxes when the detrusor muscle contracts, and emptying of the bladder occurs.

Reflex bladder control is initiated by visceral afferent impulses from volume and tension receptors in the bladder wall. At low levels of bladder distension, these visceral afferent fibers stimulate the lower motor neurons of the Onuf nucleus, resulting in contraction of the external sphincter. At high levels of bladder distension, visceral afferent impulses stimulate pontine micturition center neurons that inhibit sympathetic and Onuf somatic neurons, resulting in

relaxation of the internal and external sphincters, respectively, and elicit parasympathetic activity resulting in contraction of the detrusor and emptying of the bladder. Thus, micturition is controlled by spinopontospinal reflex mechanisms.

Interruption of this reflex results in the so-called **neurogenic bladder.** Two types of neurogenic bladders exist: reflex and nonreflex (Fig. 18–11). The **reflex neurogenic bladder** is of upper motor neuron type; the nonreflex bladder is of lower motor neuron type. The reflex neurogenic bladder may be uninhibited or automatic. The **uninhibited reflex bladder,** which is incontinent but empties fully, results from bilateral lesions of the micturition centers in the frontal lobe. Emptying of the bladder is normal because reflex control of the pontine micturition centers are intact. The **automatic reflex bladder,** which is incontinent and does not empty fully, results from bilateral spinal cord lesions above sacral levels. Emptying of the bladder is incomplete because the spinal reflex pathways that trigger the pontine micturition centers are interrupted. The **nonreflex neurogenic bladder,** which is characterized by severe urinary retention and incontinence, results from bilateral lesions of the sacral spinal cord or the spinal nerve roots in the caudal equina (Fig. 18–11).

CONTROL OF THE SEX ORGANS

The sex organs are innervated by parasympathetic, sympathetic, and visceral afferent fibers. Visceral afferent fibers from the female and male sex organs pass to the spinal cord via sympathetic and sacral parasympathetic routes and have their cell bodies located in the dorsal root ganglia of T10–L2 and S2-S4, respectively. An exception to the rule that visceral pain fibers follow the sympathetic nerves occurs in the case of pain from the cervix of the uterus and the prostate. In both cases, pain travels with the parasympathetic nerves and enters the spinal cord at S2-S4.

The preganglionic parasympathetic fibers arise from S2-S4, enter the pelvic cavity via the pelvic nerve, and synapse on ganglia in the hypogastric and the uterovaginal or prostatic plexuses. Postganglionic parasympathetic fibers

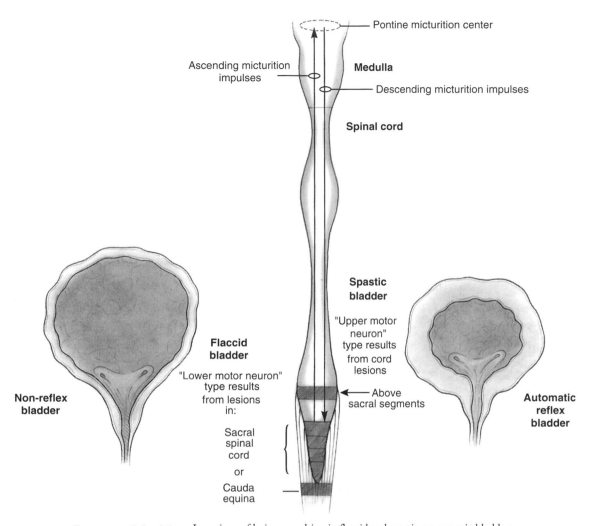

FIGURE 18-11.   Locations of lesions resulting in flaccid and spastic neurogenic bladders.

Two commonly encountered abnormalities associated with the sympathetic system are Horner syndrome and **acute sympathetic shock syndrome.** Horner syndrome is characterized by miosis, ptosis, and anhidrosis (absence of sweating) and may occur as the result of unilateral peripheral or central lesions. The peripheral lesions involve (a) preganglionic fibers chiefly in spinal nerve T1 or in the cervical sympathetic trunk or (b) postganglionic neurons and fibers in the superior cervical ganglion. Central lesions producing Horner syndrome occur chiefly as the result of (a) interrupting the pupillodilator path in the dorsolateral part of the medullary reticular formation or in the cervical spinal cord or (b) destruction of the ciliospinal center in the sympathetic nucleus at C8 and T1.

Acute sympathetic shock syndrome is characterized by bradycardia, hypotension, bilateral Horner syndrome, and difficulties in adjusting to a warm environment because sweating and cutaneous vasodilation cannot be elicited. This syndrome occurs in acute bilateral cervical spinal cord injuries due to the interruption of the descending impulses to the sympathetic nuclei. The signs usually subside after several days when reflex regulation of sympathetic activities returns.

from the uterovaginal ganglia in the female innervate the vaginal glands and erectile tissue of the clitoris. In the male, the postganglionic parasympathetic fibers arise from the cavernous and prostatic ganglia and supply the cavernous or erectile tissue of the penis.

Sympathetic preganglionic fibers arise from T10–L2 and synapse chiefly in the inferior mesenteric ganglion. Postganglionic sympathetic fibers in the female supply the blood vessels and smooth muscle of the uterus and vagina, whereas in the male sympathetic postganglionic fibers supply the ductus deferens, prostate gland, and seminal vesicle.

Parasympathetic activity in women produces secretion of vaginal glands and clitoral engorgement; in men parasympathetic impulses are necessary for penile erection. Sympathetic activity in women produces rhythmical contractions of the vagina; in men the sympathetic nerves are necessary for ejaculation.

CHAPTER REVIEW

18–1. What are the chief differences between the somatic and autonomic efferent systems?

18–2. Describe the origin of the cranial parasympathetic system.

18–3. Describe the origin of the sacral parasympathetic system.

18–4. Describe the origin of preganglionic sympathetic fibers.

18–5. Which cranial nerves contain autonomic afferent fibers and describe their connections.

18–6. What are the chief peripheral routes of visceral pain fibers?

18–7. Define and give an explanation for referred pain.

18–8. Where is the site of referral and the anatomical basis of cardiac referred pain?

18–9. Contrast the effects of stimulation of parasympathetic and sympathetic nerves on the heart, urinary bladder, and sex organs.

THE BLOOD SUPPLY OF THE CENTRAL NERVOUS SYSTEM: STROKE

■ **A 55-year-old man with diabetes, a heavy smoker, with a history of atherosclerotic coronary disease suffered several episodes of complete visual loss in his left eye described as though someone pulled a shade over his orbit. Associated with this visual loss was numbness and tingling in the right hand and fingers, drooping of the right side of the face, and significant difficulty in producing words. All of these symptoms occurred without warning and cleared completely within 20 minutes. The patient's neurologic examination was normal and the only positive finding was a loud bruit over his left carotid artery. An angiogram demonstrated severe atherosclerotic blockage at the proximal internal carotid artery (ICA) and a carotid endarterectomy was performed. No further *transient ischemic episodes* were experienced.**

Total cerebral blood flow averages approximately 750 mL/min. This 750 mL is supplied by the two carotid arteries and the basilar artery, each contributing approximately 250 mL/min. The total intracranial blood volume is 100 to 150 mL at any instant; so the intracranial circulating pool turns over five to seven times each minute. Average cerebral blood flow (CBF) is 55 mL/100 g of brain tissue per minute. If CBF falls to less than 30 to 35 mL/100 g/min ischemia occurs; if CBF falls below 20 mL/100 g/min infarction occurs. Extended flows below 15 mL/100 g/min inevitably result in massive infarction.

The neurons of the central nervous system, unlike the primary cells of most organ systems, are very dependent on aerobic metabolism. When deprived of blood flow for only 20 seconds, the brain is reduced to a state of unconsciousness; if circulation is not reestablished in 4 to 5 minutes, this state is usually irreversible. The brain itself makes up approximately 2% of the body weight (1500 gm) but uses 15% of the total cardiac output (5 L/min) and consumes 20% (50 mL/min) of the total available O_2. This enormous blood flow and O_2 consumption demands an extensive yet smoothly functioning delivery system, the cerebrovascular system.

Different areas of the cerebrum and spinal cord receive different amounts of blood depending on metabolic activity. Under most circumstances, the more metabolically active gray matter has a greater flow than the white matter (75 mL versus 25 mL/100 g/min). In addition, certain neurons in the CNS (i.e., selected layers of the hippocampus and the cerebellar and cerebral cortices) display a selective vulnerability to O_2 loss such that they are affected first in states of acute **hypoxia.**

The cerebrovasculature autoregulates to maintain a constant amount of blood flow to the neuraxis despite fluctuations in systemic blood pressure. The larger extracerebral vessels possess a readily identifiable adventitial plexus of nerves, but autoregulation persists even after their complete removal, because (unlike the peripheral vascular system) the sympathetic and parasympathetic influences on cerebrovascular tone are quite limited.

Cerebral autoregulation is closely related to local metabolic processes and many metabolites affect cerebral blood flow. The most important metabolites that affect cerebral blood flow are the local concentrations of O_2 and CO_2. Hypoxia or **hypercarbia** or both result in cerebral vasodilation and increased cerebral blood flow, whereas **hypocarbia** results in vasoconstriction and diminished blood flow.

> Clinically, the effects of O_2 and CO_2 on cerebrovascular tone can be manipulated in patients with elevated intracranial pressure. One of the common treatments of elevated intracranial pressure is hyperventilation. Hyperventilation lowers the PCO_2 and elevates the PO_2, causing cerebral vasoconstriction and diminished cerebral blood flow, thereby resulting in secondary lowering of the intracranial pressure.

Intracranial arteries differ considerably in histologic composition from those found elsewhere in the body. The intima of intracranial vessels possesses a well-developed internal elastic membrane (IEM), which is actually thicker than that found in extracranial vessels. The media (composed of muscle and elastica), however, is much less prominent than that of extracranial arteries. The adventitia is thin and contains no paravascular supporting tissue, no external elastic lamina, and no vasovasorum. Histologically, intracranial veins are thin-walled structures consisting mostly of collagen with minimal elastic tissue, little muscle, and no valves.

> In primates, small discontinuities of the media occur at the points where larger intracranial arteries branch. In these areas the adventitia actually abuts the IEM. Clinically, these so-called "media gaps" relate to the location of saccular aneurysms formed as the IEM is damaged by progressive atherosclerosis. With the congenital absence of the media and with developmental damage to the IEM, the vessel wall is supported by only the endothelium and adventitia. This weak support progressively balloons to form an aneurysm.

The intracranial extracerebral vessels are contained within the subarachnoid space (Fig. 1–8). As these vessels and their branches penetrate the brain, they become intracerebral. A small perivascular extension of the subarachnoid space is formed alongside these penetrating vessels. This **Virchow-Robin space** extends from the general subarachnoid space and gradually thins as the vessel penetrates deep into the brain substance.

> Disease processes in the subarachnoid space such as subarachnoid hemorrhage and meningitis may gain entrance into the brain tissue itself as they fill the perivascular spaces surrounding the penetrating vessels.

THE BLOOD-BRAIN BARRIER

The concept of a selective barrier between the intravascular space and the brain is suggested by the result of dyes (such as trypan blue) being introduced into the blood stream—most of the body tissues including the meninges are stained, but not the brain. The blood-brain barrier selectively prevents the penetration of certain substances into the cerebral space. The anatomical composition of the blood-brain barrier consists of the capillary endothelium, the astrocytic foot processes, and a shared basement membrane (Fig. 1–4). The selective permeability of the blood-brain barrier probably rests along the capillary endothelium. The tight junctions and nonfenestrated composition of the capillary endothelium impede the passage of many substances.

> In certain areas of the brain, circumventricular organs such as the neurohypophysis, the area postrema, the pineal, the subcommissural and subfornical organs, the optic recess, and the median eminence, have a fenestrated capillary endothelium that allows these areas to stain following intravascular dye administration. Similarly, in infants the capillary endothelium is immature and fenestrated, allowing substances such as bilirubin to enter. Elevation of bilirubin in the neonate may lead to staining in the basal ganglia, thalamus, and ependyma, a condition called **kernicterus.**

Physiologically, the passage of substances across the blood-brain barrier depends on their molecular size, lipid miscibility, and degree of ionic dissociation. Many drugs that are useful in the treatment of systemic disorders are ineffective in identical CNS disorders due to their inability to cross the blood-brain barrier. The astrocytic foot processes control the intracerebral volume by regulating the quantity of substances such as sodium, water, glucose, etc. that enter this space. Disruptions of the astrocytic foot processes generally result in leakage of fluid into the brain with the development of **cerebral edema.** This condition occurs commonly with trauma and tumors.

CEREBRAL VASCULATURE

The anterior and posterior parts of the brain receive blood from the carotid and vertebral arteries, respectively (Fig. 19–1). Hence, two cerebral circu-

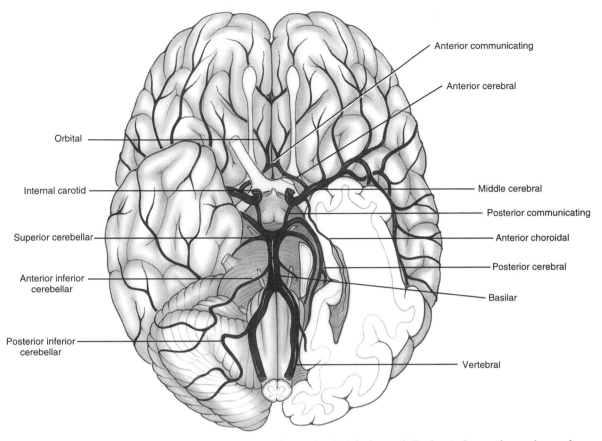

FIGURE 19-1. Major cerebral arteries on base of brain. On the left, the cerebellar hemisphere and ventral part of the temporal lobe have been removed.

latory systems are described: an anterior or carotid system and a posterior or vertebral-basilar system.

ANTERIOR OR CAROTID SYSTEM

The common carotid artery begins on the right as the brachiocephalic trunk bifurcates into the common carotid and the subclavian arteries. The left common carotid artery branches from the arch of the aorta at its highest point. Each common carotid artery lies within the carotid sheath, with the internal jugular vein lateral and the vagus nerve dorsal (lying between the artery and vein). Near the upper border of the thyroid cartilage, the common carotid artery bifurcates into the internal and external carotid arteries. The carotid sinus and carotid body, which influence blood pressure and res-

piratory regulation, respectively, are located at the bifurcation and extend along the proximal few millimeters of the ICA.

From the bifurcation, the external carotid artery proceeds medially to divide into its many extracranial branches, whereas the ICA proceeds posterolaterally (without branching) to enter the carotid canal in the petrous portion of the temporal bone.

Radiographically, the course of the ICA can

> Clinically, the carotid bifurcation is a common site of atherosclerotic narrowing and the subsequent production of **cerebral ischemia** and stroke.

> The angiographic shape of the ICA as it winds its way through the petrous canal and the cavernous sinus is termed the **carotid siphon.** The cavernous segment is not actually bathed in the venous blood of the sinus but is surrounded by sinus endothelium and supported by numerous trabeculae. Several prominent branches, including the tentorial (which supplies the tentorium), the inferior hypophysial (which supplies the posterior lobe of the pituitary gland), and the cavernous (which supplies the surrounding dura) are located along this portion of the vessel. As the ICA leaves the cavernous sinus, it pierces the dura and becomes for the first time an intracranial vessel (cerebral segment).

be subdivided into four segments: cervical, petrous, cavernous, and cerebral. The cervical segment extends from the common carotid bifurcation to the point where the artery pierces the carotid canal. The petrous segment is contained within the carotid canal of the petrous portion of the temporal bone. This portion of the artery has several small branches to the inner ear. The cavernous segment is contained within the cavernous sinus and extends from the point the artery leaves the carotid canal to the point at which it enters the dura near the anterior clinoid process.

The cerebral segment is the terminal portion of the ICA and ends as the internal carotid bifurcates into the anterior and middle cerebral arteries (Fig. 19–1). Other major branches of the cerebral segment include the ophthalmic artery, the superior hypophysial arteries, the posterior communicating artery, and the anterior choroidal artery.

Ophthalmic Artery

The ophthalmic artery leaves the ICA beneath the optic nerve and enters the orbit through the optic foramen with the optic nerve (Fig. 19–2). It gives rise to the central artery of the retina and eventually communicates freely with the external carotid artery via its lacrimal, ethmoidal, supraorbital, supratrochlear, and nasal branches.

Superior Hypophysial Arteries

The superior hypophysial arteries exit from the internal carotid arteries to form a plexus around the pituitary stalk (Fig. 19–3).

> The capillaries of these vessels aid in the formation of the hypophysial-portal system that supplies the anterior lobe of the pituitary gland (Fig. 17–3).

Posterior Communicating Artery

The posterior communicating artery leaves the dorsolateral surface of the ICA just before its terminal branching and joins the proximal portion of the posterior cerebral artery, thus connecting the anterior and posterior circulations (Figs. 19–1, 19–2).

> Clinically, one of the most frequent sites for aneurysm formation is where the posterior communicating artery arises from the ICA.

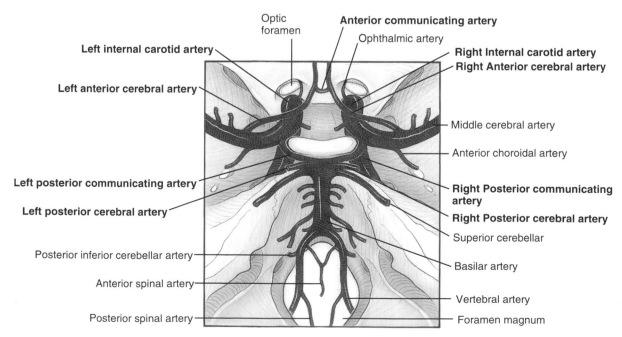

FIGURE 19–2.   The cerebral arterial circle of Willis (bold) and other major cerebral arteries as observed on the floor of the cranial cavity.

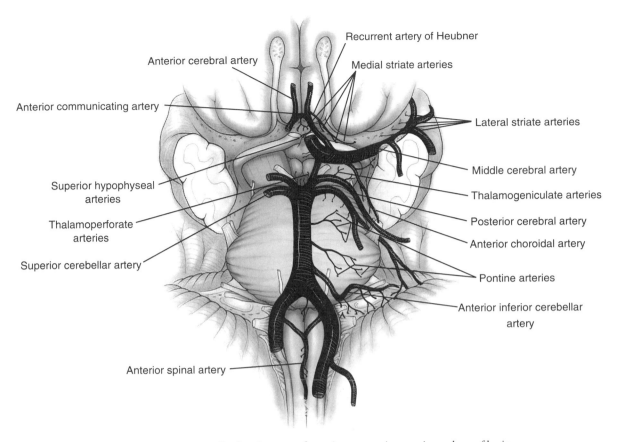

FIGURE 19-3. Perforation zones for major penetrating arteries on base of brain.

Anterior Choroidal Artery

The anterior choroidal artery usually arises from the internal carotid just proximal to its bifurcation. Sometimes, however, it arises from the MCA, the posterior communicating artery, or the bifurcation of the middle and anterior cerebral arteries. The anterior choroidal artery crosses the optic tract and passes toward the medial surface of the temporal lobe (Figs. 19–1, 19–3). The penetrating branches of the anterior choroidal artery supply the hippocampal formation, the amygdaloid nucleus, and the ventral and entire retrolenticular part of the posterior limb of the internal capsule. In addition, the anterior choroidal artery supplies the **choroid plexus** of the inferior horn of the lateral ventricle (Fig. 19–1).

Anterior Cerebral Artery

The anterior cerebral artery (ACA) is divided by the anterior communicating artery into proximal or precommunicating (A-1) and distal or postcommunicating (A-2) segments.

A-1 Segment

The A-1 segment begins at the carotid bifurcation and passes over the optic tract and chiasm to reach the anterior communicating artery (Figs. 19–1–19–3). Along its course, branches supply portions of the anterior hypothalamus.

Recurrent Artery of Heubner

The recurrent artery of Heubner is conspicuous by its large size. It arises either from the distal part of the A-1 segment or the proximal part of the A-2 segment and courses laterally along the A-1 segment to join the lateral striate arteries as they enter the anterior perforated substance (Fig. 19–3). The recurrent artery supplies the ventral parts of the head of the caudate nucleus, the anterior pole of the putamen, the anterior part of the globus pallidus, and the anterior limb of the internal capsule as far dorsal as the top of the globus pallidus.

Anterior Communicating Artery

The anterior communicating artery joins the two anterior cerebral arteries with the A-1 segments of these vessels located proximally and the A-2 segments distally (Figs. 19–1–19–3). Anatomically, the anterior communicating artery is seldom a distinct vessel but more often constitutes a complex network or web of vessels. Small perforators from the anterior communicating artery supply the genu of the corpus callosum, septum pellucidum, and septal nuclei.

> The anterior communicating artery forms an important potential source of blood flow between the two hemispheres, particularly when one ICA occludes. In addition the anterior communicating artery is another one of the frequent sites of saccular aneurysm formation.

Postcommunicating or A-2 Segment

The A-2 segment of the ACA begins at the anterior communicating artery (Figs. 19–1 to 19–3). Proximal branches of the A-2 segment include the orbital artery (Fg. 19–1), which supplies the gyrus rectus and olfactory bulb and tract, and the frontopolar artery, which supplies the anterior part of the superior frontal gyrus. The A-2 segment ends by bifurcating into the callosomarginal artery and the pericallosal trunk near the genu of the corpus callosum (Fig. 19–4).

Callosomarginal Artery

The callosomarginal artery follows the course of the callosomarginal sulcus, supplying anterior, middle, and posterior frontal branches to the superior frontal gyrus (Fig. 19–4). It ends as the paracentral artery to the paracentral lobule. All of these branches anastomose with pre-rolandic and post-rolandic branches of the MCA as they turn onto the convexity of the hemisphere.

Pericallosal Trunk Artery

The pericallosal trunk artery is regarded as a continuation of the ACA. It passes posteriorly in close relation to the corpus callosum, supplying penetrating vessels to the corpus callosum, septum pellucidum, and fornix. Terminal branches include the precuneal artery, which supplies the precuneus, and the posterior callosal artery, which supplies the splenium of the corpus callosum (Fig. 19–4).

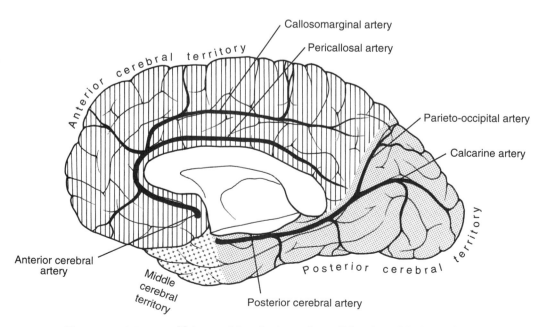

FIGURE 19–4. Major arterial territories on the medial surface of the hemisphere.

A stroke in the cortical distribution of one ACA results in sensorimotor deficit in the opposite foot and leg. Urinary incontinence and contralateral frontal lobe signs may also be observed.

Middle Cerebral Artery

The MCA is the largest branch of the ICA. It is the cerebral artery most often occluded. It is divided into a proximal (M-1) segment and a distal (M-2) segment by the MCA bifurcation.

M-1 Segment

The proximal portion of the MCA is related to the lowest portion of the insula as the artery travels to reach the lateral or **Sylvian fissure**. From this segment, 10 to 15 penetrating vessels, the lateral striate arteries or the lenticulostriate arteries, arise and supply the dorsal part of the head and the entire body of the caudate nucleus, most of the lentiform nucleus, and the internal capsule above the level of the globus pallidus. Like the recurrent artery of Heubner, these penetrating arteries run a recurrent

Clinically, the lenticulostriate vessels are the most common site of spontaneous hypertensive hemorrhage in individuals with long-standing hypertension.

course back along the M-1 segment to penetrate the lateral two thirds of the anterior perforated substance (Fig. 19–3).

The other M-1 segment branches include the anterior temporal artery, which supplies the most anterior portion of the temporal lobe, and the orbitofrontal artery, which supplies the lateral portions of the orbital surface of the frontal lobe.

M-2 Segment

The bifurcation of the MCA is located at the base of the insula and it forms the M-2 segment, which consists of the superior and inferior trunks. These trunks travel deep in the lateral (Sylvian) fissure along the insula. At the insula, branches travel along the frontal and temporal opercula to exit the lateral fissure and proceed along the convexity of the hemisphere. Generally, the superior trunk supplies branches to the frontal and parietal lobes, and the inferior trunk supplies the temporal and occipital lobes (Fig. 19–5). The angiographic shape of the superior and inferior trunks and their branches is called the **middle cerebral candelabra.** The branches of both the superior and inferior trunks are named according to the region they supply. These include the precentral or pre-rolandic, the central or rolandic, the postcentral or post-rolandic, the anterior and posterior parietal, the

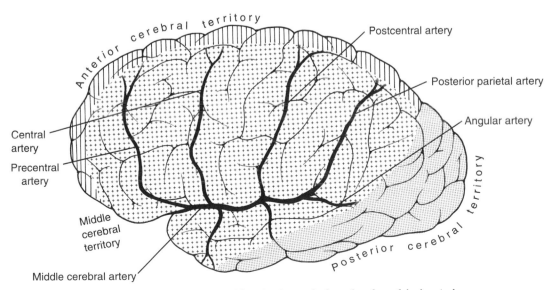

FIGURE 19–5. Major arterial territories on the lateral surface of the hemisphere.

angular, the posterior temporal, and the posterior occipital arteries. The precentral, central, postcentral, anterior and posterior parietal, and angular arteries leave the lateral fissure and supply most of the cerebral convexity, anastomosing with the branches of the ACA near the anterior and dorsal margins of the convexity. The posterior temporal and posterior occipital branches supply most of the temporal and occipital convexity, anastomosing with branches of the posterior cerebral artery at the posterior and ventral margins of the hemisphere.

> A stroke in the cortical distribution of the MCA results in a severe sensorimotor deficit in the contralateral face and upper limb. With dominant hemisphere involvement, global aphasia also results; with nondominant hemisphere involvement, the neglect syndrome or amorphosynthesis results.

POSTERIOR OR VERTEBRAL-BASILAR SYSTEM

Vertebral Arteries

The vertebral arteries are the first branches of the subclavian arteries. They generally enter the transverse foramina of CV6 and travel upward through the transverse foramina of the other cervical vertebrae to reach the superior margin of CV1, where they pierce the atlantooccipital membrane. They then enter the cranial cavity through the foramen magnum ventral to the hypoglossal nerves, travel along the anterior or lateral surfaces of the medulla, and join to form the basilar artery near the pontomedullary junction (Fig. 19–1).

After entering the cranial cavity, each vertebral artery gives rise to a posterior spinal artery that descends along the posterolateral aspect of the spinal cord. The vertebral arteries, 1 to 2 cm before joining to form the basilar artery, give rise to their largest branches, the posterior inferior cerebellar arteries (PICA).

The PICA curve around the medulla ventral to the roots of IX CN, X CN, and XI CN. The PICA reach the region of the cerebellar tonsil and proceed along the posterior inferior cerebellar surface (Fig. 19–1). Multiple penetrating vessels supplying the posterolateral medulla arise from the PICA as they curve around this region (Figs. 19–6, 19–7). Other branches supply the choroid plexus of the fourth ventricle before the PICA terminate as inferior vermian and

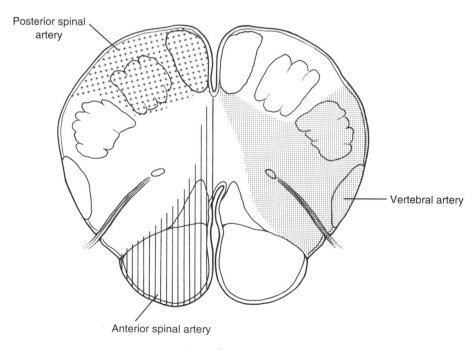

FIGURE 19–6.   Arterial territories in the caudal medulla.

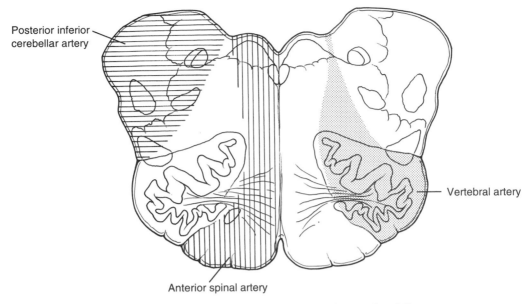

Posterior inferior
cerebellar artery

Vertebral artery

Anterior spinal artery

FIGURE 19-7. Arterial territories in the rostral medulla.

tonsillar-hemispheric branches, which supply all of the posterior and inferior parts of the cerebellum.

Immediately before the vertebral-basilar junction, anterior spinal arteries arise from both vertebral arteries and join almost immediately to form a single anterior spinal artery that runs along the anterior median fissure of the spinal cord (Figs. 19–2, 19–3).

> A stroke in the distribution of the vertebral artery (or the PICA) results in an ipsilateral loss of pain and temperature sensations in the face, contralateral loss of pain and temperature sensation in the limbs, trunk, and neck, an ipsilateral Horner syndrome, hoarseness, dysphagia, nystagmus, vertigo, diplopia, ipsilateral ataxia, and ipsilateral loss of taste. This combination of signs is the **lateral medullary** or **Wallenberg syndrome.**

Basilar Artery

The basilar artery begins near the pontomedullary junction and travels in the shallow median groove on the ventral surface of the pons to end at the midbrain. At the midbrain it divides into the posterior cerebral arteries (PCA) (Figs. 19–1–19–3). As the basilar artery travels

along the pons, it supplies multiple penetrating vessels to the pons itself. These vessels penetrate the pons as paramedian, short circumferential, and long circumferential arteries (Fig. 19–8). Symmetrical large branches arising at about the middle of the basilar artery are called the anterior inferior cerebellar arteries (AICA) (Figs. 19–1, 19–3). Similar large paired vessels arising just proximal to the termination of the basilar artery are called the superior cerebellar arteries (SCA) (Figs. 19–1–19–3).

The AICA emerge from the basilar artery and travel along the course of VII CN and VIII CN (Fig. 19–3). At times, these vessels may actually enter the internal auditory meatus for a short distance, but ultimately they reach the anterior and inferior portions of the cerebellum, their principal area of supply. The labyrinthine or internal auditory arteries may arise from the AICA or directly from the basilar artery.

Just proximal to the bifurcation of the basilar artery into the PCA, the basilar artery gives off the SCA. These vessels encircle the midbrain and end by dividing into hemispheric and superior vermian branches that supply the superior aspects of the cerebellum and most of the cerebellar nuclei and superior cerebellar peduncles (Fig. 19–8).

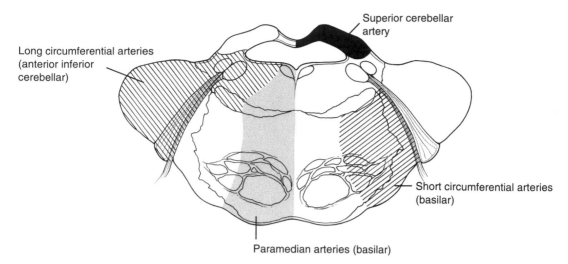

FIGURE 19–8. Arterial territories in the midpons.

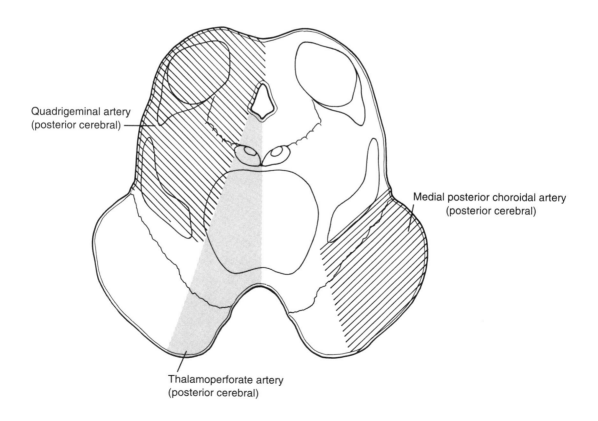

FIGURE 19–9. Arterial territories in the caudal midbrain.

Posterior Cerebral Artery

The PCA begin at the basilar bifurcation near the tip of the dorsum sellae. A short distance after arising, the PCA anastomose with the posterior communicating arteries (Figs. 19–1–19–3), thus connecting the anterior and posterior cerebral circulations. Each of the PCA swings around the anterior aspect of the oculomotor nerve, passes laterally along the surface of the cerebral crus to reach the dorsal surface of the free margin of the tentorium, and then proceeds posteriorly along the inferomedial surface of the temporal lobe (Figs. 19–1, 19–3).

The PCA give rise to brainstem and cortical branches. The chief brainstem branches are named according to their areas of supply as follows: thalamoperforate, medial posterior choroidal, and quadrigeminal, which arise medial to the anastomosis with the posterior communicating artery and supply the midbrain (Figs. 19–9, 19–10); and the thalamogenicu-late, lateral posterior choroidal, and peduncular, which arise lateral to the posterior communicating anastomosis and supply the lateral parts of the posterior diencephalon. Cortical branches arise as the PCA courses along the inferomedial surface of the temporal lobe to reach the occipital lobe, and they supply the hippocampus and the medial and inferior surfaces of the temporal and occipital lobes. The PCA ends by forming the parieto-occipital and calcarine arteries found in the respective sulci (Fig. 19–4). The calcarine artery supplies the primary visual area. The cortical branches of the PCA extend slightly onto the lateral surfaces of the temporal and occipital lobes where they anastomose with branches of the MCA.

> A stroke in the cortical distribution of the posterior cerebral artery results in a contralateral homonymous hemianopsia. With dominant (usually left) hemisphere involvement, reading and writing abnormalities also result.

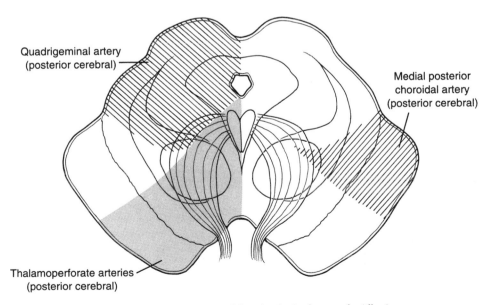

Quadrigeminal artery (posterior cerebral)

Medial posterior choroidal artery (posterior cerebral)

Thalamoperforate arteries (posterior cerebral)

FIGURE 19–10. Arterial territories in the rostral midbrain.

THE CEREBRAL ARTERIAL CIRCLE OF WILLIS

The **cerebral arterial circle,** described by Sir Thomas Willis in 1664, consists of the larger cerebral vessels and their interconnections located on the ventral surface of the brain. The arteries of the **circle of Willis** (Fig. 19–2) include anterior communicating, left anterior cerebral, left internal carotid, left posterior communicating, left posterior cerebral, basilar, right posterior cerebral, right posterior communicating, right internal carotid, and right anterior cerebral. A perfectly symmetrical circle of Willis in which each component vessel is of the same caliber occurs only in a minority of instances. More commonly, one or more of the arteries (most frequently the anterior cerebral, posterior cerebral, anterior communicating, or posterior communicating) are, to some degree, atrophic.

The function of the cerebral arterial circle of Willis is debated, but it probably serves as a potential vascular shunt, assisting in the development of collateral circulation to the brain should one of the proximal vessels (such as the carotid or basilar) become temporarily or permanently occluded.

Developmental Changes in the Circle of Willis

During embryologic development, the internal carotid arteries supply blood to the anterior, middle, and posterior cerebral arteries, the latter via a large posterior communicating artery. With development, however, the distal posterior cerebral supply comes from the basilar artery through the proximal posterior cerebral artery as the posterior communicating artery atrophies. In most people, the result of this atrophy is an anterior circulation (consisting of the anterior and middle cerebral arteries supplied by the carotid arteries) and a posterior circulation (consisting of the posterior cerebral arteries supplied by the vertebral-basilar trunk). However, in 20% of the population, the embryologic circulation persists, with one or both posterior cerebral arteries being supplied mainly by the anterior circulation through persistently large posterior communicating arteries.

In instances where one or more of the primary pathways for blood flow is lost, the maintenance of cerebral blood flow depends on collateral sources. The circle of Willis is one of the most important sources of collateral circulation to the brain, but its effectiveness depends on the size of each component. Other collateral pathways exist in connections between the anterior (carotid) and posterior (basilar) circulations (such as the primitive trigeminal, otic, and hypoglossal arteries). These vessels generally disappear with development. Other prominent sources of collateral flow include anastomoses between the external carotid and the internal carotid and vertebral arteries. Clinically, these collaterals are most frequently seen in patients who have occlusive disease of a carotid or vertebral artery in the neck. In these instances, it is not uncommon to find the intracranial portions of the occluded vessels supplied via the ophthalmic branch of the carotid artery or via the muscular branches of the vertebral artery from the external carotid ramifications about the orbit and in the neck. Similar anastomoses between the meningeal vessels and the vessels on the surface of the cerebrum may be seen. Anastomoses between the distal branches of the anterior, middle, and posterior cerebral arteries, however, are limited, and collateralization through perforating vessels is generally not seen.

Perforating Central Branches

The branches of the cerebral arterial circle of Willis that penetrate the ventral surface of the brain are called the perforating, penetrating, central, or ganglionic branches and are divided into four groups: medial striate, lateral striate, thalamoperforate, and thalamogeniculate (Fig. 19–3).

Medial Striate Arteries

The medial striate arteries arise chiefly from the A-1 segment of the ACA, although some may arise from the most proximal part of the A-2 segment, the anterior communicating artery, or the most terminal part of the ICA. Collectively referred to as the medial striate arteries, they enter the brain in the medial third of the anterior perforated substance. The largest and most lateral of these arteries to enter the brain is the recurrent artery of Heubner (Fig. 19–3). The medial striate arteries are the principal sources of the blood supply to the supraoptic and preoptic regions of the hypothalamus and to the ventral part of the head of the caudate nucleus and the adjacent parts of the anterior limb of the internal capsule and putamen.

Lateral Striate Arteries

The lateral striate arteries usually arise entirely from the M-1 segment of the MCA, although sometimes a few may come from the initial part of the ACA (Fig. 19–3). They are frequently called the lenticulostriate arteries and they enter the brain in the lateral two thirds of the anterior perforated substance. The lateral striate arteries supply the dorsal part of the head of the caudate nucleus, most of the putamen and adjacent part of the globus pallidus, and the dorsal part of the posterior limb of the internal capsule (Fig. 19–11).

As mentioned previously, these vessels are the most common sites of spontaneous hemorrhage in individuals with long-standing hypertension. For this reason, collectively they are called the "artery of cerebral hemorrhage."

Thalamoperforate Arteries

Thalamoperforate arteries arise along the posterior communicating artery and the posterior cerebral artery proximal to the point at which these two vessels join. These penetrating arteries enter the brain in the posterior perforated substance (Fig. 19–3). The more anterior vessels supply the tuberal region of the hypothalamus and the anteromedial part of the thalamus, including the anterior and medial dorsal nuclei (Fig. 19–11). The more posterior vessels supply the mamillary region of the hypothalamus, the subthalamus, the adjacent parts of the thalamus, and the medial parts of the rostral midbrain tegmentum and cerebral crus (Figs. 19–9, 19–10).

Thalamogeniculate Arteries

The thalamogeniculate arteries arise from the posterior cerebral artery distal to its anastomosis with the posterior communicating, and penetrate the brain at the geniculate bodies. They supply the most posterior parts of the thalamus, including the ventral lateral and ventral posterior nuclei and the medial three fourths of the metathalamic nuclei.

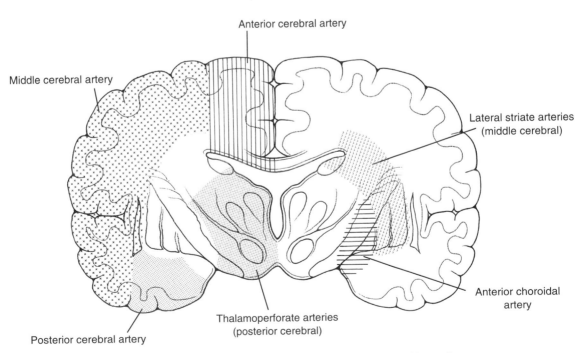

FIGURE 19–11. Arterial territories of diencephalon and hemisphere.

SPINAL CORD VASCULATURE

The spinal cord is supplied by paired posterior spinal arteries and a single larger anterior spinal artery. In addition, multiple radicular vessels arise segmentally from cervical, intercostal, lumbar, and sacral arteries. The anterior and posterior spinal arteries are not of sufficient caliber to maintain circulation throughout the entire spinal cord. Hence, they rely to a great extent on the radicular component.

The largest radicular artery is the so-called artery of Adamkiewicz, which generally enters the spinal cord in the lower thoracic or upper lumbar area. Clinically, this area of the spinal cord is susceptible to vascular insult should this radicular artery be compromised.

The anterior spinal artery descends along the surface of the cord at the anterior median fissure and supplies from five to nine sulcal arteries to each spinal cord segment. Each sulcal artery passes to the bottom of the anterior median fissure, where it swings right or left to enter the spinal cord and supply that side. In addition to the sulcal arteries, the anterior spinal supplies coronal arteries that course laterally along the surface of the cord to anastomose with similar branches from the posterior spinal

arteries. The latter are located in the posterolateral sulci and also give rise to penetrating branches that accompany the posterior roots into the spinal cord. The sulcal and coronal branches of the anterior spinal artery supply the anterior two thirds of the spinal cord, whereas the penetrating and coronal branches of the posterior spinal arteries supply the posterior third (Fig. 19–12).

A stroke in the distribution of the anterior spinal artery results in the development of total motor paralysis and dissociated sensory loss below the level of the lesion. The sensory loss if dissociated (loss of pain and temperature but no involvement of position and vibration sense) is due to sparing of the dorsal columns supplied by the posterior spinal arteries.

VEINS OF BRAIN AND SPINAL CORD

Unlike systemic veins, cerebral veins are without valves and muscle tissue. The venous system of the brain is divided into a superficial and a deep portion. The superficial veins are larger and more numerous than the corresponding cortical arteries and tend to lie alongside the arteries in the cerebral sulci. The superficial venous system empties into the more superficially located sinuses, especially the superior sagittal,

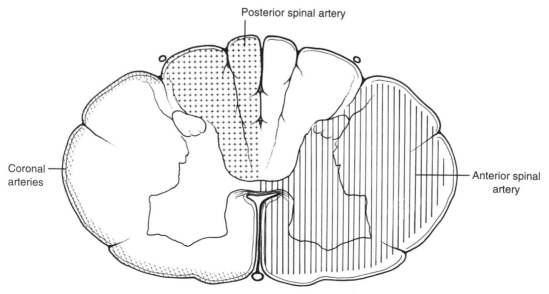

FIGURE 19–12. Arterial territories in spinal cord.

inferior sagittal, and transverse sinuses via anastomotic or draining veins. The most prominent anastomotic veins are the superficial middle cerebral vein draining into cavernous or sphenoparietal sinus, the great anastomotic vein (of Trolard) draining into the superior sagittal, and the posterior anastomotic vein (of Labbé) draining into the transverse sinus.

The deep venous system consists of the great vein (of Galen), the internal cerebral veins, the basal vein (of Rosenthal), and their tributaries including the transcerebral veins (that drain the white matter) and the subependymal veins (that drain the periventricular structures).

The great vein (of Galen) is located beneath the splenium of the corpus callosum and receives the paired internal cerebral veins, the two basal veins (of Rosenthal), and drainage from the medial and inferior parts of the occipital lobe. The internal cerebral veins lie in the roof of the third ventricle. Large tributaries include the thalamostriate veins (draining thalamus and striatum), choroidal veins (from choroid plexus of lateral ventricle), and septal veins (from septum pellucidum).

The basal vein (of Rosenthal) begins near the anterior perforate substance, encircles the cerebral crus, and ends at the great vein (of Galen). Basal vein drainage includes the medial and inferior surfaces of the frontal and temporal lobes, the insular and opercular cortices, and regions of the hypothalamus and midbrain.

The venous drainage of the spinal cord is concentrated in a dense plexus of veins located in the epidural space (Batson internal vertebral venous plexus).

This valveless spinal maze of veins communicates freely with sacral, lumbar, and intercostal veins, thus providing an open pathway for tumor and infection metastases.

CHAPTER REVIEW QUESTIONS

19–1. What are the chief morphologic features of cerebral arteries?

19–2. What is the anatomical substrate of the blood-brain barrier?

19–3. Describe the arterial circle of Willis.

19–4. What is the arterial supply of the spinal cord?

19–5. List the arterial supply of each of the following:

    a. Broca speech area
    b. Lower limb sensorimotor cortex
    c. Visual cortex
    d. Posterior limb of internal capsule
    e. Dorsolateral part of rostral medulla
    f. Anterior and lateral funiculi of spinal cord

THE CEREBROSPINAL FLUID SYSTEM: HYDROCEPHALUS

■ A 6-month-old infant is brought to the emergency room with high temperature (103° F) and irritability. On arrival, the child suffers a generalized convulsion and becomes somnolent. A spinal tap demonstrates turbid cerebrospinal fluid (CSF) with many white blood cells and a diminished glucose. A Gram-positive organism is identified. After a course of antibiotics the child makes a complete recovery. Three months later, however, the infant returns with developmental delay, an increasing head circumference, and bulging anterior fontanelle. A computed tomography (CT) scan shows severe ventriculomegaly. A ventriculoperitoneal shunt is inserted with complete restoration of normal milestones.

CSF in the ventricles and subarachnoid space surrounding the brain provides protective cushioning for the brain against the forces associated with surface contact pressure and sudden movement.

THE VENTRICULAR SYSTEM

The ventricular system consists of a lateral ventricle in each hemisphere, a third ventricle in the diencephalon, and a fourth ventricle in the hindbrain between the cerebellum and the pons and rostral medulla. The cerebral aqueduct, in the midbrain, connects the third and fourth ventricles.

LATERAL VENTRICLES

The lateral ventricles (left and right) are divided into five specific parts: anterior or frontal horn, body, trigone, posterior or occipital horn, and inferior or temporal horn (Fig. 20–1).

Anterior or Frontal Horn

The segment of the lateral ventricle anterior to the interventricular foramen (of Monro) is called the anterior or frontal horn. Medially, it is bounded by the septum pellucidum, fornix, and genu of the corpus callosum. Laterally, the head of the caudate bulges into the frontal horn. The floor of the frontal horn is the rostrum of the corpus callosum.

> Clinically, the frontal horns are devoid of choroid plexus making them an excellent place for the position of spinal fluid diversion systems (shunts).

Body

The body of each lateral ventricle extends from the foramen of Monro to the splenium of the corpus callosum. Like the frontal horn, the septum pellucidum continues as the medial border of the ventricular body, and the ventricular roof remains bounded by the corpus callosum. Laterally, the ventricular body is adjacent to the body of the caudate nucleus, and its floor is formed by the thalamus with the fornix, choroid plexus, and thalamostriate vein visible on the surface.

Trigone

The trigone or atrium is the most expanded part of the lateral ventricle. As the name implies, it is triangular in shape. Anteriorly, it is

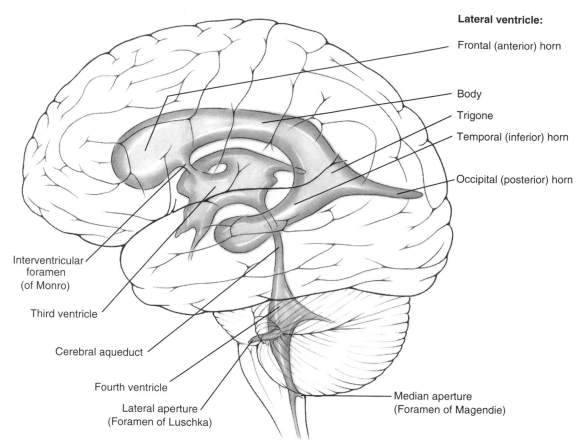

FIGURE 20-1.   The ventricles and their locations in the brain. Left lateral view.

related to the fornix and pulvinar. The trigone contains an abundant tuft of choroid plexus, the **glomus,** along its anterior wall, which is continuous with the choroid plexus of the body, and temporal horn.

Posterior or Occipital Horn

The posterior or occipital horn is within the occipital lobe and is the most variable part of the ventricular system. Medially, the calcar avis, formed by the calcarine fissure, bulges into the occipital horn. Like the frontal horn, the occipital horn is also devoid of choroid plexus.

Inferior or Temporal Horn

The inferior or temporal horn is within the temporal lobe. It ends about 3 cm behind the temporal pole. Its roof is formed by the tapetum of the corpus callosum. Medially, it is bounded by the tail of the caudate nucleus and the hippocampus, and it contains choroid plexus in its superior-medial aspect.

INTERVENTRICULAR FORAMEN OF MONRO

The interventricular foramen is the passageway between each lateral ventricle and the single third ventricle. Bordering the interventricular foramen are the anterior tubercle or nucleus of the thalamus, septum pellucidum, column of the fornix, and thalamostriate vein. Passing through the interventricular foramen is the choroid plexus.

THIRD VENTRICLE

The third ventricle is bordered bilaterally by the thalamus and hypothalamus (Fig. 4–2). Sometimes a connection between the thalami, the interthalamic adhesion or mass intermedia, bridges across the third ventricle. Anteriorly, the third ventricle is bounded by the lamina terminalis with the anterior commissure dorsal and the optic recess ventral. The floor of the third ventricle is formed by the infundibular recess and tuber cinereum with the mamillary bodies posteriorly. The roof of the third ventricle is formed by the tela choroidea and contains the internal cerebral veins and choroid plexus. Posteriorly, suprapineal and infrapineal recesses are formed around the pineal gland with the posterior commissure inferior. The third ventricle drains into a tubular canal, the cerebral aqueduct (of Sylvius).

CEREBRAL AQUEDUCT OF SYLVIUS

The cerebral aqueduct is located within the midbrain and connects the third and fourth ventricles. Its length is 1.5–1.8 cm, and its diameter is 1–2 mm. It is arched in a slightly dorsal direction.

> Clinically, the cerebral aqueduct is the narrowest part of the ventricular system. **Obstructive hydrocephalus** due to aqueductal blockage commonly occurs here.

FOURTH VENTRICLE

The fourth ventricle is a single midline cavity whose rhomboid-shaped floor is formed by the pons and rostral medulla. It expands posteriorly in an inverted kite shape, with its roof bounded by the superior and inferior medullary vela and the superior cerebellar peduncles. Choroid plexus is attached to the inferior medullary velum and extends laterally through the lateral apertures (**foramina of Luschka**) into the subarachnoid space at the origin of IX CN and X CN. The lateral borders of the fourth ventricle are the three cerebellar peduncles. A median aperture, the **foramen of Magendie,** empties into the vallecula, an anterior extension of the cisterna magnum.

SUBARACHNOID SPACE AND CISTERNS

The subarachnoid space is continuous across the cerebral and cerebellar convexities and along the spinal cord. Extracerebral arteries and veins and cranial nerves are suspended in this space by web-like arachnoid trabeculations. In vivo, this space is distended with CSF, which bathes and nourishes the structures contained within. The subarachnoid cisterns are expansions of the subarachnoid space, occurring primarily along the ventral surface of the brainstem and basal forebrain. The CSF in the cisterns provides support and buoyancy for cerebral vessels and cranial nerves.

> Under normal circumstances, no real CSF barrier exists across the ependymal surface of the ventricles or across the pialglial membranes, so that the cerebral extracellular (interstitial) space communicates freely with the CSF circulation.

The subarachnoid cisterns (Figs. 20–2A, 20–2B) are readily identifiable in vivo because they are filled with CSF. In the cadaver brain they are difficult to observe because they have collapsed.

The cisterna magna is the largest of the cisternal compartments. It is located posterior to the medulla and caudal to the cerebellum. Its forward projection between the cerebellar tonsils is the vallecula, into which the median aperture empties.

The pontomedullary cistern lies ventral to the pons and the medulla, between these structures and the clivus. It contains the basilar artery and its branches.

The lateral cerebellomedullary cistern is located lateral to the rostral medulla and surrounds IX CN, X CN, and XI CN.

The cerebellopontine (CP) cistern is located in the CP angle and surrounds V CN, VII CN, and VIII CN. It is immediately beneath the tentorium and lateral to the petrous ridge.

The quadrigeminal cistern overlies the tec-

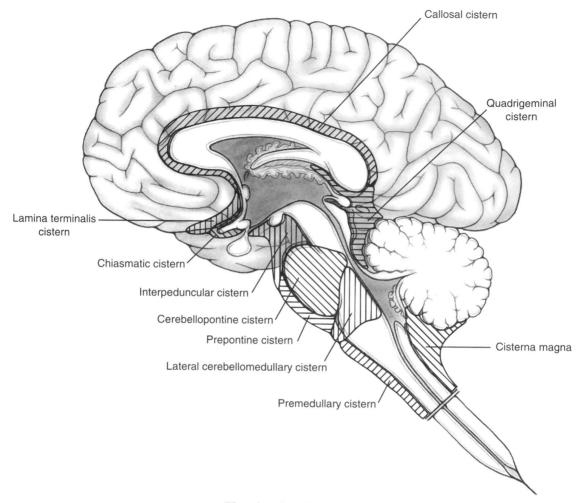

FIGURE 20–2A.   The subarachnoid cisterns at or near the median plane.

tum of the midbrain and contains the vein of Galen. Anteriorly it is bounded by the pineal gland and the pulvinar, superiorly by the splenium of the corpus callosum, posteriorly by the free edge of the tentorium, and inferiorly by the central lobule of the cerebellum.

The interpeduncular cistern straddles the interpeduncular fossa. It is triangular in shape and bounded anteriorly by the membrane of Liliquist, a tough arachnoidal trabecula between the interpeduncular cistern and chiasmatic cistern.

The crural cistern is a lateral and dorsal expansion of the interpeduncular cistern that separates the cerebral peduncles from the parahippocampal gyri.

The ambient cistern joins the interpeduncular and crural cisterns to the quadrigeminal cistern. It lies adjacent to the tentorial edge and contains the posterior cerebral artery and IV CN and VI CN.

The chiasmatic cistern surrounds the optic chiasm and the pituitary stalk, the carotid cistern surrounds the cerebral segment of the carotid artery, and the olfactory cistern surrounds the olfactory tract in the olfactory sulcus.

The lamina terminalis cistern is immediately adjacent to the lamina terminalis. It contains the anterior cerebral and anterior communicating arteries.

The Sylvian cistern fills the lateral or Sylvian fissure and contains the middle cerebral artery

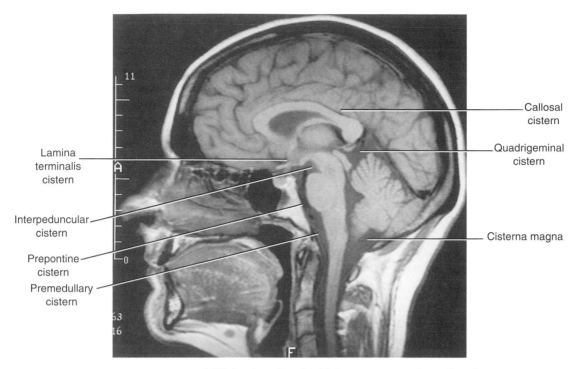

Callosal cistern

Quadrigeminal cistern

Lamina terminalis cistern

Interpeduncular cistern

Cisterna magna

Prepontine cistern

Premedullary cistern

FIGURE 20-2B. MRI showing subarachnoid cisterns at or near the median plane.

and its branches. The callosal cistern lies immediately adjacent to the corpus callosum and contains the pericallosal arteries.

CHOROID PLEXUS

Most CSF is secreted by the choroid plexus contained within the lateral, third, and fourth ventricles through an energy-dependent secretory process. Some CSF is produced by the flow of brain extracellular fluid across the ependymal lining of the ventricular system. As a result of these two methods of formation, CSF can be considered a plasma ultrafiltrate that serves a role in maintaining a constant chemical milieu for neurons.

> Total (normal) CSF volume is approximately 150 mL, with 75 mL in the cisterns, 50 mL in the subarachnoid space, and 25 mL in the ventricles. CSF is formed at the rate of about 0.5 mL/min (450–600 mL/day). Thus the total pool of CSF undergoes replacement between three to four times a day.

CEREBROSPINAL FLUID CIRCULATION

Cerebrospinal fluid circulates within the ventricles of the brain and within the cranial and spinal subarachnoid space (Fig. 20–3). It is produced in the lateral, third, and fourth ventricles and exits the ventricular system through the three openings in the fourth ventricle: the median aperture and paired lateral apertures (Fig. 20–1). After exiting the ventricular system, CSF enters the cisterns around the lower and upper brainstem. From the cisterns, CSF then flows along the convexity of the cerebrum to its absorption site in the **arachnoid granulations** chiefly in the superior sagittal sinus (Fig. 20–3).

CEREBROSPINAL FLUID TAP

CSF can be sampled from a number of locations. Most commonly a CSF tap is done in the lower back via a puncture of the dural sac into the lumbar subarachnoid space (Fig. 2–3). Lum-

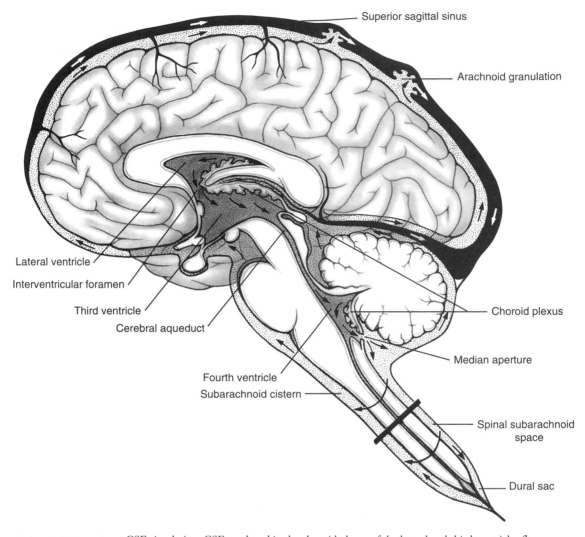

Superior sagittal sinus

Arachnoid granulation

Lateral ventricle

Interventricular foramen

Third ventricle

Cerebral aqueduct

Choroid plexus

Median aperture

Fourth ventricle

Subarachnoid cistern

Spinal subarachnoid space

Dural sac

FIGURE 20-3. CSF circulation. CSF produced in the choroid plexus of the lateral and third ventricles flows through the aqueduct, fourth ventricle, and outlet foramina into the subarachnoid cisterns. Through the cisterns the fluid passes into the subarachnoid space up over the convexities toward the superior sagittal sinus for final absorption through the arachnoid villi.

bar punctures should be performed below the LV2 lumbar spinous process, the level of spinal cord termination at the conus medullaris. Other reservoirs of CSF can also be accessed including the lateral ventricle (ventriculostomy), cervical subarachnoid space (lateral C1–C2 puncture), and cisterna magna (cisternal tap).

The chemical content of normal CSF relates to its location in the CSF pathway. For example, ventricular CSF contains 15 mm/100 mL protein and 75 mg/100 mL glucose, whereas lumbar CSF contains 45 mg/100 mL protein and 60 mg/100 mL glucose. Normally, few if

any cells are found in the CSF regardless of its removal site.

CSF is normally a clear, colorless fluid. Changes in CSF appearance often give clues as to the disease process: red—blood from recent hemorrhage, turbid—pus from infectious process, yellow—excessive protein from stagnation of flow or blood breakdown.

HYDROCEPHALUS

Obstruction of the CSF pathway can result in the stagnation of flow and the development of hydrocephalus. Hydrocephalus by current definition implies a dilation of one or more parts of the ventricular system due to an abnormal collection of CSF. This is meant to exclude the ventricular dilation that commonly occurs following cerebral atrophy as seen in dementia. The sites of hydrocephalus formation relate to the part of the CSF pathway involved in the disease process. In general, two types of hydrocephalus occur, obstructive and communicating. Obstructive hydrocephalus refers to any disease process that restricts CSF flow within or from the ventricular system. Thus, a blockage located anywhere along the ventricular pathways (such as at the interventricular foramen of Monro, at the aqueduct, or at the outlet foramina of the fourth ventricle) produces obstructive hydrocephalus with enlargement of those ventricles proximal to the obstruction. Any disruption of flow after the CSF has exited the ventricular system, on the other hand, is referred to as **communicating hydrocephalus.** Communicating hydrocephalus occurs with obstructions in the cisternal pathways, along the subarachnoid space, or at the arachnoid villi.

> Obstructive hydrocephalus is commonly associated with congenital malformations such as aqueductal stenosis or with tumors that protrude into the ventricular pathway, thereby obstructing flow. Communicating types of hydrocephalus usually result from processes that occur in the cisternal or subarachnoid space such as hemorrhage or infection. Regardless of its etiology and site, the diagnosis of hydrocephalus is readily discernible by cranial CT and magnetic resonance imaging.

INTRACRANIAL PRESSURE

Pressure within the intracranial-spinal space (ICP) is normally less than 100 mL H_2O. ICP is determined by the volumes of brain tissue, CSF, blood, and other tissue within the rigid cranial vault. An increase in the size of any single component (e.g., brain swelling, CSF collection, vasodilation) results first in a diminishment in the size of the other components (compensatory), but then in an increase in ICP.

> Headaches, nausea, vomiting, changes in level of consciousness, extraocular muscle palsies, papilledema, and head enlargement (in infants) are associated with elevated ICP.

CHAPTER REVIEW QUESTIONS

20–1. What are the functions of CSF?

20–2. Name the parts of the lateral ventricle and give their locations.

20–3. Describe the flow of CSF from its formation to its absorption.

20–4. Contrast the noncommunicating and communicating types of hydrocephalus.

PRINCIPLES FOR LOCATING LESIONS AND CLINICAL ILLUSTRATIONS

Focal lesions in the central nervous system (CNS) can be localized by the manifestations of long pathway involvement and the segmental distribution of the abnormalities. The most important long pathways in the brainstem and spinal cord are the pyramidal tract, the spinothalamic tract, the dorsal column–medial lemniscus path, and the spinal trigeminal tract. Long pathways in the cerebral hemispheres are the pyramidal and corticobulbar tracts, the somatosensory thalamic radiation, and the visual pathway.

SPINAL CORD

The major long paths in the spinal cord are the pyramidal or lateral corticospinal tract, the spinothalamic tract, and the dorsal column tracts (gracile and cuneate). The level of a spinal cord lesion may be determined by the loss of functions in dermatomes and myotomes.

The key to localizing lesions in the spinal cord is the loss of motor or sensory functions or both below the foramen magnum, i.e., in the area of distribution of the spinal nerves. (Two exceptions are Horner syndrome, which may occur after cervical or upper thoracic spinal cord lesions, and somatosensory losses on the back of the head and scalp, which may occur after lesions in spinal cord segments C2 and C3.) Spinal cord transection results in an immediate and permanent loss of all sensations and voluntary motor control below the level of the lesion (Fig. 21–1). Bilateral damage of the central part of the spinal cord (central cord syndrome) re-sults in the loss of sensations and voluntary motor control in the area of peripheral distribution of the more rostral spinal cord segments, but not the more caudal. This "sacral sparing" phenomenon occurs because of the somatotopic localization in the long ascending and descending pathways, i.e., the more rostral spinal nerves are represented internal to the more caudal (Fig. 21–2). Spinal cord hemisection causes damage to the lateral corticospinal tract and dorsal column, resulting in spastic paralysis and the loss of tactile, vibration, and limb position senses ipsilaterally, and damage to the spinothalamic tract, resulting in the loss of pain and temperature senses contralaterally (Fig. 21–3). Lesions involving the ventral white commissure result in the loss of pain and temperature sensations bilaterally in approximately the same dermatomes as the lesion. This phenomenon usually results from syringomyelia or cavitation of the spinal cord and is called the commissural syndrome (Fig. 21–4).

BRAINSTEM

The major long paths in the brainstem are the pyramidal or corticospinal tract, spinothalamic tract, medial lemniscus, spinal trigeminal tract, and the superior cerebellar peduncle. The level of a brainstem lesion is most readily identified by the cranial nerve involved in the lesion. In general, focal brainstem lesions can be divided into two groups—those located in the medial parts and those located in the lateral parts of the medulla, pons, or midbrain.

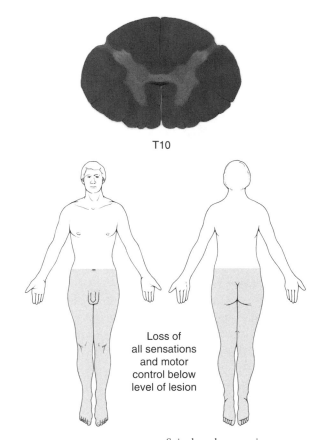

T10

Loss of
all sensations
and motor
control below
level of lesion

FIGURE 21-1.   Spinal cord transection.

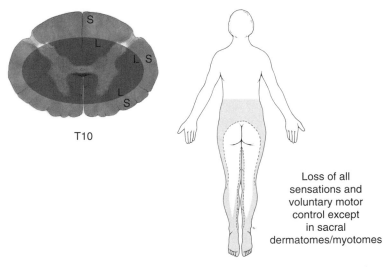

T10

Loss of all
sensations and
voluntary motor
control except
in sacral
dermatomes/myotomes

FIGURE 21-2.   Central cord syndrome: sacral sparing. (L = lumbar region, S = sacral region).

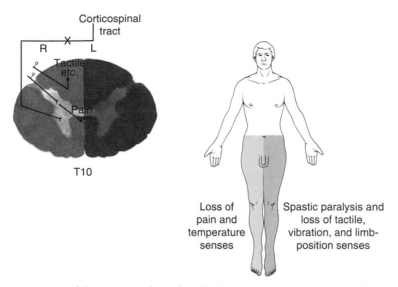

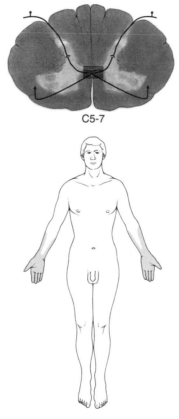

FIGURE 21–3. Left hemisection of spinal cord at T10: Spastic paralysis and loss of tactile, vibration, and limb position senses on left (ipsilateral) side and loss of pain and temperature senses on right (contralateral) side.

FIGURE 21–4. Commissural syndrome: Lesion of ventral white commissure results in bilaterally symmetrical loss of pain and temperature in dermatomal distribution of spinal cord segments involved.

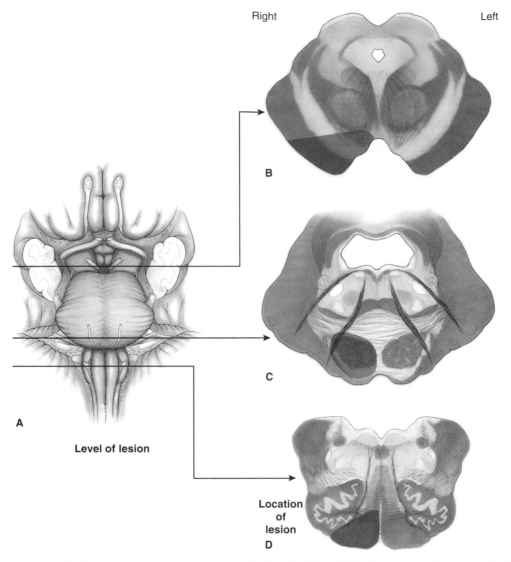

FIGURE 21–5. Medial brainstem lesions at the levels of III CN, VI CN, and XII CN. **A.** Level of lesion. **B.** III CN and pyramidal tract lesion. **C.** VI CN and pyramidal tract lesion. **D.** XII CN and pyramidal tract lesion. **E.** Oculomotor palsy. **F.** Abducent palsy. **G.** Hypoglossal palsy. **H.** Spastic weakness, more severe distally in upper and lower limbs.

MEDIAL BRAINSTEM LESIONS

Lesions located in the medial part of the brainstem involve the pyramidal tract and result in a contralateral spastic hemiplegia. The level of the lesion can be determined by involvement of the hypoglossal, abducent, or oculomotor nerve (Fig. 21–5), all of which emerge close to the pyramidal tract.

LATERAL BRAINSTEM LESIONS

Lesions involving the lateral part of the brainstem usually involve the spinothalamic tract. In the medulla and caudal pons, the spinothalamic and spinal trigeminal tracts are close to each other. When a lesion involves both tracts, pain and temperature sensations are impaired in the face ipsilaterally and the trunk and limbs contralaterally (Fig. 21–6). The level of such a lesion can be determined by involvement of cranial nerves VII, VIII, IX, or X.

Lateral brainstem lesions at more rostral levels involve, in addition to the spinothalamic tract, the motor and principal trigeminal nuclei at midpons (Fig. 21–6), the superior cerebellar peduncle at rostral pons (Fig. 21–7) and caudal midbrain, and

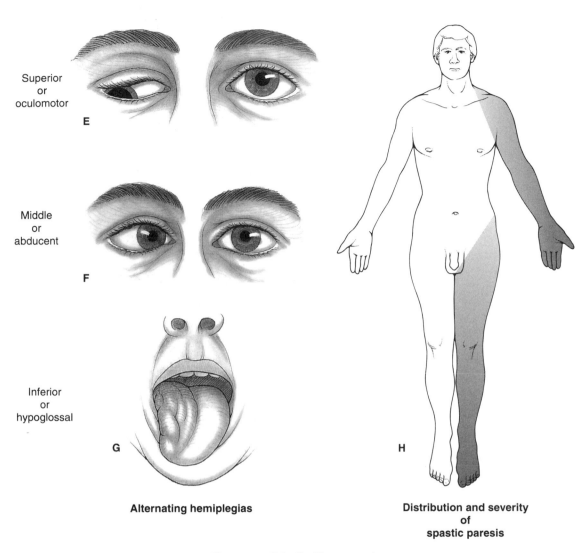

Superior
or
oculomotor

E

Middle
or
abducent

F

Inferior
or
hypoglossal

G

Alternating hemiplegias

H

**Distribution and severity
of
spastic paresis**

FIGURE 21–5 (CONTINUED).

the medial lemniscus and trigeminothalamic tracts at rostral midbrain (Fig. 21–8).

CEREBRAL HEMISPHERE

Focal lesions involving the long paths in the cerebral hemisphere are manifested on the contralateral side of the body. The most common site of long pathway involvement in the cerebral hemisphere is the internal capsule where the pyramidal tract and thalamic so-matosensory radiations are adjacent to each other, and the corticobulbar tract is nearby (Fig. 15–5A). Such a lesion results in contralateral spastic hemiplegia, contralateral hemianesthesia, and contralateral lower face weakness (Fig. 21–9), if located in the more dorsal part of the internal capsule. A more ventral capsular lesion may also involve the optic radiation (Fig. 15–5B), resulting in contralateral homonymous hemianopsia in addition to the other three abnormalities.

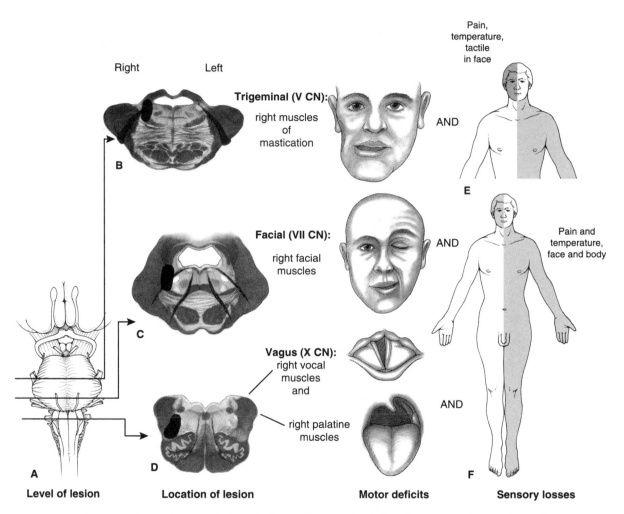

FIGURE 21-6. Lateral brainstem lesions: **A.** Level of lesion, lesion in lateral tegmentum: **B.** at midpons, **C.** at caudal pons, **D.** at rostral medulla, **E.** all somatosensations in ipsilateral face (principal nucleus and spinal trigeminal tract), pain and temperature in contralateral limbs, trunk, neck (spinothalamic tract), **F.** pain and temperature in ipsilateral face (spinal trigeminal tract), and contralateral limbs, trunk, neck (spinothalamic tract). *Dark shading:* all sensations, *Light shading:* pain and temperature only.

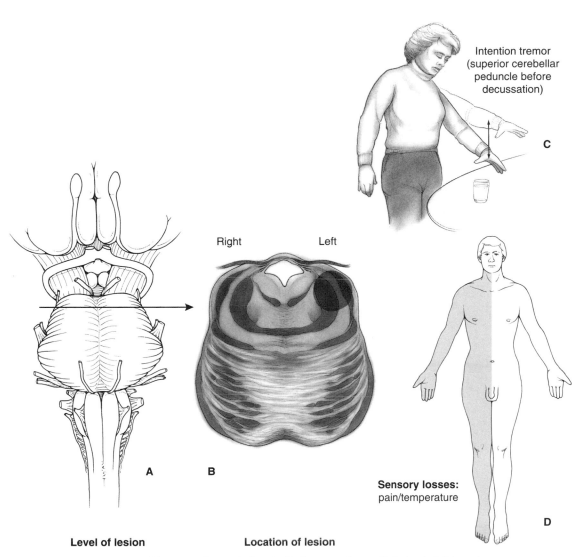

Level of lesion   **Location of lesion**

FIGURE 21–7.   Lateral brainstem lesion: **A.** Level of lesion: rostral pons. **B.** lesion in left lateral tegmentum. **C.** ipsilateral (left) intention tremor (left superior cerebellar peduncle before decussation). **D.** contralateral (right) pain and temperature losses (left spinothalamic tract).

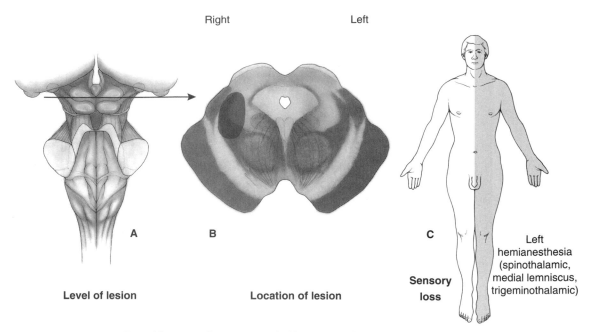

FIGURE 21-8. Lateral brainstem lesion. **A.** Level of lesion: rostral midbrain. **B.** lesion in right somatosensory paths. **C.** contralateral (left) hemisensory loss.

Right   Left

Left hemianesthesia (spinothalamic, medial lemniscus, trigeminothalamic)

Level of lesion   **Location of lesion**   **Sensory loss**

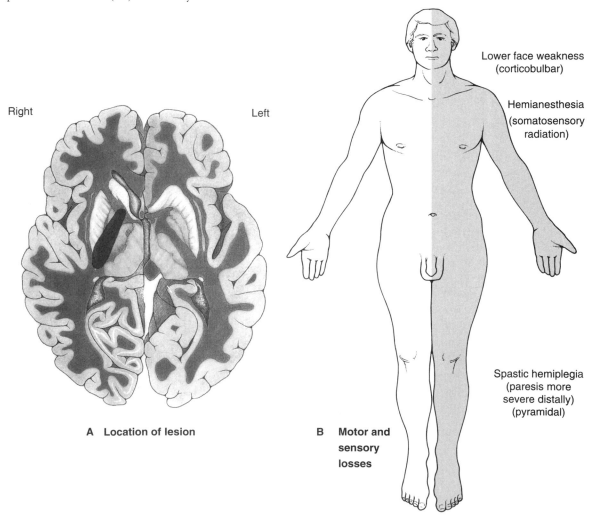

Right   Left

Lower face weakness (corticobulbar)

Hemianesthesia (somatosensory radiation)

Spastic hemiplegia (paresis more severe distally) (pyramidal)

A   Location of lesion   **B   Motor and sensory losses**

FIGURE 21-9. Lesion of long paths in internal capsule. **A.** Location of lesion in horizontal section. **B.** Motor and sensory losses.

CLINICAL ILLUSTRATIONS

1. An 11-year-old girl complained of pain in the neck and the left shoulder and had a fever of 102° to 103°F. A few days later the left arm, forearm, and hand were paralyzed; the muscles flaccid. Reflexes in the left upper limb were absent. Motor control of other parts of the body were intact. After 4 weeks, the forearm and the hand could be slightly extended by voluntary effort, but no other voluntary movement of these parts could be executed. The paralyzed muscles remained flaccid and showed marked atrophy.

    a. Localize the site of the lesion.
    b. What historical condition was frequently responsible for this clinical picture?

2. A 29-year-old woman, who since the birth of her fourth child 2 years ago had been taking birth control pills, suddenly experienced double vision and weakness in her right upper and lower limbs. Neurologic examination showed right upper and lower limb weakness accompanied by increased resistance to passive stretch, exaggerated tendon reflexes, and an extensor plantar response. In addition, she had a loss of two-point, vibration, and limb position senses on the right side in the upper and lower limbs, trunk, and neck and a loss of pin prick sensations on the right side of her face. A corneal reflex on the right could be elicited from either eye. The left side of her face sagged, and she was unable to close the left eye or retract the left side of her mouth. Although her eyes converged for near vision and she could look up and down, she could not look to the left and her left eye was deviated medially. In attempting to gaze to the right, the right eye abducted normally, but the left eye did not adduct.

    a. In a labeled sketch at the level of the lesion, name and locate precisely the structures involved and tell which abnormality is associated with each structure.
    b. Account for the loss of pain in the right eye but the presence of a corneal reflex on stimulating this eye.
    c. Account for the ability of the right eye to turn medially for near vision but not when the patient attempted to gaze to the left.
    d. Account for the adductor paralysis of the left eye during gaze to the right.
    e. If these phenomena are a result of a vascular occlusion (thrombosis), which major brain artery is most likely involved?

3. A middle-aged woman appeared in the clinic because of difficulties in walking and a sagging of the corner of her mouth. Her history showed that these abnormalities were the latest in a long series of events. About 5 years previously, the woman had a series of dizzy spells and complained of tinnitus in the right ear. Several years later the noise disappeared and the patient noticed a hearing loss in the same ear. Somewhat later she found it difficult to close her right eye tightly, and the corner of her mouth on the right side began to droop and did not rise when she smiled. Recently, she experienced intermittent painful sensations in the right side of her face, and now it has become numb. Within the past several weeks, she noticed a tendency to sway to the right, and while walking she often staggered and sometimes fell to the right. These recent events have been accompanied by difficulty in swallowing and hoarseness. Neurologic examination also revealed a loss of taste on the right side of her tongue. No corneal reflex could be elicited from the right eye.

    a. Locate the lesion.
    b. Name the structures involved and specify which abnormality is associated with each.
    c. What is the probable etiology of the lesion?

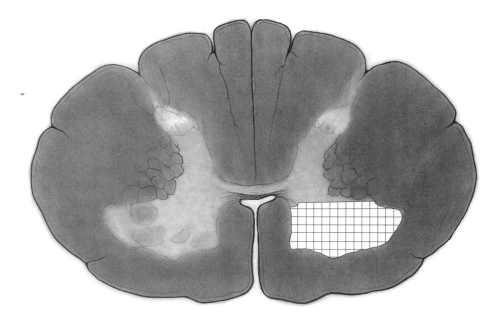

1. a. The extent of the paralysis indicates that the lesion is on the left side and extends from C5–T1 segments inclusively.
   b. Acute anterior poliomyelitis was an infective disease that resulted in degenerative lesions mainly affecting the α-motoneurons in the anterior horn of the spinal cord.

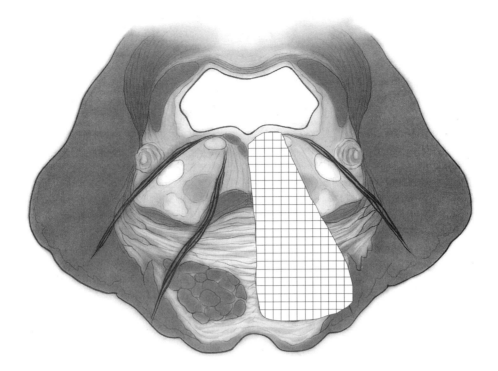

2. a. Level: caudal pons
Structures and Abnormalities: Left corticospinal—weakness in the right upper and lower limbs with increased resistance to passive stretch, exaggerated tendon re-flexes, and an extensor plantar response
Left medial lemniscus: Loss of two-point, vibration, and limb position senses in the upper and lower limbs, trunk, and neck on the right side
Left trigeminothalamic tract: Loss of pin prick on the right side of the face
Left ascending root of facial nerve: Paralysis of the left facial muscles (upper and lower)
Left abducent nucleus and nerve: Left eye esotropia and paralysis of abduction
Left paramedian pontine reticular formation (PPRF): paralysis of gaze to the left
   b. Loss of pain in right eye is due to left trigeminothalamic tract injury. The corneal reflex involves the spinal trigeminal tract and its nucleus as well as interneurons in the reticular formation that carry impulses to the facial nucleus; the trigeminothal-amic tract is not involved in the corneal reflex.
   c. The right eye turns medially during convergence, which does not involve the hor-izontal gaze center PPRF. It does not turn medially on attempting to gaze to the left because the damaged left PPRF results in paralysis of gaze to the left.
   d. The adductor paralysis of the left eye during gaze to the right is due to a lesion of left medial longitudinal fasciculus (MLF).
   e. Basilar artery

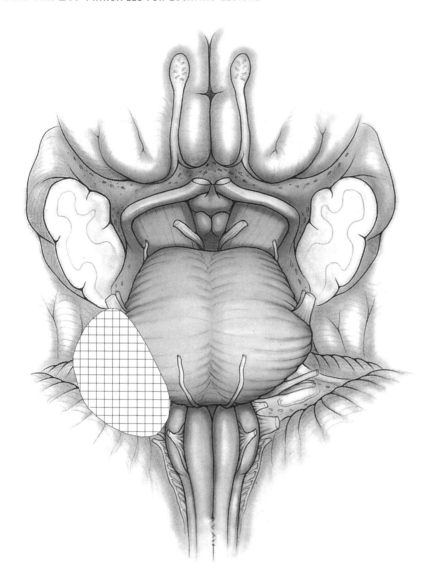

3. a. Location: cerebellar angle
   b. Structures and Abnormalities:
       1. Vestibular nerve (dizziness)
       2. Cochlear nerve (tinnitus → deafness)
       3. Facial nerve (facial paralysis)
       4. Trigeminal nerve (face pain and numbness)
       5. Cerebellum and inferior cerebellar peduncle (ataxia)
       6. Glossopharyngeal and vagus nerve (swallowing—hoarseness)
       7. Facial and glossopharyngeal nerves (taste)
       8. Facial or trigeminal nerve (corneal reflex loss)
   c. Acoustic neurinoma (starting along vestibular nerve just inside internal acoustic
      meatus—proceeding to cerebellar angle)

4. The patient is a 45-year-old hypertensive man who suddenly collapsed. He was immediately hospitalized and it was noted at that time that he had a generalized flaccid paralysis of the right limbs with no response to tendon stimulation. Examination 3 weeks later showed a spastic hemiplegia on the right side of the body. An extensor plantar response was present on the right side, and tendon reflexes of the right limbs were exaggerated, and resistance to passive movements was increased. A weakness of the lower facial muscles on the right was also noted. Pin prick was not sharp and was poorly localized and a loss of tactile and position senses on the right side of the entire body was evident. In addition, he had a right homonymous hemianopsia.

   a. In a labeled sketch at the level of the lesion, name and locate precisely the structures involved and tell which abnormality is associated with each structure.
   b. Explain the initial flaccid paralysis in the right limbs.
   c. Account for: (1) the weakness of the right lower facial muscles and not the upper and (2) the presence of decreased sensation to pin prick, but the complete absence of tactile and position senses on the right side.
   d. What is a common etiology for this clinical picture?
   e. Describe the pathologic process and common sites of involvement.

5. Locate and describe six neurologic abnormalities you would expect to find in a conscious patient immediately after the right halves of spinal cord segments C8 and T1 are destroyed by a bullet.

   a. How would the abnormalities differ 3 months after the injury?

6. A 56-year-old woman, a heavy cigarette smoker for 35 years, experienced difficulties in walking and in using her right arm, both of which became progressively worse over a period of 4 months. Examination showed an intention tremor and dysmetria in her right upper and lower limbs while she was performing the finger-to-nose and heel-to-shin tests. In addition, she had difficulty with heel-to-toe walking and tended to veer toward the right. She was unable to supinate and pronate her right arm repetitively for even short periods of time. Although the myotatic reflexes and resistance to passive movements in her right limbs were slightly reduced, neither paralysis nor sensory disturbances were found in these limbs or in any other part of her body. A chest radiograph taken immediately after the physical examination showed a mass in her left lung, and a computed tomography scan of her head showed a CNS mass.

   a. Where would you expect the CNS mass to be located, and what structure or structures would be involved?
   b. Why did the abnormalities occur only when the patient performed a volitional movement?
   c. Define the term "ataxia."
   d. What is the likely etiology?

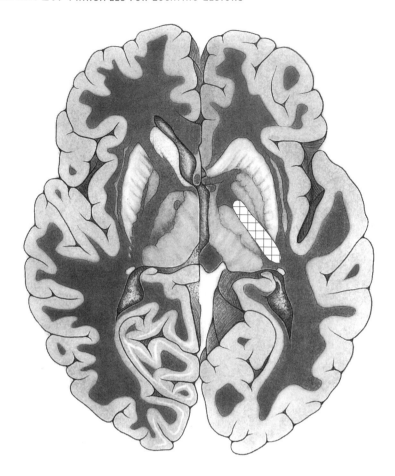

4. a. Level: posterior limb of the internal capsule
   Structures and Abnormalities:
   1. Left corticospinal tract: Right spastic hemiplegia
   2. Left corticobulbar tract: Right lower facial muscle weakness
   3. Left thalamocortical radiation: Pin prick not sharp and poorly localized and severe loss of tactile and position senses on the entire right side of the body
   4. Left geniculocalcarine tract: Right homonymous hemianopsia
   b. Initial flaccid paralysis in right limbs due to CNS shock phenomenon in right lower motor neurons immediately after sudden release from cortical control
   c. The corticobulbar tract influences the upper facial nucleus (for the upper facial muscles) bilaterally but influences the lower facial nucleus only contralaterally. Decreased sensation to pin prick occurs because the pain paths in the brainstem and forebrain are diffuse; hence, only precise localization, intensity, and sharpness of pin prick (the cortical phenomena) are lost with a lesion of the path distal to the thalamus.
   d. Hypertensive intracerebral hemorrhage related to longstanding high blood pressure
   e. Small vessel disease especially microaneurysm formation in the distribution of perforating arteries, most frequently lateral striate.

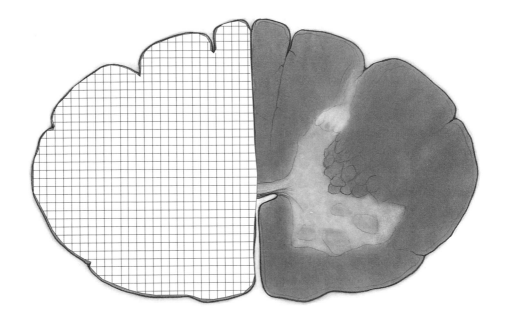

5. Abnormalities and Structures:
   a. Immediately after hemisection:
      1. Flaccid paralysis in the right hand (right anterior horn)
      2. Flaccid paralysis in right lower limb (right lateral corticospinal tract)
      3. Loss of two-point, vibration, and limb position senses on the right side from the sole of the foot up the lower limb and trunk to the axilla and medial surface of the upper limb (right gracile and cuneate tracts)
      4. Decreased pain and temperature sensations in the skin on the medial surface of the right upper limb (right tract of Lissauer)
      5. Loss of pain and temperature sensations on the left side from the sole of the foot up the lower limb and trunk to about the second rib (right spinothalamic tract)
      6. Right ptosis, miosis of the right eye and anhidrosis on the right side of the face: Horner syndrome (right ciliospinal center)
   b. 3 months later:
      1. Paralysis and severe atrophy of the intrinsic muscles in the right hand (lower motor neuron syndrome)
      2. Right lower limb paralysis accompanied by increased resistance to passive stretch, exaggerated myotatic reflexes, clonus and extensor plantar response (upper motor neuron syndrome)
      3. Would remain the same

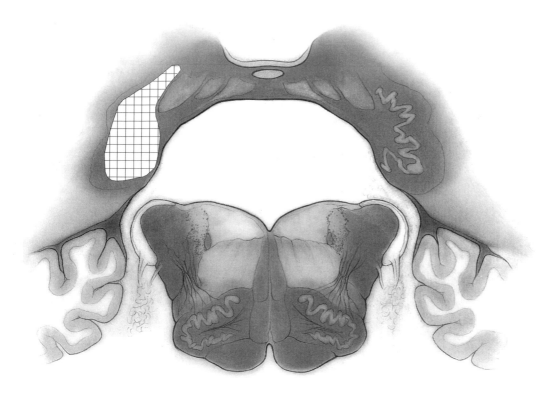

6. a. Level: cerebellum

    Structure: right dentate nucleus

   b. Cerebellar abnormalities are present only when volitional movements are commanded or initiated.

   c. Ataxia is the loss of muscular coordination.

   d. Metastatic carcinoma of lung

7. A 63-year-old man has been bothered by the shaking of his hands and generalized stiffness of his body, which have become progressively more severe over the past 3 years. On entering the examining room he moves slowly and deliberately, shuffling his feet, his shoulders and trunk are stooped forward, and his arms are at his sides and not swinging. During the ensuing history and physical examination his face remains mask-like with no changes of expression. In both hands, a resting tremor of the pill-rolling type stops only when the patient performs a voluntary movement such as lighting a cigarette or picking up a pencil. Examination reveals the presence of lead-pipe rigidity manifested by a generalized hypertonicity with greatly increased resistance to passive movement. Although the patient moves infrequently, examination reveals no paralysis or sensory disturbances in any part of the body.

   a. Locate the lesion and name the structure or structures involved.
   b. Define the term "dyskinesia."
   c. Which are the positive signs and which are the negative signs manifested by this patient?
   d. Name the likely diagnosis and the rationale for the pharmaceutical and the surgical treatments of this condition.

8. A 28-year-old man was involved in a one-car, high-speed automobile accident. There was no loss of consciousness and no known head injury at the time, and his only complaint thereafter was aching in his neck and left shoulder. He had no other problems until 5 days later when he awoke with dizziness, nausea, vomiting, and an unsteady gait. He was hospitalized 8 hours later.

   Neurologic examination revealed a left Horner syndrome. The left gag reflex was absent. Prominent ataxia was noted in the left arm and leg, but strength was normal. Sensation to pin prick was decreased over the left side of the face and over the neck, trunk, and limbs on the right side. The patient could not stand without falling to the left. His upper and lower limb reflexes were symmetric, and the plantar responses were flexor. After 6 days he was discharged from the hospital with a left Horner syndrome, mild left arm and leg dysmetria, and a mildly ataxic gait. All signs and symptoms resolved over the next 4 weeks.

   Seven weeks after the injury, he experienced sudden onset of dysphagia, unsteadiness of gait, and left ptosis—all precipitated by lifting a light load. These signs and symptoms lasted about 10 minutes. He was readmitted to the hospital and angiography revealed partial occlusion of a blood vessel. He was discharged and instructed to refrain from heavy lifting. Eight months later, examination was normal and he was asymptomatic.

   a. In a labeled sketch at the level of the lesion, name and locate precisely the structures involved and tell which abnormality is associated with each structure.
   b. What blood vessel was partially occluded?

9. A woman, 20 years of age, who had suffered from endocarditis, suddenly fainted and remained unconscious for several hours. On awakening, she was unable to speak although she could say "damn!" repetitively when she was frustrated with being unable to speak. She was able to print words to form sentences with her left hand, but not with her right hand, which was flaccid and paralyzed. Several months later, the loss of speech persisted and she showed a spastic weakness of the right arm and hand with increased resistance to passive movement and exaggerated tendon reflexes. The lower facial muscles on the right side were paralyzed.

   a. Locate the lesion, name the structures involved, and tell which abnormality is associated with each structure.
   b. If this patient's symptoms are the result of a vascular accident (hemorrhage or thrombosis), which artery is most likely involved?
   c. Define the term "aphasia."

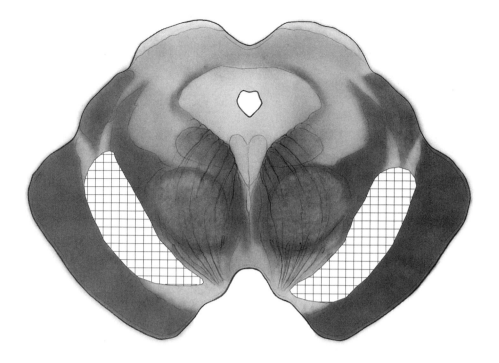

7. a. Level: midbrain

   Structure: substantia nigra (pars compacta)

   b. Dyskinesia is a disorder of movement that occurs spontaneously and is usually associated with basal ganglia disease.

   c. Positive signs: Resting tremor, lead-pipe rigidity. Negative signs: slow movements (bradykinesia), shoulders and trunk stooped forward, arms at sides and not swinging, and mask-like facial expression

   d. Paralysis agitans (Parkinson disease)—pharmaceutical treatment with levodopa replaces the dopamine in the striatum. Surgical procedures: Transplantation of fetal dopamine-producing tissue (suprarenal medulla) has shown some success. Cryosurgical lesions of the pallidothalamic path in the motor thalamus and of the medial segment of the pallidum have also been used successfully.

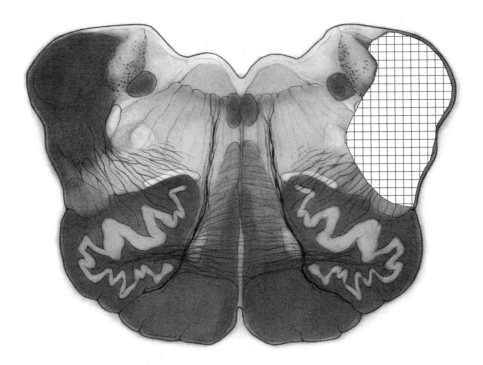

8. a. Level: Rostral medulla
   Structures and Abnormalities:
   Left spinal trigeminal tract: Decreased pin prick in left side of face
   Left spinothalamic tract: Decreased pin prick in neck, trunk, and limbs on right side
   Left inferior cerebellar peduncle: Ataxia and dysmetria in left limbs
   Left vagus nerve rootlets: Absence of left gag reflex
   Interruption of fibers in left lateral reticular formation carrying descending input to ciliospinal center: Left Horner syndrome
   b. Vertebral artery, possibly posterior inferior cerebellar artery (lateral medullary or Wallenberg syndrome)

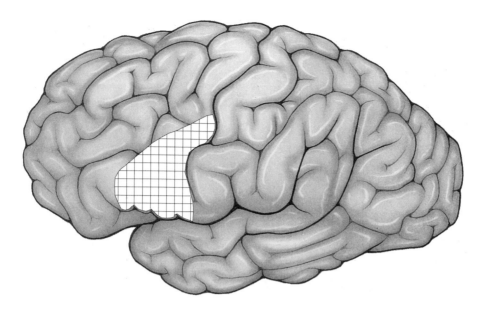

9. a. Level: Cerebral cortex
   Structures and Abnormalities:
   Broca speech area in left inferior frontal gyri: Loss of speech (motor aphasia)
   Ventral part of the left precentral gyrus: Spastic weakness of right hand and weakness of right lower facial muscles
   b. Middle cerebral artery: Branches to the inferior frontal and ventral precentral areas
   c. Aphasia is the inability to understand or communicate speech, writing, or signs.

10. A 63-year-old man complained of brief episodes lasting about a minute during which he experienced an unpleasant odor or a feeling of anxiety and fear. Immediately following these episodes, he felt as if he was in a dream-like state in which he heard and saw things that he had experienced before. He was aware that he was unable to understand what other people were saying to him during these episodes. While experiencing the puzzling episodes, he looked preoccupied, and sometimes his lips and tongue moved as if he had a hair in his mouth. Examination fails to reveal any abnormality except a visual field defect.

    a. Where is the lesion?
    b. What do the episodes represent?
    c. Locate the structures associated with the
        1. Unpleasant odor
        2. Anxiety and fear
        3. "Déjà vu" phenomenon
        4. Lip and tongue movements
    d. What visual field defect would you expect?

11. A 15-year-old girl became obese and listless during the past year. She also had episodes of high fever without apparent cause and cessation of her menstrual period for several months. She drank copious amounts of water because she was always thirsty and she urinated excessively. Neurologic examination revealed an obese girl with a visual field defect.

    a. Where is the lesion?
    b. Locate the structures associated with the
        1. Fever
        2. Obesity
        3. Listlessness
        4. Dysmenorrhea
        5. Thirst and polyuria
    c. What visual field defect would you expect?

12. A professional hockey player complained that his leg felt so tired he could hardly walk, much less play hockey. Neurologic examination showed marked weakness in the left leg and foot accompanied by an extensor plantar response, increased resistance to passive stretch, and exaggerated knee and ankle jerks. Pin prick was not as sharp or well localized below the knee in the left lower limb as compared to the rest of the body. In addition, with his eyes closed, passive flexion and extension of his left leg, foot, and toes were incorrectly described and the other more discriminative touch senses (tactile localization and two-point sense) in his leg, foot, and toes were also severely impaired.

    a. Give the level and location of the lesion and identify the structures involved in the above abnormalities.
    b. If vascular in nature, what artery would be involved?

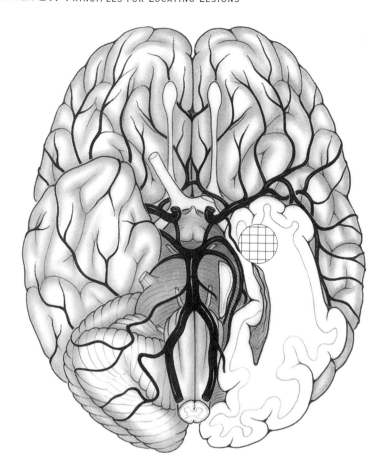

10. a. Level: Temporal lobe—tumor deep to uncus and parahippocampal gyrus
    b. Temporal lobe epilepsy
    c. Structures:
        1. Unpleasant odor—olfactory center at uncus
        2. Anxiety and fear—temporal pole
        3. Déjà vu—middle and posterior temporal cortex (memory)
        4. Lips and tongue movements—amygdala
        5. Inattention—hippocampal formation
    d. Contralateral upper homonymous quadrantic anopsia—loop of Meyer

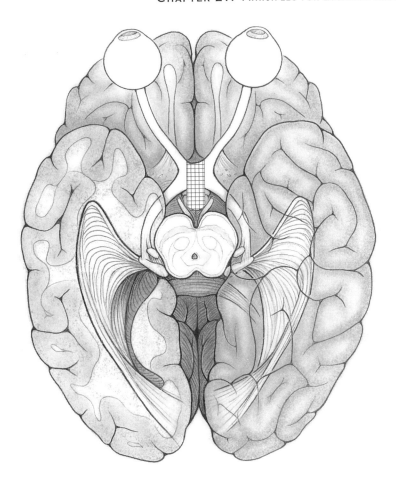

11. a. Level: Hypothalamus (case of craniopharyngioma)
    b. Abnormalities and Structures:
       1. Fever—preoptic area
       2. Obesity—tuberal area (ventromedial nucleus)
       3. Listlessness—posterior hypothalamus
       4. Dysmenorrhea—tuberal area (releasing factors for anterior pituitary)
       5. Thirst and polyuria—supraoptic and paraventricular nuclei (diabetes insipidus)
    c. Visual field defect: bitemporal heteronymous hemianopsia

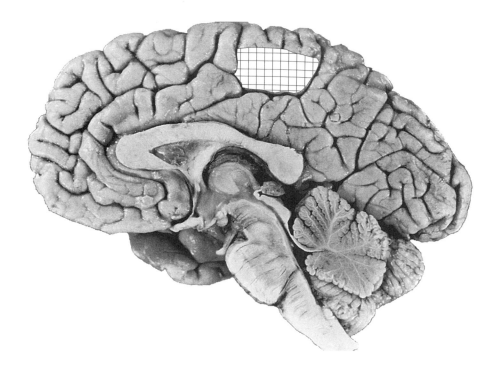

12. a. Level: Cerebral cortex
       Structures and Abnormalities:
         Anterior part of right paracentral lobule: Spastic weakness, etc. in left leg and foot
         Posterior part of right paracentral lobule: Somatosensory loss in left leg and foot
    b. Vascular supply: Right anterior cerebral artery

13. Robert's college friends noticed that his head tilted to the left. Later Robert noticed a tremor when he attempted a movement, and, when reaching for a glass of soda, he would often knock it over. Disturbed, he went to see a neurologist. On examination, his right eye did not depress fully when adducted. Intention tremor, dysmetria, and dysdiadochokinesia were noted in his right upper and lower limbs. Robert also presented the inability to adduct the left eye when he gazed to the right; but it did adduct when vision was shifted from a far object to a near object.

    a. Locate the level of the lesion and identify the structures for which each abnormality is given.
    b. Why did Robert's head tilt to the left?
    c. What is the likely diagnosis?

14. After sustaining too many blows to the head while playing racquetball, Mary presented with the following abnormalities: She had a left lower homonymous quadrantic anopsia and was unaware of the left side of her body and its surroundings.

    a. In a labeled sketch identify the level and area of the lesion, and name the structures involved and the abnormalities associated with each.
    b. A branch of which blood vessel was most likely damaged?

15. A man came into the city hospital one morning after an evening of excessive drinking. Shortly after a fall in which he struck his head, he complained of inability to use his left eye, and his left upper eyelid drooped. Later, his left eyelid was entirely closed, and, when the eyelid was lifted, the eye was turned down and out. Weakness was noted in the right upper and lower limbs. Examination revealed that muscle tone and reflexes in the right limbs were increased. A Babinski response was detected on the right side. The left pupil was fixed in the dilated position, whereas the right pupil responded normally to increased light intensity in either eye. When the patient smiled, no elevation occurred on the right side of the mouth.

    a. In a labeled sketch at the level of the lesion, name and locate precisely the structures involved and tell which abnormality is associated with each structure.
    b. Explain why the left eye was closed and turned down and out.
    c. Explain why only the right pupil responded to increased light in the left eye.

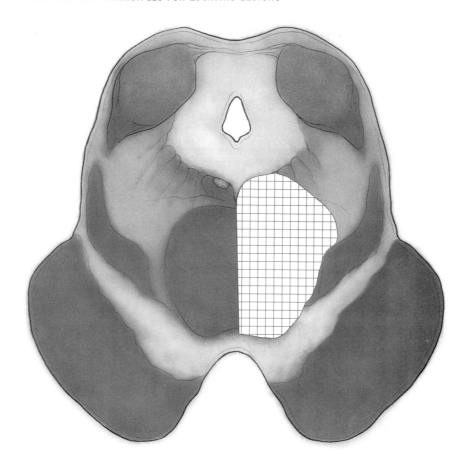

13. a. Level: Inferior colliculus (distal to the decussation of the superior cerebellar peduncle

    Left superior cerebellar peduncle: Intention tremor, dysmetria and dysdiadochokinesia in right limbs

    Left trochlear nucleus: Right eye, when adducted, has weakness in depression

    Left MLF: Left internuclear ophthalmoplegia (left eye does not adduct on gaze to right)

  b. With trochlear lesions the affected eye is slightly extorted and the person compensates by tilting the head downward to the opposite side.

  c. Demyelinating process such as multiple sclerosis

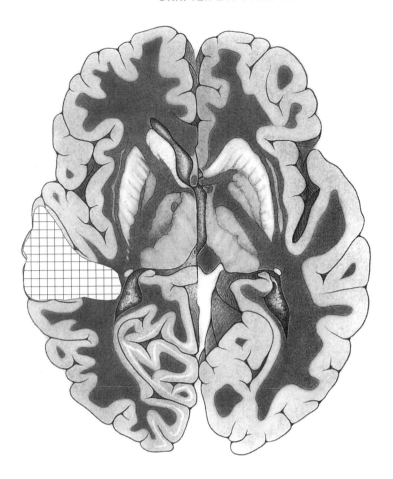

14. a. Level: Parietal lobe
    Structures and Abnormalities:
    Dorsal part of right optic radiation: Lower left homonymous quadrantic anopsia
    Right posterior parietal lobe: Neglect of left side of body and surroundings
    b. Vascular supply: Middle cerebral artery

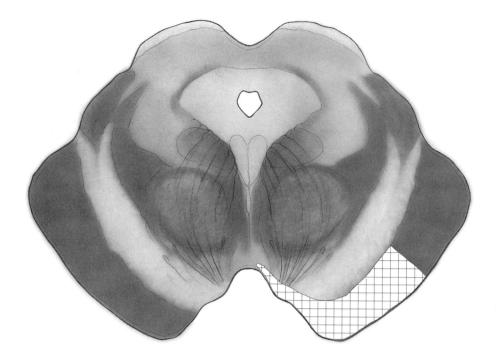

15. a. Level: Superior colliculus
    Structures and Abnormalities:
    Left corticospinal tract: Weakness in the right upper and lower limbs with increased muscle tone, reflexes, and a Babinski response
    Left corticobulbar tract: Paralysis of the right lower facial muscles
    Left oculomotor nerve: Left ptosis, left eye turned down and out, and left pupil dilated
  b. The oculomotor nerve innervates all the eye muscles except the superior oblique and the lateral rectus muscles, which depress and abduct the eye, respectively. With paralysis of the superior levator the eyelid droops severely.
  c. The left optic nerve and right oculomotor nerve are intact, but the left oculomotor nerve (containing the pupilloconstrictor fibers) is not.

Appendix A

CRANIAL NERVE COMPONENTS AND LESIONS

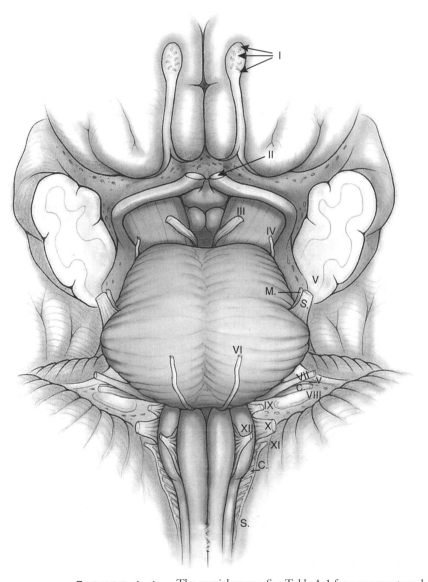

I Olfactory
II Optic
III Oculomotor
IV Trochlear
V Trigeminal
    M. Motor Root
    S. Sensory Root
VI Abducent
VII Facial
VIII Vestibulocochlear
IX Glossopharyngeal
X Vagus
XI Accessory
    C. Cranial
    S. Spinal
XII Hypoglossal

FIGURE A-1. The cranial nerves. See Table A-1 for components and distributions.

SUMMARY: SPECIAL SENSORY CRANIAL NERVES

NERVE	FUNCTION	ORIGIN	PERIPHERAL DISTRIBUTION	CENTRAL CONNECTIONS	SIGNS
I Olfactory	Olfaction or smell	Olfactory epithelium	Superior nasal concha and nasal septum	Olfactory bulb	Loss of sense of smell (anosmia)
II Optic	Vision	Retinal ganglion cells	Retinal bipolar cells	Lateral geniculate nuclei	Blindness
	Light reflex (afferent limb)	Retinal ganglion cells	Retinal bipolar cells	Pretectal nuclei	Absence of pupillary constriction bilaterally on testing blind eye
VIII Vestibular	Balance	Vestibular ganglion	Maculae of utricle and saccule	Vestibular nuclei	Dysequilibrium
	Vestibulo-ocular reflex (afferent limb)	Vestibular ganglion	Cristae of semicir-cular ducts	Vestibular nuclei	Absence of vestibulo-ocular reflex (VOR)
Cochlear	Hearing	Spiral ganglion	Spiral organ	Cochlear nuclei	Deafness

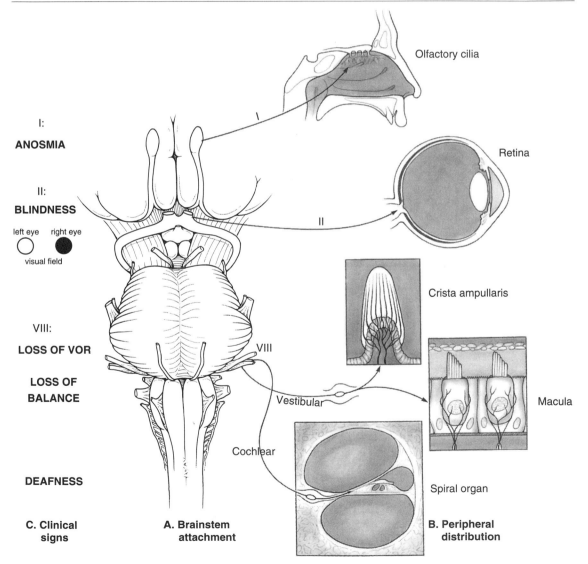

FIGURE A-2.   Special sensory cranial nerves: Olfactory, optic, and vestibulocochlear. A. Brainstem attachment; B. Peripheral distribution; C. Clinical signs.

SUMMARY: OCULAR MOTOR CRANIAL NERVES

NERVE	FUNCTION	ORIGIN	PERIPHERAL DISTRIBUTION	SIGNS
III Oculomotor	Eye movements	Oculomotor nucleus	Medial, superior, inferior recti, inferior oblique muscles	Ophthalmoplegia with eye turned down and out
	Elevation of eyelid	Oculomotor nucleus	Superior palpebral levator	Ptosis
	Pupillary constriction and accommodation	Edinger-Westphal nucleus	Ciliary ganglion; postganglionics to sphincter of pupil and ciliary muscles	Mydriasis; loss of accommodation of lens
IV Trochlear	Eye movements	Trochlear nucleus (contralateral)	Superior oblique muscle	Diplopia: extorsion of eye; weakness in depression of adducted eye
VI Abducent	Eye movements	Abducent nucleus	Lateral rectus muscle	Diplopia: medial deviation; abductor paralysis

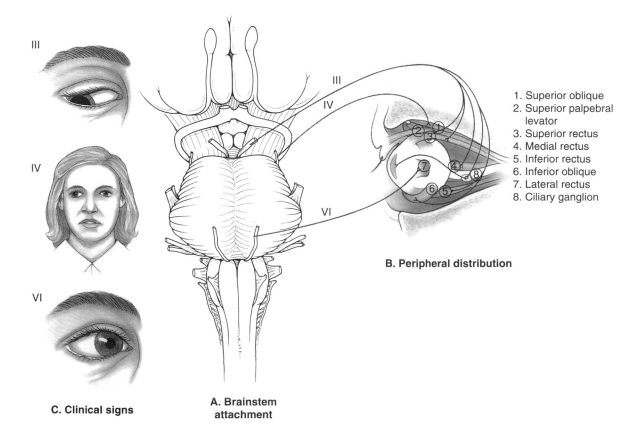

III

IV

VI

1. Superior oblique
2. Superior palpebral levator
3. Superior rectus
4. Medial rectus
5. Inferior rectus
6. Inferior oblique
7. Lateral rectus
8. Ciliary ganglion

B. Peripheral distribution

C. Clinical signs

A. Brainstem attachment

FIGURE A-3.   Ocular motor nerves: oculomotor, trochlear, and abducent. **A.** Brainstem attachment; **B.** Peripheral distribution; **C.** Clinical signs (right III, IV, VI nerves).

SUMMARY: RIGHT FACIAL HEMIANESTHESIA

NERVE	FUNCTION	ORIGIN	PERIPHERAL DISTRIBUTION	CENTRAL CONNECTIONS	SIGNS
V Trigeminal	Mastication	Motor trigeminal nucleus	Masseter, temporalis, pterygoids, mylohyoid, tensor palatini, anterior belly of digastric		Weakness of jaw; ipsilateral deviation of opened jaw
	Dampens tympanic membrane	Motor trigeminal nucleus	Tensor tympani		Insignificant
	Sensations	Trigeminal ganglion	Face, anterior scalp, oral and nasal cavities, orbit	Principal and spinal trigeminal nuclei	Facial hemianesthesia
	Proprioceptive reflexes	Mesencephalic trigeminal nucleus	Muscles of mastication, periodontal membrane, temporomandibular joint	Motor trigeminal nucleus	Insignificant

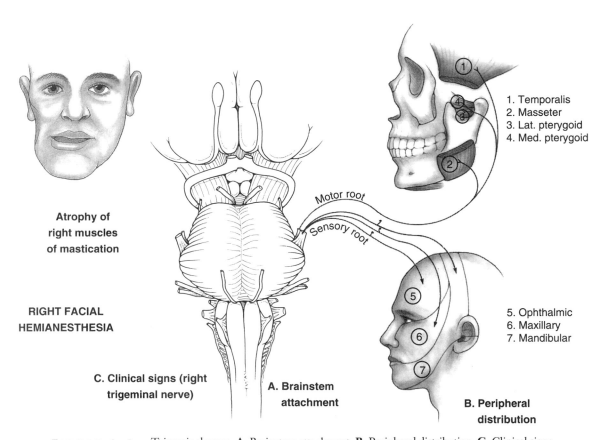

1. Temporalis
2. Masseter
3. Lat. pterygoid
4. Med. pterygoid

Motor root

Sensory root

Atrophy of right muscles of mastication

RIGHT FACIAL HEMIANESTHESIA

5. Ophthalmic
6. Maxillary
7. Mandibular

C. Clinical signs (right trigeminal nerve)

A. Brainstem attachment

B. Peripheral distribution

FIGURE A-4.   Trigeminal nerve. **A.** Brainstem attachment. **B.** Peripheral distribution. **C.** Clinical signs.

SUMMARY: FACIAL NERVE

NERVE	FUNCTION	ORIGIN	PERIPHERAL DISTRIBUTION	CENTRAL CONNECTIONS	SIGNS
VII Facial	Facial expression	Facial nucleus	Facial muscles, stylohyoid, posterior belly of digastic		Facial paralysis; loss of corneal reflex (efferent limb)
	Dampens vibrations of stapes	Facial nucleus	Stapedius		Hyperacusis
	Secretion	Superior salivatory nucleus	Pterygopalatine ganglion: secretomotor to lacrimal and nasal glands		Loss of lacrimation
			Submandibular ganglion: secretomotor to sub-mandibular and sublin-gual glands		Dry mouth
	Taste	Geniculate ganglion	Taste buds in anterior two thirds of tongue	Solitary nucleus	Loss of taste in ipsi-lateral anterior two thirds of tongue
	Sensations	Geniculate ganglion	Posterior auricular area	Spinal trigeminal nucleus	Insignificant

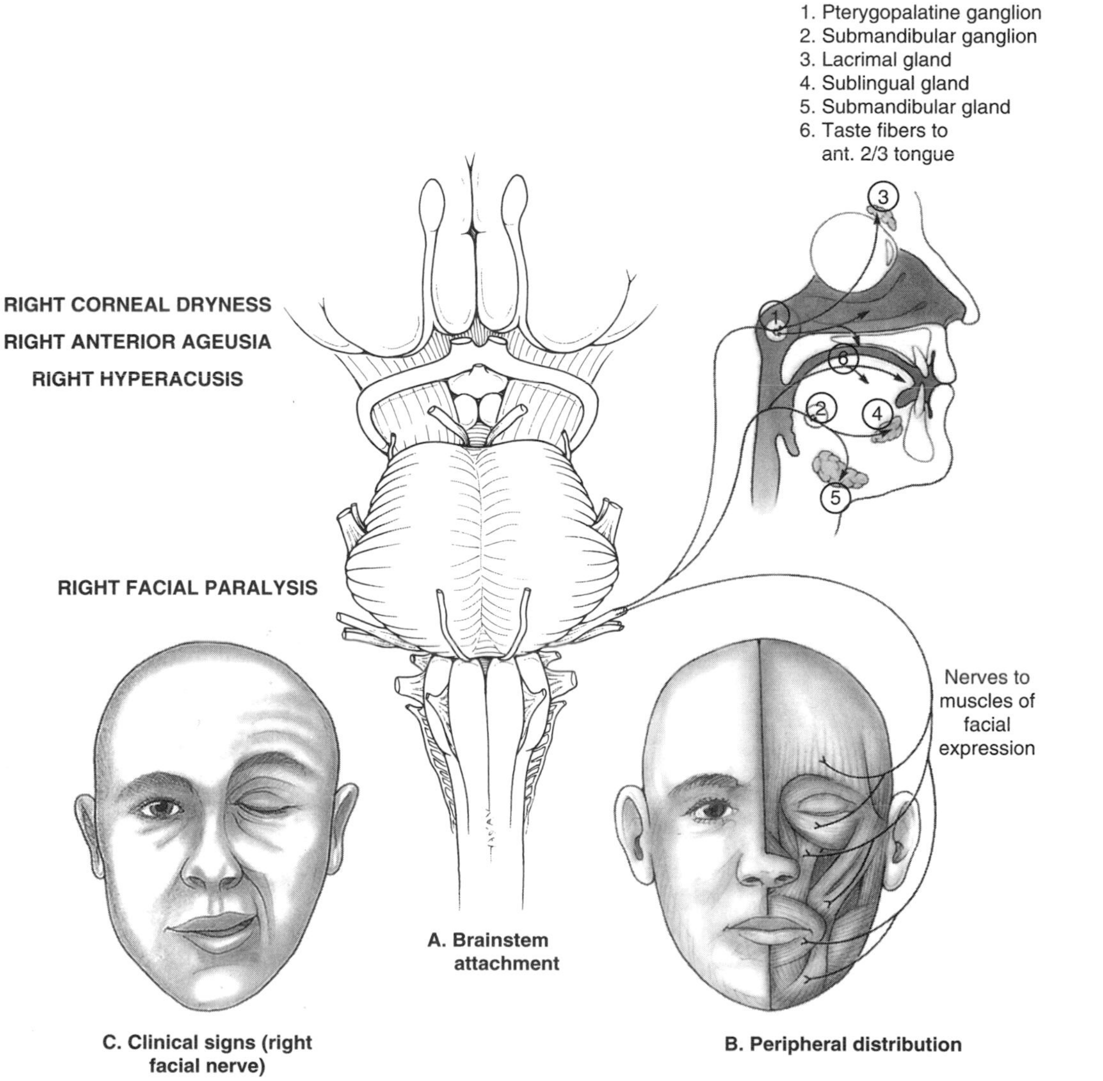

1. Pterygopalatine ganglion
2. Submandibular ganglion
3. Lacrimal gland
4. Sublingual gland
5. Submandibular gland
6. Taste fibers to ant. 2/3 tongue

RIGHT CORNEAL DRYNESS

RIGHT ANTERIOR AGEUSIA

RIGHT HYPERACUSIS

RIGHT FACIAL PARALYSIS

Nerves to muscles of facial expression

A. Brainstem attachment

C. Clinical signs (right facial nerve)

B. Peripheral distribution

FIGURE A-5. Facial nerve. **A.** Brainstem attachment. **B.** Peripheral distribution. **C.** Clinical signs.

Summary: Glossopharyngeal Nerve

Nerve	Function	Origin	Peripheral Distribution	Central Connections	Signs
IX Glosso-phanyngeal	Elevate pharynx during swallowing	Nucleus ambiguus	Stylopharyngeus and superior pharyngeal constrictor		Dysphagia
	Salivation	Inferior Salivatory nucleus	Otic ganglion: secre-tomotor to parotid		Insignificant
	Taste	Inferior (petrosal) ganglion	Posterior third of tongue	Solitary nucleus	Loss of taste in tongue posteriorly
	General sensations	Superior and inferior ganglia	Posterior oral cavity, tonsillar region, audi-tory tube, middle ear	Spinal trigeminal nucleus	Anesthesis, loss of gag reflex (affer-ent limb)
	Chemoreceptor and baroreceptor reflexes (afferent limbs)	Inferior ganglion	Carotid bulb and sinus	Solitary nucleus	Loss of carotid sinus reflex (if bilateral lesion)

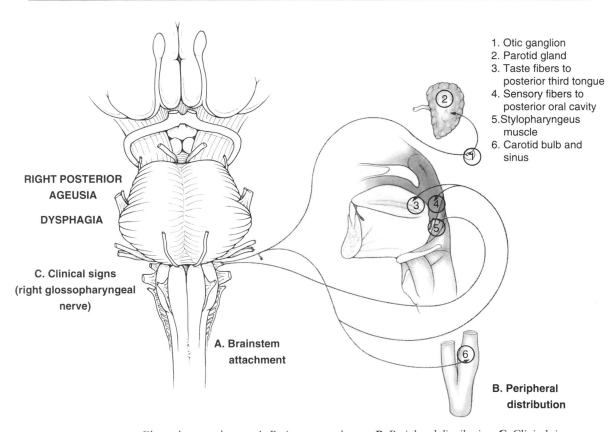

1. Otic ganglion
2. Parotid gland
3. Taste fibers to posterior third tongue
4. Sensory fibers to posterior oral cavity
5. Stylopharyngeus muscle
6. Carotid bulb and sinus

RIGHT POSTERIOR AGEUSIA

DYSPHAGIA

C. Clinical signs (right glossopharyngeal nerve)

A. Brainstem attachment

B. Peripheral distribution

Figure A-6.   Glossopharyngeal nerve. **A.** Brainstem attachment. **B.** Peripheral distribution. **C.** Clinical signs.

SUMMARY: VAGUS NERVE

NERVE	FUNCTIONS	ORIGIN	PERIPHERAL DISTRIBUTION	CENTRAL CONNECTIONS	SIGNS
X Vagus	Swallowing and vocalization	Nucleus ambiguus	Palatal muscles, pharyngeal constrictors, vocal muscles		Dysphagia, weak and hoarse voice, sagging of palatal arch, contralateral deviation of uvula
	Cardiac depressor, bronchoconstrictors, GI motility and secretion	Dorsal vagal nucleus	Terminal ganglia in cardiac, pulmonary, enteric plexuses		Insignificant if unilateral
	Taste	Inferior (nodose) ganglion	Epiglottal and palatal regions	Solitary nucleus	Insignificant
	Sensations	Inferior (nodose) ganglion	Epiglottis, larynx, respiratory tree, GI tract	Solitary nucleus	Hemianesthesia of pharynx and larynx, loss of cough reflex (afferent limb)
	Chemoreceptor and baroreceptor reflexes	Inferior (nodose) ganglion	Aortic bulb and sinus	Solitary nucleus	Insignificant if unilateral
	Sensations	Superior (jugular) ganglion	External ear and auditory canal	Spinal trigeminal nucleus	Anesthesia of external auditory canal

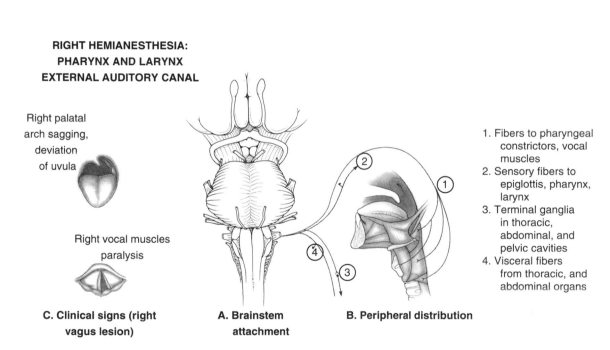

RIGHT HEMIANESTHESIA:
PHARYNX AND LARYNX
EXTERNAL AUDITORY CANAL

Right palatal
arch sagging,
deviation
of uvula

Right vocal muscles
paralysis

1. Fibers to pharyngeal constrictors, vocal muscles
2. Sensory fibers to epiglottis, pharynx, larynx
3. Terminal ganglia in thoracic, abdominal, and pelvic cavities
4. Visceral fibers from thoracic, and abdominal organs

C. Clinical signs (right vagus lesion)   **A. Brainstem attachment**   **B. Peripheral distribution**

FIGURE A-7. Vagus nerve. **A.** Brainstem attachment. **B.** Peripheral distribution. **C.** Clinical signs.

SUMMARY: ACCESORY AND HYPOGLOSSAL NERVES

NERVE	FUNCTION	ORIGIN	PERIPHERAL DISTRIBUTION	SIGNS
XI Accessory	Swallowing and vocalization	Nucleus ambiguus	Pharyngeal and vocal muscles (with vagus)	Insignificant
	Head and shoulder movements	Spinal accessory nucleus in C1-5 or C6	Sternomastoid and trapezius muscles	Weakness in turning head toward opposite side and shrugging shoulder
XII Hypoglossal	Tongue movements	Hypoglossal nucleus	Styloglossus, hyoglossus, genioglossus and intrinsic tongue muscles	Unilateral atrophy, ipsilateral deviation on protrusion, fasciculations

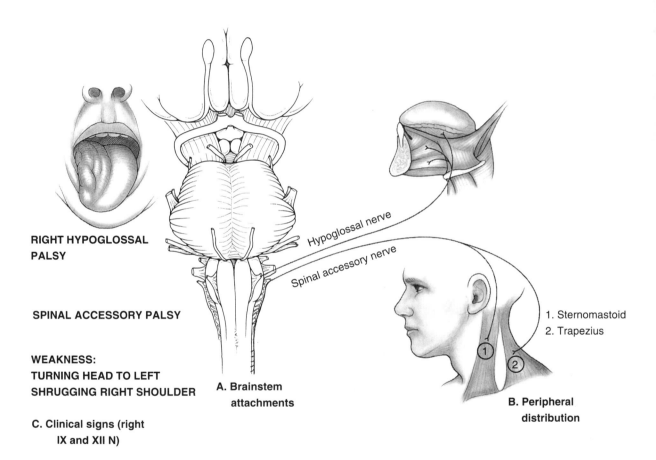

RIGHT HYPOGLOSSAL
PALSY

Hypoglossal nerve

Spinal accessory nerve

SPINAL ACCESSORY PALSY

1. Sternomastoid
2. Trapezius

WEAKNESS:
TURNING HEAD TO LEFT
SHRUGGING RIGHT SHOULDER

A. Brainstem
   attachments

B. Peripheral
   distribution

C. Clinical signs (right
   IX and XII N)

FIGURE A-8.   Accessory and hypoglossal nerves. **A.** Brainstem attachments. **B.** Peripheral distribution. **C.** Clinical signs.

TABLE A–1. CRANIAL NERVE COMPONENTS AND DISTRIBUTIONS

NERVE	CELLS OF ORIGIN	CENTRAL CONNECTIONS	PERIPHERAL DISTRIBUTION	FUNCTION	SYMPTOMS AND SIGNS OF DAMAGE
I Olfactory	Bipolar cells in olfactory epithelium (special sensory)	Olfactory bulb	Cilia at surface of olfactory epithelium in superior nasal concha and upper third of nasal septum	Smell	Anosmia
II Optic	Ganglion cells of retina (special sensory)	Lateral geniculate nuclei	Bipolar cells of retina	Vision	Blindness
		Superior colliculus and pretectal nuclei		Pupillary reflexes	Absence of light reflexes on shining light in blind eye
III Oculomotor	Oculomotor nucleus (somatic motor)		Medial, superior and inferior recti, inferior oblique, and levator palpebrae superioris	Moves the eye and elevates upper eyelid	Opthalmoplegia with eye deviated down and out, severe ptosis
	Edinger-Westphal nucleus of oculomotor complex (visceral motor)		Ciliary ganglion; postganglionics via short ciliary nerves to sphincter of pupil and ciliary muscle	Pupil constriction and accommodation of lens	Mydriasis; loss of pupillary light and accommodation reflexes in ipsilateral eye
IV Trochlear	Trochlear nucleus (somatic motor)		Superior oblique muscle	Extorsion; depression of adducted eye	Diplopia, head tilt to unaffected side; weakness in depression of ipsilateral adducted eye
V Trigeminal	Trigeminal ganglion (general sensory)	Spinal trigeminal nucleus (caudal part) and principal trigeminal nucleus	Anterior scalp, face, mucous membranes of nose and mouth, teeth, contents of orbit, tympanic membrane, supratentorial meninges	Somatosensations	Loss of facial sensations and corneal reflex on stimulation ipsilaterally
	Motor trigeminal nucleus (branchial motor)		Masseter, temporalis, pterygoids, mylohyoid, tensors tympani and palatini, anterior belly of digastric	Mastication	Weakness and wasting of muscles of mastication; deviation of opened jaw to ipsilateral side
	Mesencephalic trigeminal nucleus (general sensory)		Muscles of mastication, periodontal membrane, temporomandibular joint, and external ocular muscles	Proprioceptive reflexes	Insignificant
VI Abducent	Abducent nucleus (somatic motor)		Lateral rectus muscle	Abduction of eye	Diplopia, esotropia (convergent strabismus) and abductor paralysis of ipsilateral eye

TABLE A–1.   CRANIAL NERVE COMPONENTS AND DISTRIBUTIONS—CONTINUED

NERVE	CELLS OF ORIGIN	CENTRAL CONNECTIONS	PERIPHERAL DISTRIBUTION	FUNCTION	SYMPTOMS AND SIGNS OF DAMAGE
VII Facial	Facial nucleus (branchial motor)		Facial muscles, buccinator, stapedius, stylohyoid, posterior belly of digastric, platysma, occipitalis	Facial expression, articulation, winking, ingestion of food and drink	Paralysis of ipsilateral upper and lower facial muscles
	Superior salivatory nucleus (visceral motor)		1. Major petrosal nerve to nerve of pterygoid canal to pterygopalatine ganglion; postganglionics via maxillary nerve to lacrimal gland and mucosal glands of nasal cavity and palate	Nasal and lacrimal secretions	Loss of lacrimation
			2. Chorda tympani to lingual nerve to submandibular ganglion; postganglionics to submandibular, sublingual and lingual glands	Salivary secretion	Decreased salivation; dry mouth
	Geniculate ganglion (special sensory)	Solitary nucleus (rostral part)	Taste buds in anterior two thirds of tongue	Taste	Loss of taste in anterior two thirds of tongue ipsilaterally
	(general sensory)	Spinal trigeminal nucleus (caudal part)	Posterior auricular region, external auditory meatus, tympanic membrane	Somatosensations	Insignificant
VIII Vestibulocochlear	Vestibular ganglion (special sensory)	Vestibular nuclei and cerebellum	Hair cells of ampullary crests in semicircular ducts and maculae of saccule and utricle	Equilibrium	Vertigo, dysequilibrium, and nystagmus
	Spiral ganglion (special sensory)	Dorsal and ventral cochlear nucleus	Hair cells of spiral organ (of Corti)	Hearing	Neural deafness
IX Glossopharyngeal	Nucleus ambiguus (rostral part) (branchial motor)		Stylopharyngeus and superior pharyngeal constrictor	Elevates pharynx	Slight dysphagia
	Inferior salivatory nucleus (visceral motor)		Tympanic plexus to minor petrosal nerve to otic ganglion–postganglionics via auriculotemporal nerve to parotid gland	Salivary secretion	Partial dry mouth
	Inferior (petrosal) ganglion (special sensory)	Solitary nucleus (rostral part)	Taste buds in posterior third of tongue	Taste	Loss of taste in posterior third of tongue ipsilaterally
	(general sensory)	Spinal trigeminal nucleus	Ant. surface epiglottis, root of tongue, border of soft palate, uvula, tonsil, pharynx, auditory tube, middle ear	Somatosensations	Anesthesia of tonsillar region and loss of gag reflex from ipsilateral stimulus
	(visceral sensory)		Carotid sinus and bulb	Reflexes	Insignificant

TABLE A–1. CRANIAL NERVE COMPONENTS AND DISTRIBUTIONS—*CONTINUED*

NERVE	CELLS OF ORIGIN	CENTRAL CONNECTIONS	PERIPHERAL DISTRIBUTION	FUNCTION	SYMPTOMS AND SIGNS OF DAMAGE
X Vagus	Nucleus ambiguus (branchial motor)		Palate, pharyngeal constrictors and intrinsic muscles of larynx	Deglutition and phonation	Dysphagia, hoarseness, and paralysis of soft palate with deviation of velum and uvula to contralateral side
	Dorsal motor nucleus of vagus and region of nucleus ambiguus (visceral motor)		Cardiac nerves and plexus to ganglia of heart; pulmonary plexuses to ganglia of respiratory tree; esophageal, gastric, celiac, superior and inferior mesenteric plexuses to myenteric and submucous ganglia of digestive tract down to transverse colon	Cardiac depressor, bronchoconstrictor, GI tract peristalsis and secretion	Insignificant
	Inferior (nodose) ganglion (special sensory)	Solitary nucleus (rostral part)	Taste buds in region of epiglottis	Taste	Insignificant
	(visceral sensory)	Solitary nucleus	Posterior surface of epiglottis, pharynx, larynx, trachea, bronchi, esophagus, stomach, small intestine, ascending and transverse colon	Visceral sensations and reflexes	Anesthesia of pharynx and larynx ipsilaterally
			Aortic sinus and bulb	Reflexes	
	Superior (jugular) ganglion (general sensory)	Spinal trigeminal nucleus (caudal part)	External ear and meatus	Somatosensations	Anesthesia of ipsilateral external auditory meatus
XI Accessory cranial part:	Nucleus ambiguus (caudal part) (branchial motor)		Communicates with vagal branches to muscles of pharynx and larynx	Deglutition and phonation	Insignificant
spinal part:	Motoneurons of spinal accessory nucleus in C1–5 or C6 (somatic motor)		Sternomastoid and trapezius muscles	Movements of head and shoulder	Weakness in shrugging ipsilateral shoulder and turning head to opposite side
XII Hypoglossal	Hypoglossal nucleus (somatic motor)		Styloglossus, hyoglossus, genioglossus and intrinsic muscles of tongue	Movements of tongue	Wasting of ipsilateral tongue muscles and deviation to ipsilateral side on protrusion

Appendix B

ANSWERS TO CHAPTER QUESTIONS

CHAPTER 1 INTRODUCTION TO THE NERVOUS SYSTEM: ORGANIZATION, FUNCTIONAL UNITS, AND SUPPORTING STRUCTURES

1–1. The two main classes of cells in the CNS are neurons, the functional units, and neuroglia, the supporting units.

1–2. A synapse is the site of functional contact where impulses pass unidirectionally from one neuron to the other. Most synapses occur between axons and dendrites (axodendritic) or between axons and cell bodies (axosomatic). Histologically, most synapses consist of a terminal enlargement—the bouton—closely apposed to the surface of a dendrite or a neuronal cell body. Ultrastructurally, the bouton contains mitochondria and synaptic vesicles, and its synaptic surface (the presynaptic membrane) is separated from the target's surface (the postsynaptic membrane) by a gap, the synaptic cleft.

1–3. The integrity of axons, some of which may be 3 feet in length, is maintained by elaborate axoplasmic transport systems between the cell bodies, which are the metabolic centers of neurons, and the distant terminals of the axons. Anterograde axonal transport, i.e., movement from the cell body to the terminals, is of two main types: (*a*) fast transport of membranous organelles and synaptic vesicles or their precursors and (*b*) slow transport of cytoskeletal materials. Retrograde axonal transport brings worn-out synaptic materials and exogenous substances such as toxins or viruses from the axon terminals back to the cell body.

1–4. Functional regeneration following peripheral nerve lesions is common, whereas functional regeneration following lesions in the mature human CNS has never been substantiated.

1–5. The chief differences between astrocytes and oligodendrocytes are as follows: Astrocytes have numerous and voluminous processes that form the CNS packing material, which is metabolically very active. The ends of their processes aid in the formation of the blood-brain barrier and the external and internal limiting membranes. They are highly susceptible to CNS insults and form glial scars. Oligodendrocytes have fewer branches and their main functions are to form and maintain the CNS myelin.

1–6. a. Subdural hematoma—between the dura mater and the arachnoid membrane

b. Cerebrospinal fluid—in the subarachnoid space between the arachnoid membrane and the pia mater

c. Epidural hematoma—between the dura and the bony wall of the cranial cavity

CHAPTER 2 SPINAL CORD TOPOGRAPHY AND FUNCTIONAL LEVELS

2–1. The spinal epidural space contains adipose tissue and blood vessels, the most medically important of which is the internal vertebral venous plexus. This valveless plexus communicates freely with veins of the pelvic, abdominal, thoracic, and cranial cavities and may provide a route for the spread of infections, cancer cells, etc. from the viscera to the brain.

2–2. The dural sac contains an enlarged subarachnoid space in which is found chiefly the cerebrospinal fluid and the lumbosacral nerve roots that form the cauda equina.

2–3. Intervertebral dislocations most frequently occur at the articulations between CV5–CV6, TV12-LV1, and CV1–CV2, in order of frequency. The spinal cord–vertebral column relations at each are:

CV1–CV2 = C2
CV5–CV6 = C6 or C7
TV12-LV1 = S1–S3

2–4. The spinal cord is not endangered by lumbar puncture in adults below the LV3 level because its caudal extent is at the LV2 level.

2–5. The four spinal cord regions can be distinguished in transverse sections on the basis of gray matter size and shape as follows:

	posterior horn	*anterior horn*
sacral	massive	massive with lateral extension
lumbar	massive	massive with medial extension
thoracic	thin	thin
cervical	thin	large with lateral extension

CHAPTER 3 BRAINSTEM ANATOMY, TOPOGRAPHY, AND FUNCTIONAL LEVELS

3–1. III CN and IV CN—midbrain, V CN to VIII CN—pons, IX CN to XII CN—medulla

3–2. Ventral surface of (*a*) Medulla—pyramids, (*b*) Pons—transverse grooves of basilar part, (*c*) Midbrain—cerebral peduncles and interpeduncular fossa

3–3. Dorsal surface of (*a*) Closed medulla—gracile and cuneate tubercles, (*b*) Open medulla—hypoglossal and vagal trigones, (*c*) Pons—medial eminence and facial colliculus, (*d*) Midbrain—superior colliculus and inferior colliculus

3–4. The brainstem reticular formation is

an intermingling of nuclei and nerve fibers in the central core of the brainstem.

3–5. a. Hypoglossal trigone—open medulla, caudally
b. Motor trigeminal nucleus—midpons
c. Superior colliculus—rostral midbrain
d. Decussation of trochlear nerve—rostral pons
e. Acoustic tubercle—open medulla, rostrally
f. Gracile tubercle—closed medulla
g. Facial colliculus—caudal pons
h. Inferior colliculus—caudal midbrain

CHAPTER 4 FOREBRAIN TOPOGRAPHY AND FUNCTIONAL LEVELS

4–1. The 12 cranial nerves attach to the brain, and, hence, they travel in the cranial cavity whereas the spinal nerves attach to the spinal cord and travel in the spinal or vertebral canal. Additional differences are that cranial nerves do not have dorsal and ventral roots and their functional components vary, some being purely motor, some purely sensory, and others mixed.

4–2. Cranial nerves I and II attach to the forebrain, III and IV to the midbrain, and all the others attach to the hindbrain, V CN-VIII CN to the pons and IX CN-XII CN to the medulla.

4–3. In the forebrain are the two lateral ventricles, one in each of the cerebral hemispheres, and the third ventricle in the diencephalon. In the hindbrain is the fourth ventricle and in the midbrain is the cerebral aqueduct, which connects the third and fourth ventricles.

4–4. The terms "anterior or ventral," meaning toward the front, and "posterior or dorsal," meaning toward the back, are synonymous in all parts of the CNS except the forebrain. Because the axis of the forebrain is oriented almost perpendicular to the rest of the CNS, in the forebrain the term "ventral" is synonymous with inferior, meaning toward the base of the skull; "dorsal" is synonymous with superior, meaning toward the top of the skull.

CHAPTER 5 LOWER MOTOR NEURONS: FLACCID PARALYSIS

5–1. A motor unit is an α-motoneuron, its axon, and all the muscle fibers it innervates. Those motor units involved in coarse movements comprise as many as 2000 muscle fibers, whereas those involved in delicate movements may include as few as a dozen or so muscle fibers.

5–2. Lower motor neurons are the final common path for all influences on skeletal muscle contractions. Hence, lesions result in deficiencies in volitional movements (paralysis), muscle tone (hypotonia), and reflexes (absent).

5–3. (a) Ambiguus nucleus: Hoarse and weak voice due to paralysis of the ipsilateral vocal muscles, sagging of the ipsilateral palatal arch, and contralateral deviation of the uvula could be expected with the lesion at this level, which is the vagal part of the nucleus. (b) Oculomotor nucleus: Ipsilateral ptosis and ophthalmoplegia with the eye turned down and out; mydriasis due to interruption of visceral pupilloconstrictor components. (c) Facial nucleus: Paralysis of ipsilateral muscles of facial expression; inability to close eye tightly or retract corner of mouth. (d) Motor trigeminal nucleus: Paralysis and atrophy of ipsilateral muscles of mastication; on opening the mouth, the jaw deviates toward ipsilateral side.

CHAPTER 6 THE PYRAMIDAL SYSTEM: SPASTIC PARALYSIS

6–1. The pyramidal tract is highly susceptible to injury because it extends without interruption from the cerebral cortex to the caudal end of the spinal cord. Thus, it is subject to injury by trauma, cerebrovascular disease, neoplasms, etc. that occur at any level of the brain and spinal cord.

6–2. A lower motor neuron lesion affecting the facial muscles is due to an injury of the facial nucleus or nerve and results in paralysis of all ipsilateral facial muscles. An upper motor neuron lesion affecting the facial muscles is due to injury of the corticobulbar neurons or their axons and results in paralysis or weakness of the contralateral lower facial muscles only. The upper facial muscles are influenced by both the ipsilateral and contralateral corticobulbar tracts; hence, the upper facial muscles will not be affected by a unilateral corticobulbar tract lesion.

6–3. a. 1. Corticospinal tract: Contralateral spastic hemiplegia accompanied by exaggerated myotatic reflexes, increased resistance to passive stretch, and an extensor plantar response
      2. Corticobulbar tract: Contralateral lower facial muscle paralysis
   b. 1. Corticospinal tract: (see a. 1.)
      2. Hypoglossal nerve: Paralysis, atrophy, and deviation of protruded tongue to ipsilateral side

   c. 1. Corticospinal tract: (see a. 1.)
      2. Abducent nerve: Medial deviation (esotropia) and abductor paralysis of ipsilateral eye
   d. 1. Corticospinal tract: (see a. 1.)
      2. Corticobulbar tract: (see a. 2.)
      3. Oculomotor nerve: Ipsilateral ptosis and ophthalmoplegia with eye turned down and out (mydriasis also, due to visceromotor fibers in CN III)

CHAPTER 7 BRAINSTEM MOTOR CENTERS: DECEREBRATE POSTURING AND POSTCAPSULAR LESION RECOVERY

7–1. Impulses from the maculae of the utricles and saccules pass via the vestibular ganglion and nerve to the vestibular nuclei. From the left lateral vestibular nucleus, impulses descend via the left lateral vestibular tract to the lower motor neurons that facilitate the extensor muscles of the left limbs.

7–2. a. Decorticate posturing occurs with brainstem impairment rostral to the red nucleus.
     b. Decerebrate posturing occurs with brainstem impairment anywhere between the forebrain-midbrain junction and the rostral extent of the vestibular nuclei.

CHAPTER 8 THE BASAL GANGLIA: MOVEMENT DISORDERS

8–1. Anatomically, the corpus striatum is composed of the caudate and lentiform nuclei, the latter being further subdivided into a lateral segment, the putamen, and two medial segments, the globus pallidus. Functionally, the corpus striatum is divided into the striatum, consisting of the caudate nucleus and putamen, and the pallidum, which is the globus pallidus.

8–2. The input to the basal ganglia is directed to the striatum and is composed largely of the massive and highly topographically organized corticostriate projections from all parts of the neocortex. In addition, the thalamic intralaminar nuclei provide a small input to the basal ganglia via their thalamostriate projections.

8–3. The cardinal manifestations of basal ganglia diseases are disorders of movement and alterations in muscle tone. The disorders of movement, or dyskinesia, take the form of tremors, athetosis, chorea, or ballismus. They are more prevalent while the patient is "at rest," i.e., not intending to perform a movement. Dyskinesia can be neither prevented nor interrupted. The alteration in muscle tone in basal ganglia diseases usually takes the form of hypertonicity.

8–4. a. Structure—Bilateral compact parts of substantia nigra
     Abnormality—Parkinson disease: Mask-like facial expression, pill-rolling tremor, bradykinesia, lead-pipe rigidity, and impairment of postural adjustments.

     Decreased striatal dopamine → increased inhibition of lateral pallidum → decreased inhibition of subthalamic nucleus → increased excitation of medial pallidum → increased inhibition of ventral anterior nucleus → decreased excitation of premotor cortex (Fig. 8–13)

b. Structures—Bilateral striatal degeneration (caudate nucleus and putamen) Abnormality—Huntington chorea: Head jerking, lip and tongue smacking, gesticulations of distal parts of limbs.

(Huntington)—Striatal degeneration → decreased inhibition of lateral pallidum → increased inhibition of subthalamic nucleus → decreased excitation of medial pallidum → decreased inhibition of ven-

tral anterior nucleus → increased excitation of premotor cortex (Fig. 8–12)

c. Structures—Subthalamic nucleus Abnormality—Contralateral hemiballismus: Violent flinging of upper and lower limbs

Decreased inhibition of lateral pallidum → increased inhibition of subthalamic nucleus → decreased excitation of medial pallidum → decreased inhibition of ventral anterior nucleus → increased excitation of premotor cortex (Fig. 8–11)

CHAPTER 9 THE CEREBELLUM: ATAXIA

9–1. The inferior cerebellar peduncle emanates from the medulla and contains chiefly the olivocerebellar, dorsal spinocerebellar, cuneocerebellar, and reticulocerebellar tracts. Its more medial part, the so-called juxtarestiform body, comprises the incoming vestibulocerebellar and the outgoing cerebellovestibular connections. The middle cerebellar peduncle is largest and is made up of the pontocerebellar projections. The superior cerebellar peduncle is composed chiefly of the cerebellar output to the midbrain and thalamus, although it does contain the incoming small ventral spinocerebellar tract and descending projections to the reticular formation.

9–2. The cerebellar nuclei are, from medial to lateral, the fastigial, the interposed—composed of the globus and emboliform nuclei—and the dentate. Each receives an

excitatory input from collaterals of the climbing and mossy fibers and an inhibitory input from the Purkinje neurons.

9–3. The flocculonodular syndrome is characterized by truncal ataxia, the anterior lobe syndrome by gait ataxia, and the posterior lobe syndrome by a generalized ataxia especially noticeable in the upper limb and, if bilateral, in speech. With massive posterior lobe lesions or with damage to the dentate nucleus or superior cerebellar peduncle, intention tremor occurs. In the event of unilateral lesions of the cerebellum, the ataxia is always ipsilateral.

9–4. a. Anterior cerebellar lobe (lower limb area): Gait ataxia
b. Superior cerebellar peduncle (before decussation): Posterior lobe syndrome; ipsilaterally—intention tremor, dysmetria, dysdiadochokinesia, etc.
c. Flocculonodular lobe: Truncal ataxia

CHAPTER 10 THE OCULOMOTOR SYSTEM: VESTIBULO-OCULAR REFLEX AND CONJUGATE GAZE

10–1. The vestibulo-ocular reflex is interrupted in the central brainstem somewhere between the levels of the vestibu-

lar and oculomotor nuclei (midpons to rostral midbrain).

10–2. Right oculomotor nerve

10–3. Right abducent nerve

10–4. Internuclear ophthalmoplegia resulting from lesion of the right medial longitudinal fasciculus in the rostral pons or in the midbrain

10–5. Left frontal eye field (if transient, that is, it occurs only during the acute phase of lesion). Right horizontal gaze center in paramedian or pontine reticular formation (if permanent)

CHAPTER 11 THE SOMATOSENSORY SYSTEM: ANESTHESIA AND ANALGESIA

11–1. a. Cutaneous touch and pain sensations in dermatome L5 (first four toes and the dorsum of the foot)
  b. Tactile, vibration, and limb position and motion senses below the umbilicus on the left side and pain and temperature sensations below the inguinal ligament on the right side
  c. Pain and temperature sensations bilaterally at the level of the nipples
  d. Pain and temperature sensations in the face on the left side and pin prick and temperature in the occiput, neck, trunk, and limbs on the right side
  e. Tactile, vibration, and limb position senses in the occiput, neck, trunk, and limbs on the left side and pin prick and temperature sensations in the face on the left side
  f. Tactile, vibration, limb position senses, pin prick, and temperature senses on the entire right side
  g. Complete loss of two-point sense, stereognosis, and graphesthesia and some diminution of pin prick and temperature sensations and their precise localization, all in the left lower limb. Only precise localization and fine tactile discrimination depend on an intact primary somatosensory cortex for recognition.

CHAPTER 12 THE VISUAL SYSTEM: ANOPSIA

12–1. Detachment of the retina occurs between the pigment cells (layer 1) and the photoreceptor cells (layer 2). The detached part ceases to function because the rods and cones are metabolically dependent on the pigment cells.

12–2. Retinal layers 4, 6, and 8 contain the cell bodies of the photoreceptors, bipolar, and ganglion cells, respectively.

12–3. Night blindness is associated with vitamin A deficiency that aids in the restoration of the photopigment rhodopsin in the rods.

12–4. Color blindness is associated with the absence of the red-, green-, or blue-sensitive photopigments in the cones.

12–5. The fovea centralis is the area for most acute vision and here most of the inner layers of the retina are pushed aside so the light rays can reach the cones of the foveola with as little interference as possible. Thus, only layers 1, 2, 3, 4, and 10 are found at the fovea. The optic disc is the area where the ganglion cell axons gather together and emerge from the eye as the optic nerve. It possesses only layers 9 and 10 and is the blind spot because of the absence of photoreceptors.

12–6. As a component of the PNS, the optic nerve is unique because histologically it is similar to a CNS structure. Because it develops as an evagination of the diencephalon, the retina and its connection to the brain, the optic nerve, possess CNS morphologic characteristics. Histologically, the optic nerve resembles a spinal cord or brainstem tract in that its axons are supported by glial cells and in the absence of neurolemma cells optic nerve axons do not regenerate if injured. Moreover, like the brain and spinal cord the optic nerve is enveloped by the meninges, an arrangement that becomes medically important in the case of increased intracranial pressure, which exerts force on the optic nerve through the cerebrospinal fluid in the subarachnoid space surrounding it. Thus, increased intracranial pressure may be the cause of an edematous swelling of the optic disc, a phenomenon referred to as disc edema, papilledema, or choked disc.

12–7. a. Blindness in left eye
b. Bitemporal hemianopsia
c. Left homonymous hemianopsia
d. Right homonymous superior quadrantic anopsia
e. Left homonymous hemianopsia

12–8. The direct light reflex involves the ipsilateral optic and oculomotor nerves, whereas the consensual light reflex involves the ipsilateral optic nerve and the contralateral oculomotor nerve. Central connections are made in the light reflex center in the pretectal nuclei, which connects with the ipsilateral and contralateral Edinger-Westphal nuclei; hence, the rostral midbrain must be intact for these reflex responses to occur.

12–9. CNS and PNS structures whose damage interrupts the pupillodilation path are:

CNS—Lateral reticular formation of medulla
Lateral funiculus of cervical spinal cord
Ciliospinal center at C8 and T1
Intramedullary ventral rootlets at T1 and T2
PNS—Ventral roots of T1 and T2
T1 and T2 spinal nerves
White communicating rami of T1 and T2
Cervical sympathetic trunk
Superior cervical ganglion
Internal carotid plexus

12–10. Accommodation is the phenomenon whereby images remain in focus as the gaze shifts from far to near objects. It includes (*a*) contraction of the ciliary muscles, which allows the lens to bulge; (*b*) constriction of the pupil; and (*c*) convergence of the eyes. The center for accommodation is thought to be located in the region of the pretectum and superior colliculus. Its input comes from the visual cortex, and its output passes to the Edinger-Westphal and oculomotor nuclei. Both of these give fibers to the oculomotor nerve: those from the Edinger-Westphal nucleus are preganglionic parasympathetic axons that synapse in the ciliary ganglion from whence postganglionic fibers pass via the short ciliary nerves to the ciliary and pupilloconstrictor muscles; those from the oculomotor nuclei pass directly to the medial rectus muscle of each eye.

CHAPTER 13 THE AUDITORY SYSTEM: DEAFNESS

13–1. The bilateral representation of sound in the auditory system occurs because of the bilateral connections of (*a*) the superior olivary and trapezoid nuclei, (*b*) the nuclei of the lateral lemniscus, and (*c*) the inferior colliculi. Hence, a unilateral lesion in the auditory path anywhere from the level of the superior olivary nuclei to the cerebral cortex results in virtually no loss of hearing in either ear.

13–2. Complete ipsilateral deafness occurs after unilateral destruction of the spinal organ, the spinal ganglion, the cochlear nerve, or the dorsal and ventral cochlear nuclei.

13–3. An enlarging acoustic neurinoma causes impairment of

a. The cochlear and facial nerves in the internal acoustic meatus
b. The trigeminal, glossopharyngeal, and perhaps vagus and abducent in and near the cerebellar angle

13–4. Conduction deafness occurs as a result of external or middle ear diseases and injuries, which interfere with the conduction of sound waves or with the vibrations of the tympanic membrane or middle ear ossicles. Nerve deafness results from diseases and injuries of the spinal organ or the cochlear nerve. Conduction deafness is incomplete because sound waves are still transmitted through the cranial bones. In the event of total destruction of the spiral organ or cochlear nerve, the resulting "nerve deafness" is complete.

CHAPTER 14 THE GUSTATORY AND OLFACTORY SYSTEMS: AGEUSIA AND ANOSMIA

14–1. Three cranial nerves contain taste fibers: the facial, the glossopharyngeal, and the vagus. The taste fibers in the facial nerve supply the anterior two thirds of the tongue and have their cell bodies located in the geniculate ganglion. The glossopharyngeal nerve taste fibers are distributed to the posterior third of the tongue and their cell bodies are in the petrosal ganglion, whereas the vagal nerve taste fibers are distributed to the epiglottic and palatal regions and their cell bodies are in the nodose ganglion. The central branches of all the primary gustatory neurons enter the solitary tract and are distributed to the rostral part of the solitary nucleus sometimes called the gustatory nucleus.

14–2. The primary gustatory area is located in the opercular part of the postcentral gyrus and the adjacent part of the insula. This area is Brodmann area 43.

14–3. The olfactory membrane is 1 in² of epithelium on the superior nasal concha and the adjoining nasal septum. It contains the bipolar olfactory neurons whose peripheral processes (dendrites) extend to the surface and possess chemosensitive cilia that are bathed in mucus. The central processes of these primary olfactory neurons form the axons of the olfactory nerves.

14–4. The primary olfactory area is located in the posterolateral part of the orbitofrontal cortex. Unlike the other cortical sensory areas, it receives only ipsilateral olfactory impulses.

CHAPTER 15 THE CEREBRAL CORTEX: APHASIA, AGNOSIA, AND APRAXIA

15–1. The neocortex is comprised of six layers. Layer IV is abundant in granule cells and is the chief recipient of the afferent projection fibers. The infragranular layers are efferent in nature and give rise to the massive efferent projection fibers. The efferent projection fibers arise chiefly from the large pyramidal neurons in layer V and to a lesser extent from the fusiform neurons in layer VI. The supragranular layers are for association. Layer II is rich in granule cells and receives input from other cortical areas. Layer III contains numerous pyramidal neurons, which give rise to association and commissural fibers. Layer I provides for association between adjacent cortical areas.

15–2. a. Broca speech area in the opercular and triangular parts of the left inferior frontal gyrus
  b. Right paracentral lobule
  c. Frontal eye field in posterior part of the left middle frontal gyrus
  d. Right primary visual cortex in the parts of the cuneus and lingual gyrus along the calcarine fissure
  e. Dorsal part of the primary motor area in the left precentral gyrus
  f. Wernicke speech area in the posterior part of the left superior temporal gyrus
  g. Right posterior parietal lobe
  h. Ventral part of primary motor cortex in the left precentral gyrus

CHAPTER 16 THE LIMBIC SYSTEM: ANTEROGRADE AMNESIA AND INAPPROPRIATE BEHAVIOR

16–1. The limbic lobe borders the corpus callosum and rostral brainstem and is composed of the cingulate gyrus and its anterior extension, the septal region, and the parahippocampal gyrus. The limbic system consists of the limbic lobe as well as the hippocampal formation and amygdaloid nuclei, and the structure most strongly connected with them, the hypothalamus.

16–2. The two key functional centers of the limbic system are the amygdaloid nucleus and hippocampal formation, both of which are located in the medial part of the temporal lobe. The amygdaloid nucleus is deep to and continuous with the uncus, whereas the hippocampal formation is deep to and continuous with the posterior part of the parahippocampal gyrus.

16–3. The Papez circuit begins in the hippocampal formation and passes via the fornix to the mamillary body, from whence the mamillothalamic tract travels to the anterior thalamic nucleus. This nucleus then sends impulses to the cingulate gyrus, which projects via the cingulum to the parahippocampal gyrus; this then completes the circuit by connecting with the subiculum. Although the Papez circuit was initially thought to be concerned with emotions, it is now thought to play a role in memory and learning.

16–4. Bilateral lesions of the hippocampal formations (or posterior parts of the parahippocampal gyri) result in profound impairment of the ability to recall recent events and to form new memories. Bilateral lesions of the amygdaloid nuclei result in behavioral alterations usually described as profound apathy or docility.

16–5. Alzheimer disease: Hippocampal formation or parahippocampal gyri—recent memory—cholinergic neurons of basal nucleus of Meynert—disorientation and long-term memory

Klüver-Bucy syndrome: Amygdaloid nuclei

Korsakoff psychosis: Medial parts of medial dorsal thalamic nuclei

CHAPTER 17: THE HYPOTHALAMUS: VEGETATIVE AND ENDOCRINE IMBALANCE

17–1. The hypothalamus is divided, from anterior to posterior, into supraoptic, tuberal, and mamillary regions.

17–2. The neural hypothalamic output passes chiefly to the anterior thalamic nucleus via the mamillothalamic tract, to the midbrain reticular formation via the mamillotegmental and the medial forebrain bundle, and to the medial dorsal thalamic nucleus via the periventricular fiber system.

17–3. The hypophysial portal system is a vascular connection between the tuberal region of the hypothalamus and the anterior pituitary. Hypothalamic regulatory hormones, called excitatory and inhibitory releasing factors, produced chiefly in the arcuate and ventromedial nuclei, are secreted into the hypothalamic capillaries and transported through this portal system to target secretory cells in the anterior pituitary, thus allowing for the widespread hypothalamic influence on endocrine activity.

17–4. a. Heat loss center in anterior or preoptic part, heat gain center in posterior part
b. Parasympathomimetic activity in anterior and preoptic parts
c. Sympathomimetic activity in posterior part
d. Hypothalamic regulatory hormones in tuberal part
e. Water balance in anterior part
f. Sleep-wake cycle in anterior part
g. Sleep center in anterior and posterior parts
h. Emotion in middle and posterior parts

CHAPTER 18 THE AUTONOMIC SYSTEM: VISCERAL ABNORMALITIES

18–1. The somatic efferent system is under voluntary control and comprises the α-motoneurons and their axons, which directly innervate skeletal muscle. The autonomic or general visceral efferent system is involuntary and is composed of two efferent neurons: a preganglionic neuron, located in the central nervous system, whose axon synapses in a ganglion; and a postganglionic neuron, located in a ganglion, whose axon innervates smooth muscle, cardiac muscle, or glandular tissue.

18–2. The cranial parasympathetic system consists of the following:

a. Preganglionic neurons in the Edinger-Westphal nucleus whose axons are in the oculomotor nerve;
b. Preganglionic neurons in the superior salivatory nucleus whose axons travel in the facial nerve;
c. Preganglionic neurons in the inferior salivatory nucleus whose axons are in the glossopharyngeal nerve;
d. Preganglionic neurons in the dorsal vagal nucleus whose axons travel in the vagus nerve.

18–3. The preganglionic sacral parasympathics arise from the intermediolateral nucleus of S2,S3,S4.

18–4. All preganglionic sympathetic fibers arise from the sympathetic nucleus, which extends from about C7 or C8 to L2 or L3. This nucleus comprises an intermediolateral part in the lateral horn, an intermediomedial part in the medial part of lamina VII, an intercalated part that bridges the previous two, and neurons scattered in the lateral funiculus near the lateral horn.

18–5. Autonomic afferent fibers are very abundant in the glossopharyngeal and vagus nerves. The glossopharyngeal nerve distributes them chiefly to the oral cavity, the pharynx, and the carotid body and sinus. Through the vagus nerve, autonomic afferents are distributed to the thoracic and abdominal viscera. The autonomic afferents in these nerves synapse in the solitary nucleus and are distributed to visceral and somatic nuclei subserving cardiovascular, respiratory, and gastrointestinal reflexes.

18–6. As a general rule, pain fibers from the thoracic, abdominal, and pelvic viscera reach the spinal cord via the sympathetic nerves and trunks and the T1–L2 spinal nerves and their dorsal roots. Exceptions to this are the sigmoid colon and rectum, the neck of the bladder, the prostate gland, and the cervix of the uterus, from which pain fibers reach the spinal cord via the pelvic nerves and the S2,S3,S4 spinal nerves and their dorsal roots.

18–7. Referred pain is the phenomenon in which pain is localized in a part of the body remote from its source. The basis for the referral is the convergence within the spinal cord of visceral impulses onto somatic neurons, thereby eliciting spinothalamic tract activity that is erroneously interpreted by the cerebral cortex as having originated in cutaneous sites. Thus, referred pain is always located in the somatic area supplied by the spinal cord segments common to both the visceral afferent and the somatic afferent input.

18–8. Cardiac pain fibers travel centrally in the cardiac nerves to the sympathetic trunk.

They then descend in the trunk and travel via the white communicating rami to the spinal nerves and their dorsal roots (where their cell bodies are located) and into the spinal cord. The chief central connections are made at T2–T4; hence, the retrosternal location of cardiac pain. As the intensity of the pain increases, the T1 and T2 segments become involved and the pain then radiates to the inner aspect of the left arm.

18–9. Parasympathetic stimulation results in decreased heart rate (bradycardia), emptying of the urinary bladder, and erection of the clitoris or penis. Sympathetic stimulation results in increased heart rate (tachycardia), relaxation of the bladder and contraction of the internal urethral sphincter, and vaginal contractions or ejaculation.

CHAPTER 19 THE BLOOD SUPPLY OF THE CENTRAL NERVOUS SYSTEM: STROKE

19–1. The chief morphologic features of cerebral arteries are a thin intima with many elastic fibers and a prominent internal elastic membrane, a thin media that is frequently absent where the vessels branch, and a thin adventitia with no external elastic membrane. Thus, as compared to extracranial arteries, the cerebral arteries are extremely thin and their structure is conducive to the formation of aneurysms.

19–2. The anatomical substrate of the blood-brain barrier is the nonfenestrated capillary endothelium with its tight junctions, the astrocytic perivascular foot processes, and the basement membrane between the two.

19–3. The arterial circle of Willis is an anastomosis between the anterior and posterior cerebral circulations, which is found on the ventral surface of the brain surrounding the hypothalamus and interpe-

duncular fossa. It is formed by the right and left internal carotid arteries laterally and the basilar artery and its right and left posterior cerebral branches posteriorly. The circle is completed posterolaterally by the posterior communicating branches of the internal carotid arteries, which anastomose with the posterior cerebral arteries, anterolaterally by the anterior cerebral branches of the internal carotids, and anteriorly by the anterior communicating arteries that connect the right and left anterior cerebral arteries. The circle is rarely symmetrical; in most cases, one of the communicating arteries or a posterior cerebral artery is atrophic. Functionally, the circle serves as a potential vascular shunt.

19–4. The spinal cord is supplied by a single large anterior spinal artery and paired small posterior spinal arteries. These vessels are supplemented along the length of the spinal cord by the radicular branches of the cervical, intercostal, lumbar, and sacral arteries.

19–5. a. Middle cerebral
b. Anterior cerebral
c. Posterior cerebral
d. Dorsal part by lateral striate branches

of middle cerebral and ventral part by anterior choroidal
e. Vertebral or posterior inferior cerebellar
f. Anterior spinal

CHAPTER 20 THE CEREBROSPINAL FLUID SYSTEM: HYDROCEPHALUS

20–1. CSF functions as protection for the brain and spinal cord against surface contact pressure and sudden motion, as support for cerebral vessels and cranial nerves, and as sustenance for the neuronal internal milieu.

20–2. The lateral ventricle is composed of (*a*) an anterior or frontal horn that is anterior to the interventricular foramen, (*b*) a body located beneath the trunk of the corpus callosum, (*c*) a posterior or occipital horn whose size is highly variable, and (*d*) an inferior or temporal horn that ends about 3 cm behind the temporal pole. The largest part of the lateral ventricle is at the trigone, a triangular space at the confluence of the body and the occipital and inferior horns. It is located beneath the splenium of the corpus callosum and contains the glomus, a large tuft of choroid plexus.

20–3. CSF is secreted by the choroid plexuses into the lateral, third, and fourth ventricles. It flows from the lateral ventricles into the third ventricle through the paired interventricular foramina (of

Monro) and from the third to the fourth ventricle through the cerebral aqueduct. It flows out of the ventricular system through three openings in the fourth ventricle: a median aperture (foramen of Magendie) and paired lateral apertures (foramina of Luschka). It enters the subarachnoid space and then flows around the ventral and dorsal surfaces of the brainstem and over the cerebellum. It eventually passes along the convexity of the cerebral hemispheres toward the superior sagittal sinus into which it is absorbed through the pressure-dependent arachnoid villi and their one-way valves.

20–4. Noncommunicating or obstructive hydrocephalus refers to the blockage of CSF flow anywhere within the ventricular system whereby flow is obstructed from one ventricle to another or from the ventricular system into the subarachnoid space. Communicating hydrocephalus refers to any disruption to the flow of CSF through the subarachnoid space and cisterns or across the arachnoid villi.

Appendix C

GLOSSARY

accommodation center neurons in the tectum of the rostral midbrain that receive input directly from the occipital cortex and integrate the actions of the ciliary muscles, iris muscles, and medial rectus muscles in order to maintain a focused image on the retina during near or far vision.

acoustic neurinoma benign tumor arising from Schwann cells of the VIII CN. As the tumor grows within the internal acoustic meatus it progressively affects the cochlear, vestibular, and facial nerves; with further enlargement it invades the cerebellopontine angle affecting the cerebellum and eventually the V, IX, X, and XI CN; syn. acoustic neuroma, neurilemoma or Schwannoma; cerebellopontine angle tumor.

acute sympathetic shock syndrome characterized by bradycardia, hypotension, bilateral Horner syndrome; occurs in acute bilateral cervical spinal cord injuries due to the interruption of the descending impulses to the sympathetic nuclei.

afferent conducting impulses toward.

α-motoneuron neuron located in anterior horn of spinal cord and in certain brainstem nuclei whose axon passes directly to extrafusal fibers of voluntary muscle; syn. lower motor neuron.

alternating hemiplegia combined upper and lower motor neuron brainstem lesion affecting pyramidal tract, which results in contralateral spastic hemiplegia, and affecting oculomotor, abducent, or hypoglossal nerve rootlets, which results in ipsilateral palsies in the respective nerves.

Alzheimer disease presenile dementia in which large numbers of neurofibrillary tangles and neuritic (senile) plaques occur in the cortex. This disease is associated with neuronal degeneration in the hippocampus and parahippocampal gyrus and decreased cortical levels of choline acetyl transferase due to degeneration of neurons in such basal forebrain structures as the basal nucleus of Meynert and the diagonal band nuclei.

amacrine cell local circuit neuron in the internal nuclear layer of the retina that influences synaptic transmission between the bipolar and the ganglion cells.

ampullary crest (L., crista = crest + ampulla = a jug) sensory organ of kinetic equilibrium occurring as an elevation on the inner aspect of the membranous ampulla of each semicircular duct.

amygdala (G., almond) collection of nuclei within and deep to the uncus of the temporal lobe, forming an important behavior and emotions center of the limbic system; syn. amygdaloid nucleus.

analgesia (G., insensibility) relief of pain without loss of consciousness.

anesthesia loss of sensation as a result of pharmacologic depression of nerve function or of neurologic disease.

aneurysm dilation in the wall of a blood vessel.

anhidrosis (G., an = without + hidros = sweat) absence of sweating.

annulospiral stretch receptor afferent nerve ending, located at central portion of a muscle spindle, which responds to muscle stretch.

anosmia (G., an + osmesis = sense of smell) absence of sense of smell.

anterior commissure complex fiber system crossing midline in lamina terminalis; interconnects middle and inferior temporal gyri, olfactory bulbs, amygdalae, and other nuclei.

anterior limb of internal capsule that part of the internal capsule between the head of the caudate nucleus medially and the lentiform nucleus laterally.

anterior lobe syndrome cerebellar disorder characterized by loss of coordination initially in the lower limbs (gait ataxia) frequently as a result of Purkinje cell degeneration due to chronic alcoholism.

anterior perforated substance region behind orbital surface of frontal lobe and medial and lateral olfactory striae, through which numerous small arteries reach internal structures.

anterograde axonal transport passage from the cell body; two rates occur: (1) fast transport, 400 mm/day; requires neurotubules; membranous organelles, synaptic vesicles, and their precursors are carried this way; (2) slow transport, several millimeters per day; carries entire cytoskeleton and non-packaged macromolecules.

anterolateral cordotomy surgical sectioning of anterolateral quadrant of spinal cord for relief of chronic pain

anterolateral quadrant area of spinal white matter between attachment of dentate ligaments and emergence of anterior roots; the spinothalamic tract is located here.

antidiuretic hormone (ADH) hormone produced by neurosecretory cells in the supraoptic and paraventricular nuclei of the hypothalamus that stimulates water reabsorption from kidney.

apraxia (G., a + pratto = to do) inability to carry out a voluntary movement in the absence of paralysis, sensory loss, and ataxia.

arachnoid (G., spider) middle of three membranes covering the central nervous system (CNS).

arachnoid granulations groups of arachnoid villi, found predominantly in lacunae of the superior sagittal sinus, through which cerebrospinal fluid (CSF) is absorbed into the venous system; syn. arachnoid villi.

archicerebellum (G., archi = beginning) oldest part of cerebellum; the flocculonodular lobe or vestibulocerebellum located inferiorly, anterior to the posterolateral fissure.

arcuate fasciculus large association bundle connecting the inferior and middle frontal gyri with the superior temporal gyrus; sometimes also considered to include the superior longitudinal fasciculus.

arcuate fibers short association fibers that lie immediately beneath the cortex adjacent to a cerebral sulcus and connect adjacent gyri; syn. U-fibers.

ascending reticular activating system (ARAS) components of the brainstem reticular formation that project to parts of the thalamus and subthalamus and pace the activity of the cerebral cortex; if interrupted at the midbrain, coma results; associated with

the sleep-wake cycle; sleep centers in the pons, medulla, and hypothalamus project to the ARAS to turn it off to induce sleep; syn. reticular activating system.

astereognosis (G., a + stereos = solid + gnosis = knowledge) inability to identify an object by touch; syn. tactile amnesia.

astrocyte (G., astron = star) star-shaped neuroglial cell with cytoplasmic processes whose terminal expansions or "end-feet" ensheathe blood vessels and the surfaces of the brain and spinal cord.

ataxia (G., a + taxis = order) loss of muscular coordination.

athetosis (G., athetos = without position or place) disorder of movement involving slow writhing movements of the limbs, particularly the fingers and hands; associated with basal ganglia disorders.

auditory ossicles the small bones of the middle ear—malleus, incus, and stapes—articulated to form a chain for the transmission of sound-induced vibrations from the tympanic membrane to the oval window.

auditory radiation fibers carrying auditory impulses from the medial geniculate nucleus via the sublenticular part of the internal capsule to the transverse temporal gyri of Heschl.

automatic reflex bladder incontinence and retention; occurs after spinal cord lesions above sacral levels.

autonomic plexus ganglion sympathetic neurons located in plexuses along abdominal aorta and its branches; syn. prevertebral or collateral ganglion.

axon nerve cell process conducting impulses away from cell body.

Babinski response abnormal upward extension (dorsiflexion) of great toe in response to stroking outer border of the sole; usually indicates pyramidal tract damage; syn. extensor plantar reflex or response.

ballismus (G., ballismos = a jumping about) violent jerking or flinging movements of proximal parts of limbs and shoulders and pelvic girdle musculature; associated with lesions of the subthalamic nucleus.

basal nucleus (of Meynert) extensive group of neurons located in the substantia innominata of the anterior perforated substance; major source of cholinergic projections to neocortex and implicated in Alzheimer disease.

basilar membrane membrane supporting the organ of Corti; stretches between the osseous spiral lamina and spiral ligament; syn. membranous spiral lamina.

basket cell inhibitory neuron found deep in molecular layer of cerebellar cortex, whose axon forms a basket-like ramification around the base of a Purkinje cell body.

Bell palsy weakness of upper and lower facial muscles and inability to close the eye completely; usually caused by inflammation of facial nerve in the facial canal.

bitemporal hemianopsia loss of temporal vision in both eyes; results from median lesion of optic chiasm.

blind spot area in the retina at the origin of the optic (II) nerve in which there are no photoreceptor cells.

blood-brain barrier permeability control system governing the passage of substances between capillaries and the CNS parenchyma; partially related to such morphologic features as tight junctions between endothelial cells and perivascular astrocytic end-feet.

bone conduction sound vibrations conducted to the internal ear by the temporal bone.

bony labyrinth series of cavities within the petrous portion of the temporal bone forming the vestibule, cochlea, and semicircular canals of the inner ear; syn. osseous labyrinth.

bradycardia slowness of the heart beat, usually defined as a rate under 60 beats per minute.

Broca area opercular and triangular parts of inferior frontal gyrus in dominant hemisphere; associated with motor programs for production of words; nonfluent (motor or expressive) aphasia is attributed to its injury.

Brodmann numerical areas numerical subdivisions of the cerebral cortex, originally based on cytoarchitectural characteristics but now related to functions.

Brown-Séquard syndrome hemisection of the spinal cord; causes ipsilateral spastic paralysis and loss of touch, pressure, and position sense and contralateral loss of pain and temperature sensations below the level of the lesion.

capsular cell supporting cells surrounding the cell bodies of dorsal root and autonomic ganglion cells.

carotid plexuses postganglionic sympathetic fibers traveling along carotid arteries to smooth muscle and glands of head.

carotid siphon hairpin bend formed by internal carotid artery within the petrous canal and cavernous sinus.

cauda equina (L., cauda = tail + equus = horse) roots of lumbosacral nerves as they travel in the vertebral canal below the spinal cord to their respective lumbar intervertebral or sacral foramina.

cerebellar angle area on ventrolateral surface of brainstem where cerebellum, pons, and medulla meet; VII, VIII, and IX CN attach at this point.

cerebellar peduncle fiber bundles connecting the cerebellum to the brainstem.

cerebral aqueduct midbrain channel connecting third and fourth ventricles; syn. aqueduct of Sylvius, iter.

cerebral arterial circle arterial ring found on base of brain and formed by branches of the internal carotid and basilar arteries; connects the anterior and posterior circulations; syn. circle of Willis.

cerebral crus ventral part of cerebral peduncle of midbrain; contains corticospinal and corticobulbar fibers in its middle part and corticopontine in its medial and lateral parts.

cerebral edema brain swelling due to increased uptake of water in the neuropil and white matter.

cerebral ischemia decreased blood supply in the brain.

cerebral peduncle ventral part of midbrain that connects the forebrain to the hindbrain and consists of the cerebral crus, substantia nigra, and tegmentum.

cerebrocerebellum posterior lobe of the cerebellum having strong connections with the cerebrum; syn. neocerebellum.

cerebrospinal fluid (CSF) clear, colorless liquid secreted by the choroid plexuses and found in the ventricular system and subarachnoid space; total volume is approximately 150 mL; rate of formation is approximately 500 mL/day.

chorea (G., dance) jerky, spasmodic involuntary movements of limbs or facial muscles; associated with lesions of the caudate nucleus and putamen.

choroid plexus epithelium and blood vessels of the lateral, third, and fourth ventricles; secretes CSF.

ciliospinal center neurons in the upper one or two thoracic segments giving rise to sympathetic preganglionic fibers that convey impulses to the superior cervical ganglion from whence postganglionic sympathetic fibers elicit pupillary dilation.

ciliospinal reflex dilation of pupils in response to pain usually elicited by stroking the side of the head or neck; dependent on intact path that includes descending central autonomic path, ciliospinal center neurons, and their preganglionic sympathetic fibers, which ascend in the cervical sympathetic trunk, and includes superior cervical ganglion cells whose postganglionic fibers reach the dilator muscle of the iris.

cingulum (L., girdle) a large association bundle passing longitudinally in the white matter of the cingulate gyrus; connects frontal, parietal, and occipital lobes with parahippocampal gyrus and adjacent temporal cortex.

circadian rhythm biologic activity (such as sleep) that occurs in approximately 24-hour periods or cycles; the "clock" resides in the suprachiasmatic nucleus of the hypothalamus.

circle of Willis arterial ring found on base of brain and formed by branches of the internal carotid and basilar arteries; syn. cerebral arterial circle.

circumventricular organs highly vascularized areas with fenestrated capillaries; found chiefly in the diencephalon and lacking the blood-brain barrier.

clasp-knife response sudden relaxation or decrease in resistance to passive stretch of a limb after initial increased resistance; involves Golgi tendon organ (Ib) activity and is seen in pyramidal tract damage.

climbing fibers axons arising from the contralateral inferior olivary nucleus and carrying excitatory impulses to the Purkinje neurons of the cerebellar cortex; collaterals also excite cerebellar nuclei.

clonus series of alternating contractions and relaxations of flexors and extensors produced by passive stretch of a limb; seen in pyramidal tract damage.

cochlea (L., snail shell) spiral part of internal ear concerned with audition; located in anterior part of labyrinth in petrous part of temporal bone.

cogwheel rigidity type of rigidity in which passive movements exhibit intermittent resistance as if cogwheels were moving on one another; a manifestation of tremor superimposed on rigidity, frequently seen in Parkinsonism.

commissural syndrome loss of pain and temperature bilaterally, due to lesion of ventral white commissure of spinal cord.

communicating hydrocephalus disruption of CSF flow outside the ventricular system, usually in the cisterns, subarachnoid space, or arachnoid villi.

conduction aphasia associative aphasia; a form of aphasia in which the patient can speak and write in a way, but skips or repeats words or substitutes; associated with lesions in arcuate fasciculus.

conduction deafness incomplete deafness due to interference with passage of sound waves through the external ear or sound-induced vibrations through the middle ear.

conjugate eye movements movements of both eyes together.

consensual light reflex pupillary constriction of one eye in response to light reaching the retina of the other eye; dependent on intact optic nerve ipsilaterally and oculomotor nerve contralaterally.

corneal reflex closure of the eye on stimulation of the cornea; dependent on afferent impulses in ophthalmic division of trigeminal nerve and spinal trigeminal tract and efferent impulses through facial nucleus and nerve.

corona radiata (L., corona = crown) fibers fanning out from the internal capsule to the cortex.

corpus striatum caudate and lentiform nuclei.

cortical columns columns of neurons in cerebral cortex oriented perpendicular to six layers of cortex; make up the vertical functional units of the cortex.

corticofugal fibers axons carrying impulses away from the cortex.

corticopetal fibers axons carrying impulses toward the cortex.

cough reflex coughing response elicited by irritation of larynx or tracheobronchial tree; dependent on intact afferent fibers in vagus nerve.

cupula of ampullary crest (L., domeshaped cup; cupa = a tub) the gelatinous substance lying over the hair cells of the ampullary crest.

decerebrate posturing describes one whose brain has been injured between the vestibular nuclei and the red nucleus; characterized by extension of upper and lower limbs.

decorticate posturing describes one whose brain has been injured above the red nucleus; characterized by extension of lower limbs and flexion of upper limbs.

dendrite (G., dendron = tree) a branching neuronal protoplasmic process carrying impulses to the cell body.

dendritic spine cytoplasmic bud on surface of a dendrite for synaptic contact; syn. gemmule.

dentate ligament fibrous sheath attached medially to the pia at the lateral surface of the spinal cord, midway between the dorsal and ventral roots; anchors the spinal cord to the dura mater by its lateral serrated part consisting of 21 tooth-like processes.

dermatome (G., derma = skin + tome = a cutting) an area of skin supplied by one spinal nerve and its ganglion.

detrusor muscle muscle in the wall of the urinary bladder.

diabetes insipidus condition caused by hyposecretion of ADH and characterized by thirst and the excretion of large amounts of urine.

diaphragma sellae dural fold covering the pituitary gland; extends across sella turcica.

direct light reflex pupillary constriction in one eye in response to increased light reaching the retina of the same eye; dependent on intact ipsilateral optic and oculomotor nerves.

disc edema edema of the optic disk; may be due to raised intracranial pressure; syn. papilledema, choked disc.

doll's eye movements turning of the eyes in the direction opposite to that of rotation of the head; signifies intact vestibulo-ocular reflex in comatose patient; syn. oculocephalic reflex.

dominant hemisphere the hemisphere responsible for speech, usually the left.

dorsal rhizotomy section of the dorsal roots of spinal nerves for the relief of pain or spasticity.

dorsal root entry zone (DREZ) area in spinal cord where the dorsal roots attach, just external to dorsal horn; DREZ lesions are surgical procedures to abolish chronic deafferentation pain.

dorsal root ganglion groups of unipolar afferent neurons in the dorsal root of each spinal nerve; syn. spinal ganglion.

dorsolateral fasciculus spinal cord tract located between the posterior horn and the posterolateral sulcus; composed of short ascending and descending branches of dorsal root fibers carrying pain and thermal impulses and axons of substantia gelatinosa neurons; syn. tract of Lissauer.

Down syndrome mongolism; trisomy 21 syndrome; a syndrome of mental retardation associated with a variable constellation of abnormalities caused by representation of at least a critical portion of chromosome 21 three times instead of twice in some or all cells.

dura mater (L., dura = hard + mater = mother) the thick outer layer of the meninges.

dural sac continuation of dura mater from LV2–SV2 containing CSF and the cauda equina.

dural sinus valveless, venous channel found in dural attachments and folds.

dysdiadochokinesia (G., dys + diadochos = succeeding + kinesis = movement) a cerebellar disorder manifested by difficulty in rapidly alternating diametrically opposite movements, e.g., pronation and supination.

dyskinesia (G., dys + kinesis) disorder of voluntary movement frequently associated with basal ganglia disease.

dysmetria (G., dys + metron = measure) a cerebellar disorder manifested by difficulty in controlling the range and force of movement.

dysphagia (G., dys + phagein = to eat) difficulty in swallowing.

dysphasia (G., dys + phasis = speech) impairment of speech, characterized by a lack of coordination and failure to arrange words in proper order.

endolymph fluid of the membranous labyrinth of the inner ear.

entorhinal area part of the parahippocampal gyrus immediately posterior to the uncus; area 28.

ependyma (G., epi = upon + endyma = garment) epithelium lining the central canal of the spinal cord and the ventricles of the brain.

epidural space area external to dura; potential in cranial dura, actual in spinal dura.

esotropia (G., eso = inward + trope = turn) inward deviation of the eye; frequently caused by abducent nerve lesion; syn. convergent or internal strabismus.

expressive aphasia see *nonfluent aphasia*.

extensor plantar response abnormal upward extension of great toe in response to stroking outer border of the sole; indicates pyramidal tract damage; syn. Babinski reflex.

extrafusal muscle fibers large skeletal muscle fibers that produce muscular contraction and are innervated by α-motoneurons; to be distinguished from intrafusal muscle fibers within muscle spindles, which are innervated by γ-motoneurons.

falx cerebelli dural fold lying between the cerebellar hemispheres.

falx cerebri dural fold lying between the cerebral hemispheres.

fasciculus (L., fascis = bundle) a bundle of nerve fibers within the CNS.

fasciculus retroflexus see *habenulointerpeduncular tract*.

fast pain sharp, pricking pain that is well localized.

fimbria (L., fringe) longitudinal band of fibers coming from the alveus of hippocampus and continuing as the fornix.

final common pathway term used for the α-motoneurons through which are funneled all impulses from multiple sources to the skeletal muscles; only connections between CNS and extrafusal muscle fibers.

fissure of Sylvius deep groove on lateral surface of cerebral hemisphere; separates temporal lobe below from frontal and parietal lobes above; syn. lateral fissure.

fixation point point on which vision is focused.

flaccid paralysis muscle paralysis with hypotonicity; the cardinal sign of a lower motor neuron lesion.

flocculonodular lobe syndrome disorder characterized by instability of the trunk (truncal ataxia) usually due to tumors near the midline of the vestibulocerebellum; syn. vestibulocerebellar midline syndrome.

fluent aphasia type of language disorder in which words are formed rapidly but they do not make sense because of the loss of ability to comprehend spoken or written words; associated with lesion of Wernicke area; syn. sensory or receptive aphasia.

folium (L., a leaf) one of the folds of the cerebellar surface.

foramen of Luschka see *lateral aperture of the fourth ventricle.*

foramen of Magendie see *median aperture of the fourth ventricle.*

foramen of Monro opening between third ventricle and lateral ventricle; syn. interventricular foramen.

fornix (L., arch) bundle of fibers continuous with fimbria of hippocampus that is the main output of the hippocampal formation; runs in the free margin of the septum pellucidum and divides at the anterior commissure into a small precommissural bundle (from the hippocampus proper) and a larger postcommissural bundle (from the subiculum), which end in the anterior hypothalamus and mamillary body, respectively.

fovea centralis depression in the center of the macula lutea of the retina caused by displacement of the inner layers; contains only cones and is the area of most acute vision.

foveola minute pit in the center of the fovea centralis.

frontal eye field area 8 of the cerebral cortex located mainly in the posterior part of the middle frontal gyrus and concerned with voluntary eye movements.

GABA γ-aminobutyric acid, an inhibitory neurotransmitter.

gag reflex contraction of pharyngeal muscles on stimulation of the lateral part of the oral pharynx; dependent on intact afferent fibers in glossopharyngeal nerve and efferent fibers in vagus nerve.

gait ataxia ataxia affecting the muscles of the lower limbs.

γ-loop three-neuron reflex arc, consisting of a γ-motoneuron and its fusimotor axon, which causes intrafusal muscle fibers to contract; an Ia afferent fiber and its dorsal root ganglion cell; and an α-motoneuron and its motor end-plates, which cause extrafusal muscle fibers to contract. Allows for initiation or influence of movements and tone by γ-motoneurons.

γ-motor neuron neurons located in same places as α-motoneurons but which innervate intrafusal muscle fibers; maintain muscle spindle sensitivity.

genu of internal capsule that part of the internal capsule between the posterior part of the head of the caudate nucleus and anterior part of the thalamus medially and the lentiform nucleus laterally.

glomus (L., a ball) the choroid plexus in the trigone of the lateral ventricle; probably the most prolific producer of CSF.

glutamate excitatory neurotransmitter.

Golgi neuron (of cerebellum) nerve cell of granular layer of cerebellar cortex whose dendrites in the molecular layer are excited by the granule cell axons and whose axon inhibits granule cells.

Golgi tendon organ proprioceptive ending found in tendons; its appropriate stimulus is an increase in tendon tension.

granule cell (1) nerve cell of the inner or granular layer of the cerebellar cortex; axon enters molecular layer and forms the parallel plexus; only excitatory neuron in the cerebellar cortex. (2) intracortical neurons found predominantly in layers II and IV of the neocortex.

graphesthesia ability to recognize and identify figures drawn on the skin.

gustatory nucleus rostral part of the solitary nucleus receptive for taste fibers.

habenula cell mass found at dorsal and posterior edge of the third ventricle near the pineal body; part of the epithalamus.

habenulointerpeduncular tract compact bundle of fibers arising in the habenula and passing ventrally to the interpeduncular nucleus of the midbrain and the adjacent reticular formation; syn. fasciculus retroflexus.

heat gain center neurons in posterior hypothalamus that initiate cutaneous vasoconstriction, piloerection, and shivering.

heat loss center neurons in anterior hypothalamus that initiate sweating and cutaneous vasodilation.

helicotrema (G., helix = coil + trema = hole) area at the apex of the cochlea where the scala vestibuli and scala tympani communicate with one another.

heteronymous (G., having a different name) different visual fields of both eyes.

hindbrain pons, cerebellum, and medulla; syn. rhombencephalon.

hippocampal formation curved band of archipallium located in temporal lobe between choroidal fissure and parahippocampal gyrus; consists of hippocampus proper, dentate gyrus, and subiculum; responsible for memory and processing of new information.

homonymous (G., of the same name) same visual field of both eyes.

horizontal cell local circuit neuron in the internal nuclear layer of the retina that influences synaptic transmission between the photoreceptor cells and the bipolar neurons.

horizontal gaze center see *lateral gaze center*.

Horner syndrome disorder characterized by ptosis, miosis, and anhidrosis; due to central or peripheral interruption of sympathetic impulses to face and eye.

Huntington disease hereditary disorder characterized by progressive increase in choreoid movements and dementia; inherited by a dominant gene that causes degeneration of striatal and cortical acetylcholine and GABA neurons.

hydrocephalus (G., hydro = water + kephale = head) excessive accumulation of CSF due to obstruction of flow, interference with drainage, or increased formation.

hyperacusis abnormal loudness of hearing.

hypercarbia increased CO_2 at the tissue level.

hyperkinetic disorders increase or excessive speed in the initiation or performance of a movement.

hyperthermia fever or increased body temperature.

hypertonia, hypertonicity (G., hyper + tonos =

tension) excessive tone in skeletal muscles; manifested by increased resistance to passive stretch.

hypocarbia decreased CO_2 at the tissue level.

hypokinetic disorders (G., hypo = under + kinesis = movement) decrease or slowing in the initiation or performance of a movement.

hypophysial portal system vascular connection between the median eminence and adjacent infundibular stalk and the anterior lobe of the pituitary by means of which the hypothalamic releasing factors are transported.

hypothalamic regulatory hormones substances formed in hypothalamic neurons that are transported to pituitary gland to regulate the release of its hormones.

hypothalamic syndrome disorder manifested by diabetes insipidus, endocrine disorders, impairment of temperature regulation, abnormalities in sleep patterns, and behavior changes; results from a lesion of the hypothalamus.

hypothalamohypophysial tract unmyelinated fibers from the supraoptic and paraventricular nuclei of the hypothalamus, which reach the posterior pituitary.

hypoxia lack of adequate O_2 at the tissue level.

Ia nerve fiber axons of dorsal root ganglion cells that supply muscle spindles and excite α-motoneurons; form afferent limb of myotatic reflex.

Ib nerve fiber axons of dorsal root ganglion cells that supply tendon organs and inhibit α-motor neurons via spinal interneurons; form afferent limb of inverse myotatic reflex and clasp-knife response.

inferior cerebellar peduncle fiber bundle connecting the cerebellum and medulla; syn. restiform body.

infranuclear lesion lower motor neuron lesion involving axon in peripheral nerve.

infundibulum (L., a funnel) median eminence and infundibular stem of neurohypophysis; syn. neural stalk.

insula (L., island) lobe of the cerebrum located deep to the lateral fissure; syn. island of Reil.

intention tremor to and fro shaking that occurs when a voluntary movement is made; associated with posterior cerebellar lobe dysfunction.

internal arcuate fiber secondary touch, pressure, and position sense axons from the dorsal column nuclei that arch around the central gray in the caudal half of the medulla.

internal capsule white matter between the caudate nucleus and diencephalon medially and the lentiform nucleus laterally; continuous rostrally with corona radiata, caudally with cerebral crus.

internuclear ophthalmoplegia (G., ophthalmos = eye + plege = stroke) disorder of eye movements due to damage to the medial longitudinal fasciculus between the abducent and oculomotor nuclei; manifested during horizontal conjugate movements by lack of adduction in eye on same side as lesion.

interpeduncular fossa deep depression on the ventral surface of the midbrain between the cerebral peduncles.

intrafusal muscle fiber muscle fiber part of a muscle spindle, innervated by γ-motoneurons.

inverse myotatic reflex contraction of a muscle causes an increase in tension, which fires a Golgi tendon organ that carries this information by Ib fibers to excite the antagonists and inhibit the synergists.

iodopsin visual pigment of the cones.

juxtarestiform body medial portion of inferior cerebellar peduncle carrying primarily vestibular fibers.

kernicterus nuclear jaundice in which yellow pigment is formed in certain basal ganglia and limbic nuclei.

kinesthesia (G., kinesis = movement + aisthesis = sensation) awareness of position and movement of body parts.

kinocilium (G., kineo = to move + cilium) longest cilium found on hair cell in crista ampullaris; bending of stereocilia toward or away from kinocilium results in excitation or inhibition (respectively) of vestibular nerve fibers.

Klüver-Bucy syndrome disorder characterized by docility, oral tendencies, bulimia, and bizarre sexual behavior; results from bilateral ablation of anterior temporal lobes.

Korsakoff syndrome disorder involving memory loss, confusion, and confabulation; lesions frequently found in the walls of the third ventricle involving the mamillary bodies, medial dorsal thalamic nuclei, or anterior thalamic nuclei.

lateral aperture lateral opening connecting fourth ventricle with subarachnoid space; syn. foramen of Luschka.

lateral fissure most prominent cleft on lateral surface of cerebral hemisphere; begins anteriorly and proceeds posteriorly separating the frontal and parietal lobes from the temporal lobe; syn. Sylvian fissure.

lateral gaze center neurons in the paramedian pontine reticular nucleus that elicit horizontal eye movements to the ipsilateral side; formerly called parabducent nucleus; syn. horizontal gaze center.

lateral lemniscus tract in the lateral part of the pontine and midbrain tegmentum from the pontomedullary junction to the inferior colliculus; comprised of the central acoustic fibers, although sometimes the spinothalamic tract is included.

lateral medullary syndrome disorder characterized by loss of pain and thermal sensations over ipsilateral half of face and contralateral half of body; nausea; vertigo; ipsilateral ataxia; ipsilateral paralysis of soft palate, pharynx, and vocal cord; and Horner syndrome. Due to vascular lesion involving the vertebral or the posterior inferior cerebellar artery; syn. Wallenberg syndrome.

lead-pipe rigidity bidirectional hypertonicity resulting from increased tone in all of the muscles acting on a joint; associated with basal ganglia disorders.

lemniscus (G., lemniskos = ribbon or fillet) a secondary sensory tract ascending through the brainstem to the thalamus.

leptomeninges (G., leptos = slender or delicate + meninx = membrane) arachnoid and pia mater, the two thin membranes covering the brain and spinal cord.

light reflex constriction of pupil on increased light reaching the retina.

limbic lobe (L., limbus = border) structures on medial surface of cerebral hemisphere bordering the corpus callosum and rostral brainstem; includes the cingulate and parahippocampal gyri.

limbic system (L., limbus = border) cortical and subcortical structures that influence behavior and autonomic responses chiefly through the hypothalamus; includes the limbic lobe, amygdaloid nucleus, hippocampal formation, septal region, and hypothalamus and some also include the anterior thalamic nucleus, medial part of the midbrain tegmentum, orbitofrontal cortex, and anterior cingulate gyrus.

loop of Meyer those fibers of the optic radiation, which, after leaving the lateral part of the lateral geniculate nucleus and passing into the temporal lobe, arch over the inferior horn of the lateral ventricle before turning back toward the occipital lobe.

lower motor neuron brainstem or spinal cord α-motoneuron; axon carries impulses to extrafusal muscle fibers; syn. final common pathway.

lower motor neuron syndrome disorder characterized by flaccid paralysis, decreased or absent reflexes, and severe atrophy; due to loss of the final common path, i.e., the loss of the α-motoneurons or their axons innervating a muscle.

lumbar puncture procedure by which the dural sac is entered by inserting a needle usually between LV3-LV4 or LV4-LV5 in adults and always below LV4 in infants.

macula lutea (L., macula = spot + luteus = saffron-yellow) yellowish area of retina lateral and slightly below the optic disc at a point corresponding to posterior pole of retina.

macula of saccule sensory neuroepithelium in anteromedial part of wall of saccule.

macula of utricle sensory neuroepithelium in anterolateral part of wall of utricle.

mechanoreceptor receptor that is excited by its distortion due to touch, pressure, muscle, or tendon stretch, etc.

medial forebrain bundle diffuse system of fibers located in the lateral hypothalamus; interconnects with septal region rostrally and midbrain reticular formation caudally.

medial lemniscus tract located medially in the medulla, ventrally in the pontine tegmentum, and dorsolaterally in the midbrain tegmentum; carries touch, pressure, and position sense impulses from the contralateral gracile and cuneate nuclei to the ventral posterolateral nucleus of the thalamus.

medial longitudinal fasciculus bundle of fibers extending from the midbrain to the spinal cord; located close to the midline in the dorsal part of the tegmentum adjacent to the nuclei of the external ocular muscles; composed largely of fibers ascending to motor neurons of the external ocular nuclei, and descending to spinal motoneurons innervating the paravertebral musculature.

median aperture midline opening between posterior part of frontal ventricle and subarachnoid space; syn. foramen of Magendie

median eminence part of neurohypophysis that is frequently considered to be the raised portion of the tuber cinereum; together with the infundibular stem and process (neural lobe), forms the neurohypophysis.

medulloblastoma glioma consisting of neoplastic cells that resemble the undifferentiated cells of the primitive medullary tube.

Meissner corpuscle encapsulated tactile receptor in dermal papilla.

melanin dark brown or black pigment found in cytoplasm of neurons in some nuclei (substantia nigra, locus ceruleus, etc.).

membranous labyrinth system of endolymph-containing ducts and chambers of the inner ear; includes utricle, saccule, semicircular ducts, cochlear ducts, and their connections.

meningioma (G., meninges + oma = tumor) benign tumor of arachnoid origin; tends to occur along superior sagittal sinus, sphenoid ridges, and near optic chiasm.

microsmatic (G., mikros + osmasthia = to smell) having a feeble sense of smell.

middle cerebellar peduncle fiber bundle connecting the cerebellum and the pons; syn. brachium pontis.

middle cerebral candelabra shape of trunks and branches of middle cerebral artery in lateral fissure as seen radiographically.

miosis (G., meiosis = a lessening) constriction of the pupil.

monoplegia (G., mono + plege = stroke) paralysis or paresis in one limb.

mossy fibers afferent axons arising from cerebellar input nuclei other than the inferior olive; branch repeatedly in white matter and granule layer and are excitatory to granule cells and cerebellar nuclei.

motor aphasia see *nonfluent aphasia.*

motor end-plate acetylcholine synapse of α-motor neuron on extrafusal muscle fiber; syn. myoneural junction.

motor unit α-motoneuron, its axon, and the extrafusal muscle fibers it innervates.

Müller cell glial-like cells chiefly in the bipolar cell layer of the retina whose processes form the external and internal limiting membranes.

muscle spindle mechanoreceptor in skeletal muscle.

myasthenia gravis (G., mys = muscle + asthenia = weakness) autoimmune disease characterized by muscular weakness, beginning usually in the orofacial region, due to increased turnover of acetylcholine receptors at the neuromuscular junction.

mydriasis extreme dilation of the pupil.

myotatic reflex (G., myo = to shut + tasis = stretching) contraction of a muscle induced by stretching; syn. stretch, deep, or tendon reflex.

myotome skeletal muscles supplied by a single spinal cord segment.

negative signs functional deficits resulting from a lesion.

neglect syndrome perceptual disorder related to lack of recognition of the opposite side of the body and its surroundings.

neospinothalamic system newer spinothalamic system, which carries fast pain to the ventral posterolateral thalamic nucleus; its peripheral fibers are of the A delta type and it arises chiefly from marginal neurons in the dorsal horn of the spinal gray.

nerve deafness perception deafness due to damage to sensory cells of inner ear or to cochlear nerve; degree of hearing loss depends on amount of damage.

neurinoma benign tumor arising from Schwann cells.

neuroepithelium epithelial cells that serve as the special receptors in the auditory, vestibular, olfactory, and gustatory systems; syn. neurepithelium.

neurogenic bladder abnormal functioning of the urinary bladder as a result of a CNS or PNS lesion.

neuroglia (G., glia = glue) non-neuronal support cells of the CNS; 10 times more numerous than neurons; four types: astrocytes, oligodendrocytes, microglia, and ependymal cells; syn. glia.

neurolemma cytoplasmic sheath of Schwann cells surrounding a peripheral nerve fiber.

neuroma nerve cell or nerve fiber tumor.

neurotransmitter (L., neuro + transmitto = to send across) any specific chemical agent released by a presynaptic cell on excitation, which crosses the synaptic cleft to stimulate or inhibit the postsynaptic cell.

Nissl body plates of rough endoplasmic reticulum and free ribosomes found in cytoplasm of nerve cell perikaryon and large dendrites.

nociceptor (L., noceo = to injure, hurt + capio = to take) receptor that is stimulated by actual tissue injury or anticipated injury; a receptor for pain.

node of Ranvier discontinuity in the myelin sheath of a nerve fiber where one Schwann cell in peripheral nerves or one oligodendrocyte in central nerves meets the next.

nonfluent aphasia language disorder characterized by difficulty in forming words; associated with lesion of Broca speech area; syn. motor or expressive aphasia.

nonreflex neurogenic bladder incontinence and severe retention; a "lower motor neuron" type resulting from lesions of sacral spinal cord or cauda equina.

nuclear lesion lower motor neuron lesion involving cell body.

nystagmus (G., nystagmus = a nodding) involuntary rapid movements of the eyeballs consisting of fast and slow phases; named according to direction of fast phase.

obstructive hydrocephalus blockage of CSF flow within the ventricular system.

occipital eye field areas 17, 18, 19 of the cerebral cortex, which are concerned with eye movements chiefly of a reflex nature.

oculocephalic reflex turning of the eyes in the direction opposite to that of rotation of the head; signifies intact vestibulo-ocular reflex in comatose patient; syn. doll's eye movement.

oligodendrocytes (G., oligos = few + dendron = tree + glia = glue) neuroglial cells with small electron–dense oval nuclei and scanty cytoplasm; form myelin sheath of CNS.

operculum (L., cover or lid) those parts of the cerebrum that cover the insula and form the margins of the lateral fissure.

ophthalmoplegia (G., ophthalmos = eye + plege = stroke) paralysis of the eye muscles.

optic disc or papilla area where the optic nerve fibers leave the retina.

optokinetic nystagmus nystagmus induced by looking at a moving object; syn. railroad nystagmus.

organ of Corti sensory end organ for hearing found in cochlear duct of internal ear; syn. spiral organ.

osseous labyrinth (L., osseus = bony) spaces found in petrous part of the temporal bone comprising cochlea, vestibule, and semicircular canals; syn. bony labyrinth.

otoconia (G., otos = ear + konis = dust) crystalline particles of calcium carbonate and a protein adhering to the gelatinous otolithic membrane of the maculae of the utricle and saccule; syn. statoconia or otoliths.

otolith (G., otos + lithos = stone) one of the particles constituting the otoconia; syn. statoconium, otoconium, statolith.

otolithic membrane gelatinous substance overlying the maculae of utricle and saccule into which their cilia are embedded; contains calcium carbonate crystals, the otoliths.

oval window opening between tympanic cavity and scala vestibuli of cochlea; syn. fenestra vestibuli.

oxytocin hormone secreted by magnocellular neurons in the supraoptic and paraventricular nuclei of the hypothalamus that stimulates contraction of the smooth muscle fibers (cells) in the pregnant uterus and contractile cells around the ducts of mammary glands.

paleospinothalamic system older spinothalamic system, which carries slow pain to a broader area including the reticular formation and intralaminar thalamic nuclei, therefore less localized than the neospinothalamic system; peripheral fibers are of the C type; arise from neurons chiefly in laminae IV, V, and VI of the dorsal horn.

palsy weakness or paralysis of muscles.

Papez circuit neural circuit concerned with short-term memory and learning and thought to be reverberating; includes hippocampus, fornix, mamillary bodies, mamillothalamic tract, anterior thalamic nucleus, cingulate gyrus, cingulum, and parahippocampal gyrus.

papilledema (papilla + edema). choked disc; papillary stasis; edema of the optic disc; may be due to raised intracranial pressure; syn. disc edema.

paralysis agitans see *Parkinson disease*.

paraplegia (G., para = beside + plege = a stroke) paralysis of the lower limbs.

paresis (G., a letting go, slackening, relaxation) partial paralysis or weakness.

Parkinson disease neurologic syndrome characterized by tremors at rest and rigidity ascribed to lesions of the substantia nigra; syn. paralysis agitans.

photopic vision vision when eye is light adapted.

pia mater innermost layer of the meninges.

plasticity phenomenon whereby neurons alter or modify their connections; occurs freely in the developing nervous system and in response to injury in the mature nervous system; mechanisms include collateral sprouting, paraterminal axonal sprouting, and contact synaptogenesis; thought to be responsible for some of the behavioral changes following CNS lesions.

poikilothermy (G., poikilos = varied + therme = heat) a condition in which the body temperature varies with the environment; can result from a lesion in the posterior hypothalamus.

positive signs spontaneous, uncontrollable activity resulting from a lesion.

posterior lobe syndrome disorder characterized by ataxia, hypotonia, intention tremor, dysmetria, dysdiadochokinesia, and, if bilateral, explosive speech; results from a lesion in the posterior lobe of the cerebellum, dentate nucleus, or dentatothalamic tract; syn. neocerebellar syndrome.

projection fibers axons that connect the cerebral cortex with subcortical neurons.

propriospinal neurons spinal cord cells whose axons make up the fasciculi proprii adjacent to the gray matter.

prosopagnosia difficulty in recognizing familiar faces.

ptosis (G., fall) drooping of the upper eyelid.

Purkinje neuron large efferent neuron of the cerebellar cortex whose massive dendritic tree spreads chiefly transverse to the long axis of the folium in the molecular layer, and whose axon inhibits neurons chiefly in the cerebellar nuclei.

pyramidal cell large triangular neuron of cerebral cortex having apical dendrite extending toward pial surface as well as horizontally directed basal dendrites; axon emerges from base of cell and passes to the white matter as an association, commissural, or projection fiber.

quadriplegia (quadri + G. plege, stroke) tetraplegia; paralysis of all four limbs.

receptive aphasia see *fluent aphasia*.

referred pain pain that is perceived as coming from a site other than its origin.

reflex neurogenic bladder "upper motor neuron" type resulting from CNS lesions rostral to sacral spinal cord.

Reissner membrane see *vestibular membrane*.

retrograde axonal transport passage toward the cell body; worn-out material is brought back toward the soma by a rapid (200 to 300 mm/day) transport; toxins, e.g., tetanus, and viruses, e.g., herpes, polio, and rabies, can also be brought back.

rhodopsin visual pigment of the rods.

rigidity (L., rigidus = rigid, inflexible) stiffness or inflexibility manifested by pervasive resistance to passive movement.

Rinne tuning fork test vibrating tuning fork heard longer and louder when in contact with the skull (usually the mastoid process) than when held near the pinna—indication of some disorder of the sound-conducting apparatus.

Romberg sign if a patient standing is more unsteady with the eyes closed, dorsal column ataxia rather than cerebellar ataxia is indicated.

round window opening between tympanic cavity and scala tympani of cochlea.

saccade small, quick eye movements on changing point of fixation.

sacral sparing normal motor and sensory functions in sacral region following spinal cord injury more rostrally.

Schwann cell cell of ectodermal origin that forms

the neurolemma of a peripheral nerve fiber and contains the myelin if the axon is myelinated.

scotopic vision (G., skotos = darkness + opsis = vision) vision when the eye is dark adapted.

sensory aphasia see *fluent aphasia*.

septal region limbic system area anterior and lateral to lamina terminalis; includes subcallosal area and septal nuclei deep to it; associated with reward or pleasurable feelings.

sheath of Schwann see *neurolemma*.

slow pain dull, burning pain that is diffuse rather than localized, resulting from tissue injury.

somatosensory system pertaining to the general somatic senses: somatic pain and temperature, touch, vibration, and limb position and motion sensibility.

spasticity condition of increased muscle tone and exaggerated tendon reflexes.

spinal shock spinal cord areflexia due to sudden interruption of cortical input.

spiral organ sensory end organ for hearing found in cochlear duct of internal ear; syn. organ of Corti.

splenium (G., splenion = bandage) posterior portion of corpus callosum.

split brain brain in which the corpus callosum and sometimes the anterior and hippocampal commissures have been severed in the median plane.

stereocilia groups of extremely long, slender, nonmotile microvilli projecting from epithelial cells.

stereognosis (G., stereos = solid + gnosis = knowledge) ability to recognize an object by touch alone.

strabismus deviation of an eye due to impaired function of an extraocular muscle or nerve.

subarachnoid space beneath the arachnoid, refers to space filled with CSF.

subdural space beneath the dura, between the dura and the arachnoid; refers to a potential space containing a serous fluid.

substantia innominata gray matter of the anterior perforated substance; contains basal nucleus of Meynert.

substantia nigra pigmental nuclear mass located in the midbrain; one of the basal ganglia; malfunction associated with Parkinson disease.

subthalamic nucleus nuclear mass located in subthalamus; one of the basal ganglia; malfunction associated with ballismus.

subthalamus part of the diencephalon found be-

tween the thalamus dorsally, the cerebral peduncle ventrally, and the hypothalamus medially; composed of subthalamic nucleus, zona incerta, and prerubral field; syn. ventral thalamus.

superior cerebellar peduncle fiber bundle connecting the cerebellum and the midbrain; syn. brachium conjunctivum.

superior longitudinal fasciculus large association bundle connecting cortex on the lateral surfaces of the frontal, parietal, and occipital lobes; sometimes described as dorsal part of arcuate fasciculus.

superior medullary velum thin lamina of white matter between the superior cerebellar peduncles; forms the roof of the pontine part of the fourth ventricle in the midline, beneath the lingula of the cerebellum; syn. anterior medullary velum.

supranuclear lesion upper motor neuron lesion.

Sylvian fissure see *lateral fissure*.

sympathetic (G., syn = with + pathos = suffering) that division of the autonomic system having the origin of its preganglionic component in the thoracic and lumbar cord segments and playing a role in the preparation of the organism for emergency situations.

synapse (G., syn = together + haptein = to touch) site of functional contact between neurons where impulses pass from one neuron to another.

syndrome (G., concurrence of symptoms) the aggregate of signs and symptoms associated with any morbid state.

syringomyelia (G., syrinx = tube + myelos = marrow) spinal cord abnormality in which cavitation occurs.

tabes dorsalis (L., tabes = a wasting away) deterioration of dorsal spinal roots and dorsal columns of the spinal cord resulting from syphilis and manifested by pain and paresthesia, impairment of postural and vibratory sensibility, ataxia, and decreased stretch reflexes; syn. locomotor ataxia.

tachycardia heart hurry; rapid beating of the heart, usually applied to rates over 100 per minute.

tic douloureux trigeminal neuralgia.

transcutaneous electric nerve stimulation (TENS) selective electrical stimulation of large cutaneous afferent fibers in order to inhibit slow pain conduction in spinothalamic neurons; used for treatment of chronic pain.

transient ischemic episodes brief periods of focal cerebral dysfunction lasting less than 24 hours; caused by carotid or vertebrobasilar ischemia.

tremor (L., tremere = to shake) involuntary trembling or shaking.

trigeminal neuralgia pain of a severe, throbbing, or stabbing character in the course or distribution of the trigeminal nerve.

truncal ataxia ataxia affecting the muscles of the trunk; most often caused by a lesion of the vestibulo-cerebellar midline.

uncinate fasciculus (L., uncinatus = hook shaped) association bundle connecting the frontal and temporal lobes.

uncus (L., hook) thickening on the medial side of the parahippocampal gyrus overlying the amygdala and resting near the free edge of the tentorium cerebelli.

uninhibited reflex bladder incontinence but no retention; occurs after bilateral frontal lobe lesions.

upper motor nerve syndrome disorder characterized by spastic paralysis, exaggerated myotatic reflexes, and abnormal superficial and deep reflexes; due to lesion of corticospinal system although some include other corticofugal paths also.

vasopressin see *antidiuretic hormone* (ADH).

vermis (L., worm) the midline portion of the cerebellum; its connections are primarily with the fastigial nucleus, which affects the vestibular nuclei for equilibrium and eye movements.

vertical gaze center neurons at the levels of the superior colliculus and pretectal area, which control vertical eye movements; upward movements represented more dorsally, downward more ventrally.

vestibular membrane (Reissner membrane) membrane within the cochlea that separates the scala vestibuli and the cochlear duct.

vestibulo-ocular reflex three-neuron reflex resulting in turning of eyes in a direction opposite to that of head rotation: (1) vestibular ganglion, (2) vestibular nuclei, (3) III, IV, VI nuclei.

vibration sense awareness of deep touch and pressure tested with a vibrating tuning fork.

Virchow-Robin space spaces that surround blood vessels where they enter the CNS.

Wallenberg syndrome see *lateral medullary syndrome*.

Weber syndrome disorder characterized by contralateral spastic hemiplegia with ipsilateral ophthalmoplegia (with the eye turned down and out, ptosis, and mydriasis); results from a lesion of the cerebral crus and oculomotor nerve of one side in the midbrain; syn. superior alternating hemiplegia or alternating oculomotor hemiplegia.

Weber tuning fork test application of a vibrating tuning fork to the midline of the forehead to ascertain in which ear the sound is heard better; the better heard ear being abnormal in conduction deafness or normal in sensorineural deafness.

Wernicke area posterior part of the superior temporal gyrus of the dominant hemisphere, which functions as a receptive speech center.

Wernicke zone triangular zone in retrolenticular part of the internal capsule lateral to the lateral geniculate nucleus containing the optic radiations.

Appendix D

SUGGESTED READINGS

Apuzzo MLJ. Surgery of the third ventricle. Baltimore: Williams & Wilkins, 1987.

Barr ML, Kiernan JA. The human nervous system. 6th ed. Philadelphia: Lippincott-Raven, 1993.

Burt AM. Textbook of neuroanatomy. Philadelphia: WB Saunders, 1993.

Brodal A. Neurological anatomy in relation to clinical medicine. 3rd ed. New York: Oxford University Press, 1981.

Brodal P. The central nervous system. New York: Oxford University Press, 1992.

Carpenter MB. Core text of neuroanatomy. 4th ed. Baltimore: Williams & Wilkins, 1991.

Carpenter MB, Sutin J. Human neuroanatomy. 8th ed. Baltimore: Williams & Wilkins, 1983.

Crosby EC, Humphrey T, Lauer EW. Correlative anatomy of the nervous system. New York: Macmillan, 1962.

Heimer L. The human brain and spinal cord. Functional neuroanatomy and dissection guide. New York: Springer-Verlag, 1983.

Kandel ER, Schwartz JH, Jessell TM. Principles of neural science. 3rd ed. New York: Elsevier, 1991.

Martin JH. Neuroanatomy text and atlas. New York: Elsevier, 1989.

Nauta WJH, Feirtag M. Fundamental neuroanatomy. New York: WH Freeman, 1986.

Noback CR, Strominger NL, Demarest RJ. The human nervous system: introduction and review. 4th ed. Philadelphia: Lea & Febiger, 1991.

Nolte J. The human brain: an introduction to its functional anatomy. 3rd ed. St. Louis: Mosby–Year Book, 1993.

Westmoreland BF, Benarroch EE, Daube JR, Reagan TJ, Sandok BA. Medical neurosciences. 3rd ed. Boston: Little, Brown & Co., 1994.

Willis WD Jr, Grossman RG. Medical neurobiology. Neuroanatomical and neurophysiological principles basic to clinical neuroscience. 3rd ed. St. Louis: Mosby–Year Book, 1981.

Yasargil MG. Microneurosurgery. Vol. 1 Anatomy. Stuttgart: Georg Thieme, 1984.

Appendix E

ATLAS OF MYELIN STAINED SECTIONS

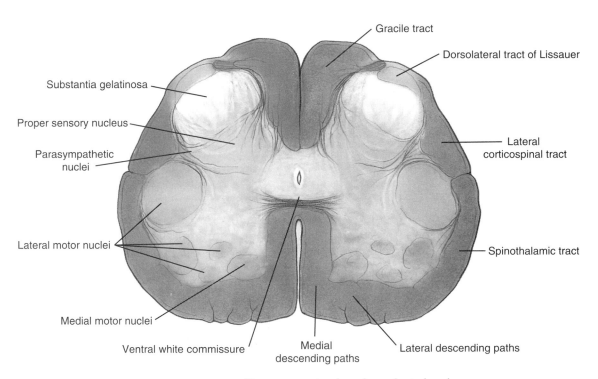

FIGURE E−1. Transverse section through sacral spinal cord.

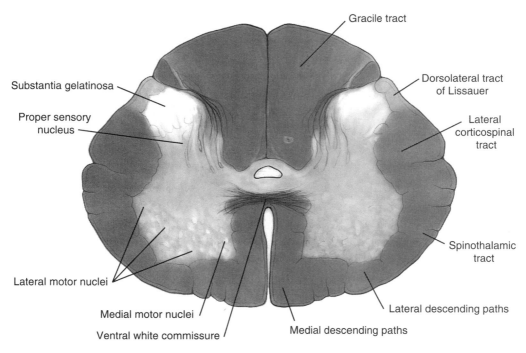

Gracile tract

Substantia gelatinosa

Proper sensory nucleus

Dorsolateral tract of Lissauer

Lateral corticospinal tract

Spinothalamic tract

Lateral motor nuclei

Medial motor nuclei

Ventral white commissure

Medial descending paths

Lateral descending paths

FIGURE E‑2. Transverse section through lumbar spinal cord.

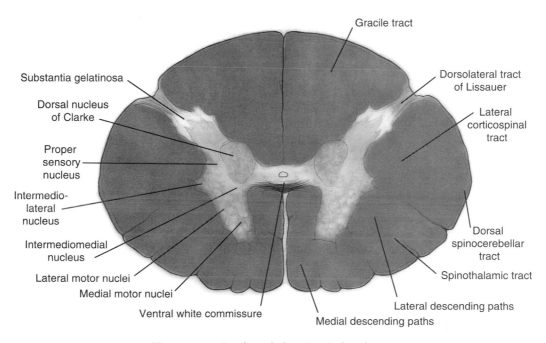

Gracile tract

Substantia gelatinosa

Dorsal nucleus of Clarke

Proper sensory nucleus

Intermedio‑lateral nucleus

Intermediomedial nucleus

Lateral motor nuclei

Medial motor nuclei

Ventral white commissure

Dorsolateral tract of Lissauer

Lateral corticospinal tract

Dorsal spinocerebellar tract

Spinothalamic tract

Lateral descending paths

Medial descending paths

FIGURE FIGURE E‑3. Transverse section through thoracic spinal cord.

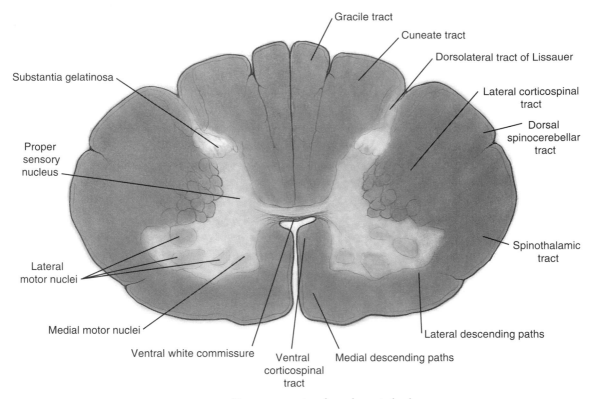

FIGURE E–4. Transverse section through cervical enlargement.

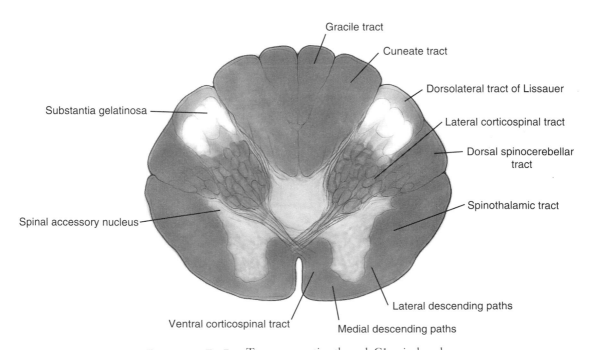

FIGURE E–5. Transverse section through C1, spinal cord.

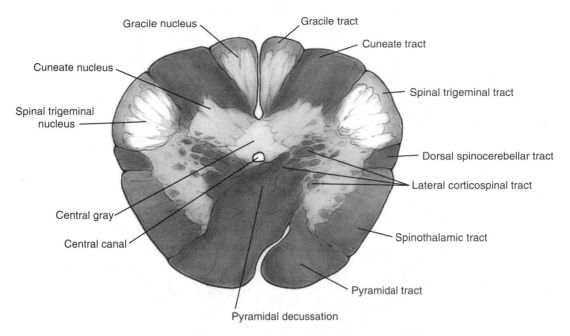

FIGURE E-6. Transverse section through medulla at pyramidal decussation.

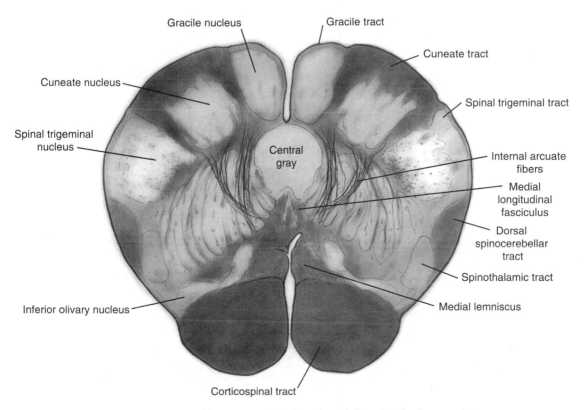

FIGURE E-7. Transverse section through medulla at dorsal column nuclei.

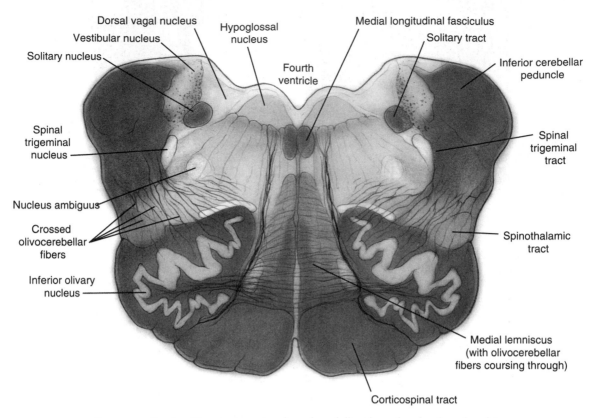

FIGURE E-8. Transverse section through medulla at hypoglossal and vagal nuclei.

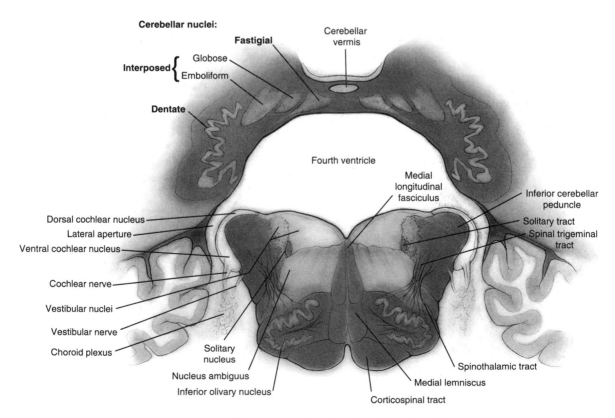

FIGURE E-9. Transverse section through medulla at lateral aperture.

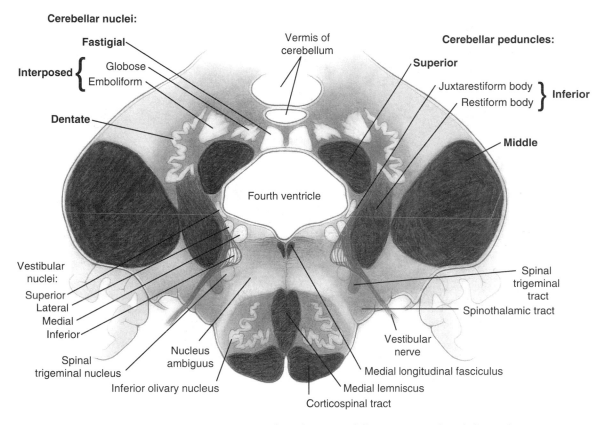

Cerebellar nuclei:

Fastigial

Interposed { Globose / Emboliform }

Dentate

Vermis of cerebellum

Cerebellar peduncles:

Superior

Juxtarestiform body

Restiform body } **Inferior**

Middle

Fourth ventricle

Vestibular nuclei:
Superior
Lateral
Medial
Inferior

Spinal trigeminal nucleus

Nucleus ambiguus

Inferior olivary nucleus

Corticospinal tract

Medial lemniscus

Medial longitudinal fasciculus

Vestibular nerve

Spinothalamic tract

Spinal trigeminal tract

FIGURE E–10. Transverse section through pontomedullary junction and cerebellar nuclei.

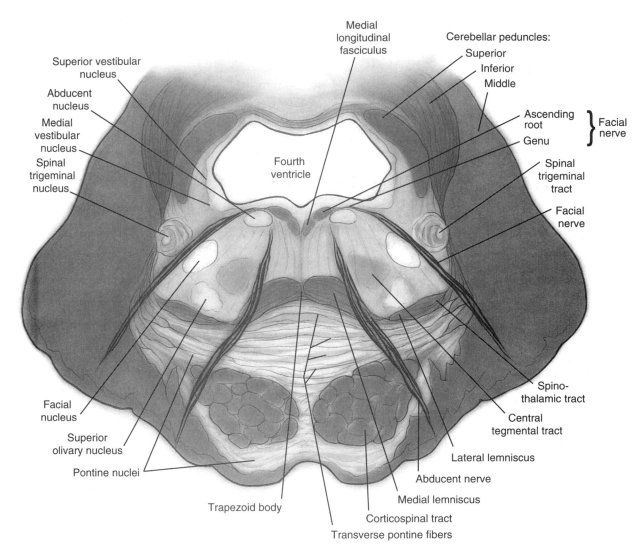

FIGURE E-11. Transverse section through caudal pons at abducent and facial nuclei.

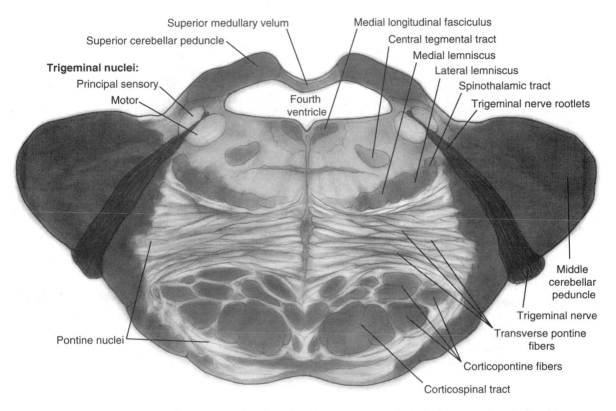

FIGURE E-12. Transverse section through midpons at motor and principal sensory trigeminal nuclei.

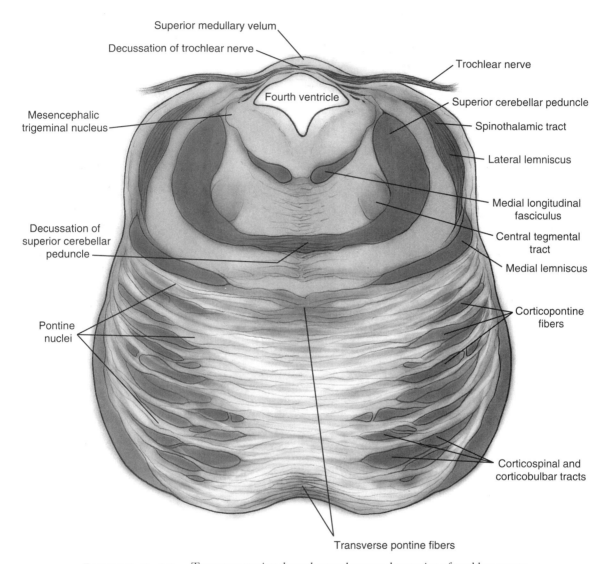

Superior medullary velum

Decussation of trochlear nerve

Trochlear nerve

Fourth ventricle

Superior cerebellar peduncle

Mesencephalic trigeminal nucleus

Spinothalamic tract

Lateral lemniscus

Medial longitudinal fasciculus

Decussation of superior cerebellar peduncle

Central tegmental tract

Medial lemniscus

Pontine nuclei

Corticopontine fibers

Corticospinal and corticobulbar tracts

Transverse pontine fibers

FIGURE E–13. Transverse section through rostral pons at decussation of trochlear nerves.

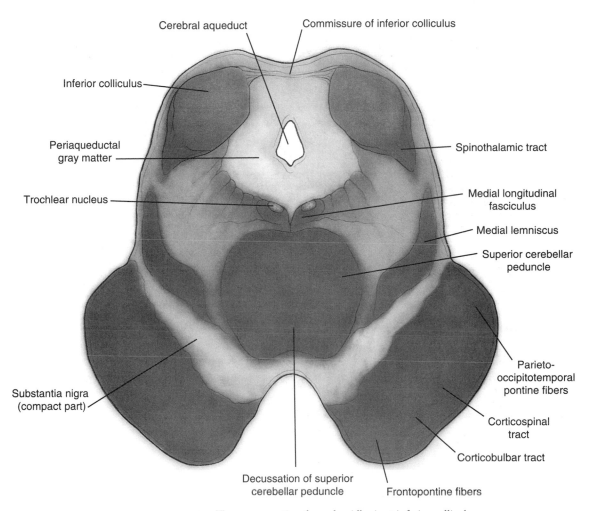

Cerebral aqueduct

Commissure of inferior colliculus

Inferior colliculus

Periaqueductal
gray matter

Spinothalamic tract

Trochlear nucleus

Medial longitudinal
fasciculus

Medial lemniscus

Superior cerebellar
peduncle

Substantia nigra
(compact part)

Parieto-
occipitotemporal
pontine fibers

Corticospinal
tract

Corticobulbar tract

Decussation of superior
cerebellar peduncle

Frontopontine fibers

FIGURE E−14. Transverse section through midbrain at inferior colliculus

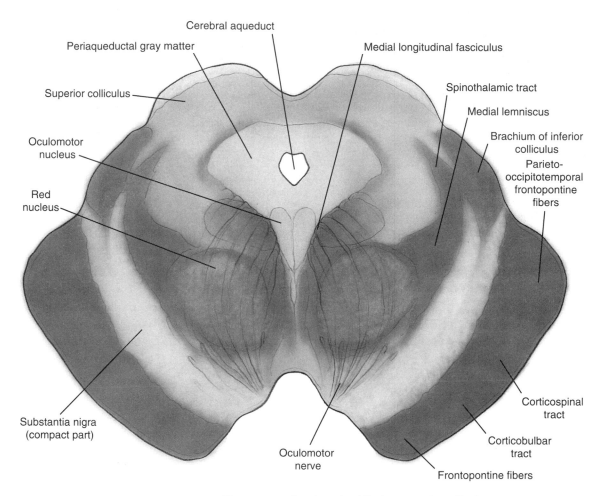

Cerebral aqueduct

Periaqueductal gray matter

Medial longitudinal fasciculus

Superior colliculus

Spinothalamic tract

Medial lemniscus

Brachium of inferior colliculus

Oculomotor nucleus

Parieto-occipitotemporal frontopontine fibers

Red nucleus

Substantia nigra (compact part)

Oculomotor nerve

Corticospinal tract

Corticobulbar tract

Frontopontine fibers

FIGURE E–15. Transverse section through midbrain at superior colliculus.

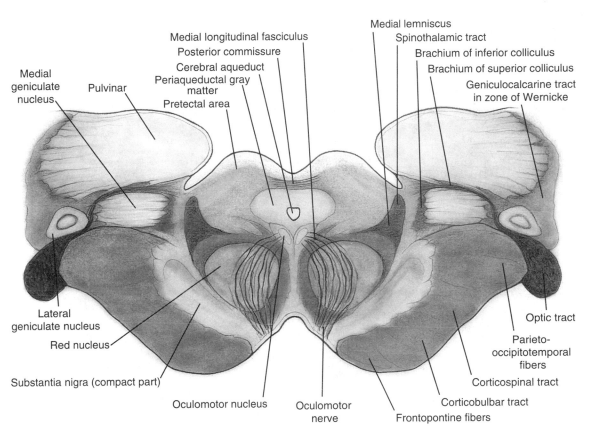

Medial geniculate nucleus

Pulvinar

Medial longitudinal fasciculus

Posterior commissure

Cerebral aqueduct

Periaqueductal gray matter

Pretectal area

Medial lemniscus

Spinothalamic tract

Brachium of inferior colliculus

Brachium of superior colliculus

Geniculocalcarine tract in zone of Wernicke

Lateral geniculate nucleus

Red nucleus

Substantia nigra (compact part)

Oculomotor nucleus

Oculomotor nerve

Frontopontine fibers

Corticobulbar tract

Corticospinal tract

Parieto-occipitotemporal fibers

Optic tract

FIGURE E-16. Transverse section through midbrain at pretectal region and overlapping posterior thalamus.

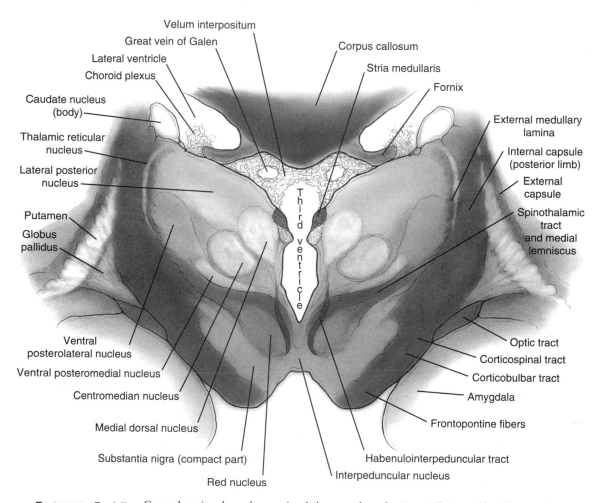

FIGURE E-17. Coronal section through posterior thalamus and overlapping midbrain and lentiform nuclei.

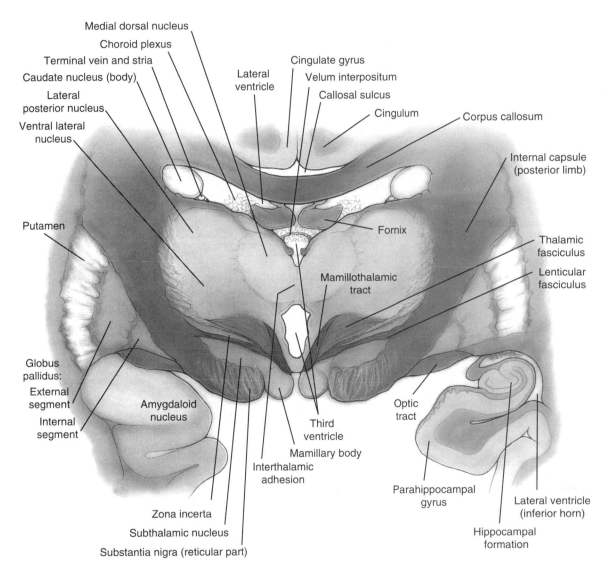

FIGURE E-18. Coronal section through deep forebrain at mamillary bodies level.

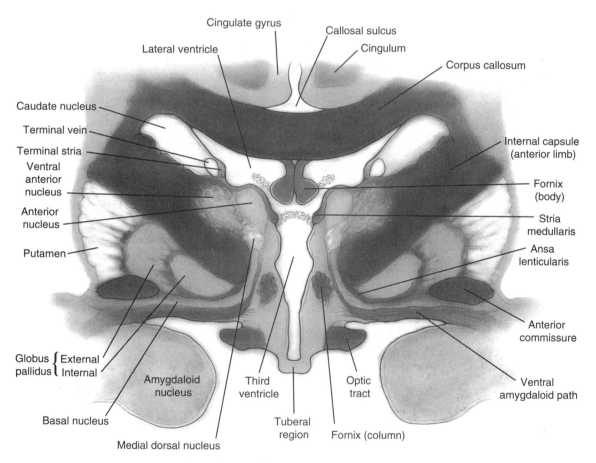

FIGURE E-19. Coronal section through deep forebrain at tuberal level of hypothalamus.

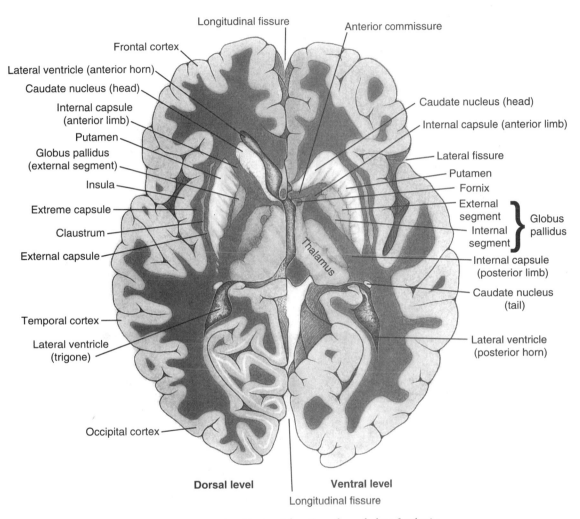

FIGURE E-20. Horizontal sections through deep forebrain.

Index

Note: Page numbers in *italics* refer to illustrations; page numbers followed by *t* refer to tables.

A

Abducent hemiplegia syndrome, alternating, 70
Abducent nerve (VI), 50–52, *51*
  lesions of, 50, *51*, *262–263*, 289, 289t, 295t
Abducent nucleus, *48*, 50–52, *51*, *330*
Abducent palsy, *263*
Accessory nerve (XI), *26*, *28*, 53, *53*, *294*, 294t, 297t
Accommodation center, *163*, 164
Accommodation reflexes, 163–164, *163*
Acoustic neurinoma, 169, 267, *270*
Acoustic striae, 169, *170*, *171*, *172*
Acute sympathetic shock syndrome, 231, 232
Afferent signals, 2
Akinesia, in basal ganglia disease, 90
Alternating abducent hemiplegia syndrome, 70
Alternating hypoglossal hemiplegia syndrome, 70
Alternating oculomotor hemiplegia, 70
Alzheimer disease, 204, *205*
Amacrine cells, *154*, 155
Ambient cistern, 254
Ambiguus nucleus, *48*, 53, *53*, *328*, *329*
Ampulla, 117, *119*
Ampullary crest, 117, *119*
Amygdala, 201, *202*, 205–207
  connections of, 205, *206*
  functions of, 205, 207
  lesions of, 207
Amygdaloid nucleus, *85*, *86*, 205–207, *206*, *337*, *338*
Anhidrosis, 162
Annulospiral stretch receptors, *58*, 59
Anopsia, 159, *160*
Anosmia, 179
Ansa lenticularis, *89*, 90
Anterior cerebral artery, *237*, *238*, 239–240, *239*
Anterior choroidal artery, *237*, 239, *239*
Anterior communicating artery, *237*, *238*, *239*, 240
Anterior inferior cerebellar arteries, *237*, *238*, *239*, 243
Anterior lobe syndrome, 111, *111*

Anterior median fissure, of spinal cord, 17–18, *18*
Antidiuretic hormone, 212
Aphasia, 275, *278*
  conduction, 199
  motor, *192*, 198
  sensory, *192*, 198–199
Apraxia, 190
Arachnoid, *8*, 9, *10*
Area(s)
  Broca speech, 193t, 194, 197–199, *198*, 198
  Brodmann, 190
  entorhinal, 201, *202*, 204
  premotor, 190
  primary gustatory, 194
  primary motor (MI), 61, 190
  primary somatosensory (SI), 134, 194
  secondary somatosensory, 194
  subcallosal, *202*, 207
  supplemental motor, 190
  vestibular, 26, 27, 74
  Wernicke speech, 193t, 198–199, *198*
Area, 1, *191*, 193t, 194, *196*
  2, *191*, 193t, 194, *196*
  3, *191*, 193t, 194, *196*
  4, 190, *191*, 193t, *196*
  5, *191*, 193t, 194
  6, 190, *191*
  7, *191*, 193t, 194
  8, 190, *191*, 193t, *196*
  17, *191*, 193t, 194
  18, *191*, 193t, 195
  19, *191*, 193t, 195
  20, *191*, 195
  21, *191*, 195
  22, *191*, 193t, 195, 198
  39, 193t, 194
  40, 193t, 194
  44, 193t, 194
  45, 193t, 194

Archicerebellum, 99, *100*
Arcuate fasciculus, *185*, 186, 188
Arcuate fibers, internal, 132, *133*, *134*, *135*
Argyll Robertson pupil, 164
Artery(ies)
    of Adamkiewicz, 248
    angular, *241*
    anterior cerebral, *237*, *238*, *239*, *239*, *240*, 247
        stroke, 241
    anterior choroidal, *237*, *238*, *238*, *239*, *239*, 247
    anterior communicating, *237*, *238*, *239*
    anterior inferior cerebellar, *237*, *239*, 243
    anterior spinal, *238*, *239*, *242*, 243, *243*, 248
        stroke, 248
    basilar, *237*, *238*, 243, *243*
    calcarine, *240*
    callosomarginal, *240*, *240*
    common carotid, 237
    coronal, 248, *248*
    internal auditory, 243
    internal carotid, *237*, *237*, *238*
    labyrinthine, 243
    lateral striate, *239*, 247, *247*
    lateral posterior choroidal, 245
    lenticulostriate, 241
    medial posterior choroidal, *244*, 245, *245*
    medial striate, *239*, 246
    middle cerebral, *237*, *238*, *239*, 241, *241*, 247
        stroke, 242
    ophthalmic, 238, *238*
    parieto-occipital, *240*
    peduncular, 245
    pericallosal, *240*
    pontine, *239*
    postcentral, *241*
    posterior cerebral, *237*, *239*, *240*, *244*, 245, *245*,
        247
        stroke, 245
    posterior communicating, *237*, *238*, *238*
    posterior inferior cerebellar, *237*, 242, *243*
        stroke, 243
    posterior parietal, *241*
    posterior spinal, *238*, 242, 248, *248*
    precentral, *241*
    quadrigeminal, *244*, 245, *245*
    radicular, 248
    recurrent of Heubner, *239*, *239*
    Rolandic, 241
    superior cerebellar, *237*, *238*, 243, *244*
    thalamogeniculate, *239*, 245, 247
    thalamoperforate, *239*, *244*, 245, *245*, 247, *247*
    vertebral, *237*, 242, *242*, 243
        stroke, 243
Association fibers, 186
Astereognosis, 194

Astrocytes, 6–7, *6*
Ataxia
    gait, 111, *111*
    truncal, 113–114, *113*
Athetosis, in basal ganglia disease, 91
Auditory cortex, *191–192*, 195
Auditory modulation, 173
Auditory ossicles, 167, *168*
Auditory pathways, 169–173, *170*, *171*, *172*
    bilateralism in, 169–170
Auditory radiation, 169
Auditory receptors, 168–169, *171*
Auditory system, 167–173
    ear of, 167–169, *168*
    lesions of, 169, 170, 173
    modulation of, 173
    pathways of, 169–173, *170*, *171*, *172*
        bilateralism in, 169–170
    receptors of, 168–169, *171*
Automatic reflex bladder, 230, *231*
Autonomic system, 217–232
    afferents of, 222–226
        brainstem, 222, 224, *224*
        spinal, 224
        visceral, 222–224, *223*, *224*
    bladder control centers of, 228–230, *229*, *231*
    cardiac control centers of, 227–228, *228*
    control centers of, 226–232, *227t*, *228*, *229*, *231*
    efferents of, 217–222, *218*, *218t*
        functions of, 221–222, *221t*
        parasympathetic division of, 217–219, *218*, *218t*,
            219, *221t*
        sympathetic division of, *218*, *218t*, 219–221, *219*,
            220, *221t*
    referred pain mechanisms of, 225–226, *225*, *226*
    sex organ control centers of, 230–232
Axon(s), 2, *3*, *4*, *4t*, 5
    myelinated, 5, 7, *7*, 9
    regeneration of, 5
    vs. dendrites, *4t*
Axonal transport, 5

B
Babinski response, in upper motor neuron syndrome,
    67, 70
Ballismus, in basal ganglia disease, 91
Basal ganglia, 83–96, *84*, *85*, *86*, *87*
    in cerebral palsy, 93
    in cognition, 96
    coronal section of, *86*
    in Huntington disease, 92, *92*
    input to, 85, 88, *88*
    interconnections of, 84–85, 88–90, *88*, *93*
    lesions of, 83, 90–96, *92*, *94*
    malfunctions of, 90–91

neurotransmitters of, 93–94, *93*
nigrostriatal projection of, *88,* 89
output of, 89–90, *89*
pallidothalamic projection of, 89–90, *89*
in Parkinson disease, 91–92, *91*
striatonigral projection of, *88,* 89
striatopallidal projection of, *88,* 89
in tardive dyskinesia, 93
Basal nucleus of Meynert, 204
Basal vein of Rosenthal, 249
Basilar artery, *237, 238, 239,* 243, *244*
Basilar membrane, 168
tonotopic localization in, 168, *168*
Basket cells, 102, *102*
Bell palsy, 52
Bitemporal hemianopsia, 159, *160*
Bladder, innervation of, 221*t,* 228–230, *229, 231*
Blind spot, 156
Blood-brain barrier, 6, 236, *237*
Bone conduction, 167
Bony labyrinth, 167, *168*
Brachium
of inferior colliculus, 169, *170, 171, 172*
of superior colliculus, *157,* 159, 160, *161, 163*
Brachium conjunctivum, 27, *101,* 102
Brachium pontis, *101,* 102
Bradykinesia, in basal ganglia disease, 90
Brainstem, 23–33
anatomy of, 23–25, *24*
anterior surface of, 25, *26*
functional levels of, 28–33, *29, 30, 31, 32, 33*
horizontal gaze center of, *120,* 122, *123*
lesions of, 23, 76–77, *76, 77*
lateral, *264, 265, 266* 262–263
medial, 262, *262–263*
motor nuclei of, *48,* 73–76, *74, 75*
in postcapsular lesion recovery, 78–80
posterior surface of, 25, *27*
reticular formation of, 27, *28,* 75
rubral nuclei of, 75–76, *76*
solitary nucleus of, 222, 224, *224,* 328
solitary tract of, 222, 224, *224*
topography of, 25–27, *26, 27*
vergence gaze center of, 122
vertical gaze center of, *120,* 122
vestibular nuclei of, 73–75, *74, 75, 328, 329, 330*
Broca area, 194, 197–199, *198*
Brodmann numbered areas, of cerebral cortex, 190,
191–192, 196–197
Bronchi, innervation of, 221*t*
Brown-Séquard syndrome, *140,* 141, 271, *273*

C
Calcarine sulcus, 157, *158*
Callosal cistern, *255*

Callosal sulcus, 39, *40*
Callosomarginal artery, 240, *240*
Capsular cells, 9
Capsular stroke, 66–69, *68, 69, 70*
Carotid artery
common, 237–242, *238, 239, 240, 241*
internal, 237–238, *237*
Carotid plexuses, 162, *162*
Carotid siphon, 237
Cauda equina, *16,* 17
Caudate nucleus, *41, 42,* 83, *84, 85, 336, 337, 338, 339*
Cell body, *3*
Central cord syndrome, *260*
Central sulcus, 39, *40*
Cerebellar angle, lesions of, 267, *270*
Cerebellar arteries, *237, 238, 239,* 243
Cerebellar cortex, 102–106
circuitry of, *101, 102,* 103, 106
climbing fibers of, *102,* 103
histology of, *102,* 102–103
mossy fibers of, *102,* 103
vs. cerebral cortex, 103
Cerebellar peduncle(s), 99, *101,* 102, *329*
Cerebellar peduncle(s), *329*
inferior, 99, *101,* 102
superior, *101,* 102
lesions of, 283, *284*
Cerebellomedullary cistern, 253, *254*
Cerebellopontine cistern, 253, *254*
Cerebellum, *24,* 99–114
anatomical subdivisions of, 99, *100*
anterior lobe of, 99, *100,* 108–111
connections of, *108, 109,* 110–111
lesions of, 111, *111*
flocculonodular lobe of, 99, *100,* 111–114
connections of, 111–113, *112*
lesions of, 113–114, *113*
folium of, 102, *102*
inferior peduncle of, 99, *101,* 102
lesions of, 99, 107–108, *107,* 111, *111,* 113–114,
113, 271, *274*
metastatic tumor of, 271, *274*
middle peduncle of, *101,* 102
nuclei of, *101, 103,* 106
peduncles of, 99, *101,* 102
posterior lobe of, 99, *100*
connections of, *104, 105,* 106–107
lesions of, 107–108, *107*
superior peduncle of, *101,* 102
Cerebral aqueduct of Sylvius, *24,* 25, 253
Cerebral arterial circle, *238,* 246–247
Cerebral artery (arteries), 236–247, *237*
anterior, *237, 238,* 239–240, *239*
carotid (anterior) system of, 237–242, *238, 239,*
240, 241

Cerebral artery (arteries)—*continued*
  middle, *237, 239*, 241–242, *241*
  posterior, *244*, 245, *245*
  vertebral-basilar (posterior) system of, 242–247, *242, 243, 244, 245, 247*
Cerebral blood flow, 235–236
Cerebral cortex, 183–199
  association fibers of, *185*, 186, 187
  auditory area of, *191–192*, 195
  basal ganglia input from, 85, 88, *88*
  Broca area of, 194, 197–199, *198*
  Brodmann numbered areas of, 190, *191–192, 196–197*
  commissural fibers of, *185, 186, 187*, 188
  connections of, *185*, 186–190, *187, 189*
  cortical columns of, 184, *185*
  frontal eye field of, 190, *191–192*
  frontal lobe of, 190–194, *191–192*, 193*t*, *196–197*
    lesions of, *192*, 193*t*
  functional areas of, 190–199, *191–192, 196–197*
  functional histology of, 184–186, *184, 185*
  gaze centers of, 122–125, *124*
  granule cells of, 183, *184*
  gustatory cortex of, *191–192*, 194
  histologic features of, 183–186, *184, 185*
  internal capsule of, 188, *189*, 190
  intracortical fibers of, *185*, 186
  language areas of, *192*, 197–198, *198*
  lateralization of, 195–197
  lesions of, 275, 278, 279, 282
  neurons of, 184–186, *184, 185*
  occipital lobe of, 193*t*, 195, *196–197*
    lesions of, 193*t*, 195, *196–197*
  orbitofrontal area of, 192–193
  parastriate cortex of, 195
  parietal association area of, *191–192*, 194, *196*
  parietal lobe of, *191–192*, 193*t*, 194, *196–197*
    lesions of, *192*, 193*t*, 283, *285*
  prefrontal cortex of, 191–194, *191, 196*
    lesions of, 193–194
  premotor cortex of, 190
  primary motor area of, 190, *191–192, 196–197*
  primary somatosensory area of, *191–192*, 194, *196–197*
  projection fibers of, *185*, 188–190, *189*
  pyramidal cells of, 183, *184*
  secondary somatosensory area of, 194
  somatosensory area of, *191–192*, 194, *196–197*
  subdivisions of, 183
  supplementary motor area of, 190, *196*
  temporal lobe of, *191–192*, 193*t*, 194–195
    lesions of, 193*t*, 195
  visual cortex of, 195, *196–197*
  vs. cerebellar cortex, 103
Cerebral edema, 236

Cerebral hemisphere(s), 38–40, *39*
  lateral surface of, 38–39, *39*
  lesions of, 263, *266*
  medial surface of, 39–40, *40*
Cerebral hemorrhage, 190
Cerebral ischemia, 66–70, *68, 69, 70*, 237
Cerebral palsy, 93
Cerebral peduncle, *41*
Cerebral veins, 248–249
Cerebrocerebellum, 99, *100*
Cerebrospinal fluid system, 9, *16*, 17, 251–257
  cerebral aqueduct of Sylvius of, *24, 25*, 253
  choroid plexus of, 255
  fluid circulation within, 255, *256*
  fluid composition of, 256
  fluid tap of, *16*, 17, 255–256
  fluid volume of, 255
  fourth ventricle of, 253
  interventricular foramen of Monro of, 252
  lateral ventricles of, 251–252, *252*
  obstruction of, 256–257
  pressure of, 257
  subarachnoid cisterns of, 253–255, *254*
  subarachnoid space of, 253–255, *254*
  third ventricle of, 253
  ventricular system of, 251–253, *252*
Chiasmatic cistern, 254, *254*
Chorea
  in basal ganglia disease, 91
  Huntington, 92, *92*
Choroidal artery
  anterior, *237, 239, 239*
  posterior, *244*
Ciliospinal center, 162, *162*
Cingulate gyrus, *42*
Cingulate sulcus, *39, 40*
Cingulum, 186
Circadian rhythm, hypothalamic regulation of, 213
Circle of Willis, *238*, 246–247
Circumferential arteries, *244*
Circumventricular organs, 211
Cisterna magna, 253, *254*, 255
Clasp-knife response, in upper motor neuron syndrome, 66–67, *68*
Clonus, in upper motor neuron syndrome, 67, *69*
Cochlea, 168, *170*
Cochlear nerve, 169, *172*. *See also* Vestibulocochlear nerve
Cognition, basal ganglia in, 96
Cogwheel rigidity, in basal ganglia disease, 90–91
Colliculus
  facial, 26, 27, 50, *51*
  inferior, 169, *170, 171, 172*
    lesions of, 283, *284*

superior, 125
   lesions of, 283, *286*
      fibers, 188
Commissural syndrome, 136, *140, 147, 261*
Commissure, anterior, *186, 187,* 188
Communicating artery
   anterior, *237, 238, 239,* 240
   posterior, *237,* 238, *238*
Communicating hydrocephalus, 257
Conduction aphasia, 199
Conduction deafness, 170
Cones, 153, *154*
Consensual light reflex, 159–160, *161*
Conus medullaris, *16*
Cordotomy, anterolateral, 136, 149
Corneal reflex, 145
Corona radiata, 61, *62, 63*
Coronary arteries, innervation of, 221*t,* 228, *228*
Corpus callosum, *186, 187*
Corpus striatum, 83–84, *84*
   horizontal sections through, *86*
   lateral view of, *84, 85*
   medial view of, *85*
Cortex
   auditory, 169, 170, 173
   cerebellar, 102, *102,* 103
   cerebral, 183–185
   gustatory, 176, *176,* 194
   motor (MI), 90, *104,* 106, 190
   orbitofrontal, 180, 207
   prefrontal, 191
   premotor, *88,* 190
   somatosensory (SI), *133, 134,* 134, *137, 138,* 138,
      145, 147, 194
   striate (see visual)
   visual, 157, *158,* 158, 159, *160, 163,* 195
Corticonuclear tract, *62, 63, 65,* 65–66
Cranial accessory nerve (XI), *26, 28,* 53, *53*
   lesions of, *294,* 294*t,* 297*t*
Cranial nerve(s), *287*
   I (olfactory), lesions of, *288,* 288*t,* 295*t*
   II (optic), lesions of, 160, 161, *288,* 288*t,* 295*t*
   III (oculomotor), 46, 49, *49*
      lesions of, *28,* 49, *49, 262–263,* 285, *286, 289,*
      289*t,* 295*t*
   IV (trochlear), 27, *28,* 49, 50, 50–52, *51*
      lesions of, 49, *50,* 289, 289*t,* 295*t*
   V (trigeminal), *28,* 50, *51,* 141–142, *142, 143, 144–*
      145
      lesions of, 50, *51, 264,* 290, 290*t,* 295*t*
      somatosensory pathways from, 141–142, *142,*
      143, 144–145
   VI (abducent), *26, 28,* 50–52, *51*
      lesions of, 50, *51, 262–263,* 289, 289*t,* 295*t*
   VII (facial), *26, 28,* 52, *53*

      lesions of, *52, 52, 264, 291,* 291*t,* 296*t*
   VIII (vestibulocochlear), *26, 28,* 73–74, *74, 75*
      lesions of, *288,* 288*t,* 296*t*
   IX (glossopharyngeal), *26, 28,* 53, *53*
      lesions of, *292,* 292*t,* 296*t*
   X (vagus), *26, 28,* 53, *53*
      lesions of, *264,* 293, 293*t,* 297*t*
   XI (accessory), *26, 28,* 53, *53*
      lesions of, *294,* 294*t,* 297*t*
   XII (hypoglossal), *26, 28,* 53, *54*
      lesions of, 53, *54, 262–263, 294,* 294*t,* 297*t*
Craniopharyngioma, of hypothalamus, 279, *281*
Crural cistern, 254, *254*
Cuneate nucleus, 110, *327*
Cuneate tract, 132, *133*
Cuneus, 195, *196*

D
Deafness, 170
Decorticate posturing, 76–77, *76, 77*
Deiters nucleus, 74
Dendrites, 2, *3, 4,* 4*t,* *5*
   vs. axons, 4*t*
Dentate gyrus, 201, *202*
Dentate ligament, *15,* 17
Dentate nucleus, *101, 103,* 106, *328, 329*
Dermatomes, 129, *130–131*
Diabetes insipidus, 212
Diaphragma sellae, *8, 9*
Diencephalon, 35–38, *36, 37*
   epithalamus of, *37,* 38
   hypothalamus of, *37,* 38
   subthalamus of, 38
   thalamus of, 36–37, *37, 38*
Direct light reflex, 159–160, *161*
Directional terms, for central nervous system, 35, *36*
Doll's eye movement, 118
Dopamine
   deficiency of, in Parkinson disease, 92, 94–96, *95*
   in hypokinetic disorders, 94–96, *95*
Dorsal rhizotomy, 136
Dorsal root entry zone, 136
Dorsal root ganglion, *15*
Down syndrome, 183
Dura mater, *8, 9, 10, 15, 16,* 17
Dural fold (falx cerebri), *8, 9*
Dural sac, *16,* 17
Dural sinuses, 17
Dysdiadochokinesia, 108
Dyskinesia
   in basal ganglia disease, 90, 91
   tardive, 93
Dysmetria, 108
Dysphagia, 53
Dystonia, in basal ganglia disease, 90

E

Ear, 167–169, *168*
  bony labyrinth of, 73
  membranous labyrinth of, 73
Eating, hypothalamic regulation of, 213
Edema
  cerebral, 236
  optic disc, 155
Efferent signals, 2
Emotion, hypothalamus in, 214
Epidural space, 9, *10*
Epithalamus, 37, *38*
Esotropia, 50, *51*
Expressive aphasia, *192*, 198
External ear, 167, *168*
Extrafusal muscle fibers, 45, *47*, 57, *57*, *58*
Extraocular muscles, 117, *118*
Eyes. *See also* Ocular motor system
  abnormalities of
    abducent nerve lesions and, *51*, 52, *124*
    oculomotor nerve lesion and, *49*, *124*
    trochlear nerve lesion and, 49, *50*
  conjugate deviation of, 123, *124*

F

Facial nerve (VII), *26*, *28*, 52, *53*
  lesions of, 52, *52*, 167, *264*, 291, 291t, 295t, 296t
Facial nucleus, *48*, 52, *53*, 330
Falx cerebelli, *8*, 9
Falx cerebri, *8*, 9
Fasciculus
  arcuate, *185*, 186, *198*, 199
  dorsolateral, 136, *138*, *139*
  medial, longitudinal, 75, *75*, *112*, 113, *119*, *120*, *121*, 122, *123*, *124*
  superior, *185*, 186, 199
  uncinate, *185*, 186, 205, *206*
Fasciculus retroflexus, 207
Fastigial nucleus, *101*, *103*, 106, *328*, *329*
Filum terminale, *16*, 17
Fissure (sulcus) of Rolando, 39
Fissure (sulcus) of Sylvius, 38–39
Fixation point, of vision, 159
Flocculonodular lobe syndrome, 113–114, *113*
Fluent aphasia, *192*, 198–199
Folium, of cerebellum, 102, *102*
Foramen of Magendie, 253
Foramina of Luschka, 253
Foramina of Monro, 35
Forebrain, *24*, 35–42. *See also* Cerebral hemisphere(s); Diencephalon
  coronal section of, *337*, *338*
  directional terminology for, 35, *36*
  functional levels of, 40–42, *41*
    horizontal section of, *339*
    lesions of, 35
    mamillary level of, 40–42, *41*
    posterior thalamic level of, 40, *41*
    tuberal level of, 42, *42*
Forebrain bundle, medial, 207
Fornix, 42, *42*, 201, *203*, 204
Fovea centralis, 155
Foveola, 155
Frontal association cortex, 191–192, *191*, *196*
Frontal eye field, 190, *191–192*
Frontal horns, of lateral ventricle, 251, *252*
Frontal lobe, 190–194, *191–192*, 193t, *196–197*
  lesions of, *192*, 193t
Functional path, 1, *2*

G

Gait ataxia, 111, *111*
Gamma aminobutyric acid (GABA), of basal ganglia, 93–94, *93*
Geniculate nucleus, *38*, *156*, 157, *157*, 169, *170*, *171*, *172*, 335
Glial cells, 5–9, *6*, *7*
Globus pallidus, *41*, *42*
Glomus, of lateral ventricle, 252
Glossopharyngeal nerve (IX), *26*, *28*, 53, *53*
  lesions of, 292, 292t, 293t, 296t
Glutamate, of basal ganglia, 93–94, *93*
Golgi neurons, *102*
Golgi tendon organs, 57–58, *58*
Gracile tract, 132, *133*
Granule cells, 106
  of cerebellar cortex, 102, *102*
  of cerebral cortex, 183, *184*
Graphesthesia, 127
Great vein of Galen, 249
Gustatory cortex, *191–192*, 194
Gustatory nucleus, 175, *176*, *177*, *178*
Gustatory system, 175–176
  pathway of, 175–176, *176*, *177*, *178*
  receptors of, 175, *176*
Gyrus(i)
  angular, *191*, 194
  cingulate, 201, *202*, *203*, 204
  dentate, *202*
  frontal
    inferior, *191*, 194, 198, *198*
    middle, 190, *191*
    superior, 190, *191*
  lingual, 195
  parahippocampal, 201, *202*, *203*, *206*
  paraterminal, *202*, 207
  postcentral, 39, *39*, *191*, 194
  precentral, 39, *39*, 190, *191*
  supramarginal, *191*, 194

temporal
  middle, *191*
  superior, *191*, 195, 198, *198*
  transverse temporal (of Heschl), 195

H
Habenula, *41*
Habenulointerpeduncular tract, 207
Hair cells, 168–169, *171*
Handedness, 195–197
Head
  movement of, 73
  sensations from, 141–142, *142*
Hearing. *See also* Auditory system
  abnormal loudness of, 52
Hearing loss, 170, 173
Heart, innervation of, 221*t*, 227–228, *228*
Hemianesthesia, contralateral, *147*, 148
Hemianopsia, bitemporal, 159, *160*
Hemiballismus, contralateral, 92–93
Hemiplegia, spastic, in upper motor neuron syn-
    drome, 66, *68*
Hemisection, of spinal cord, 71, 271, *273*
Heteronymous anopsia, 159, *160*
Heubner, recurrent artery of, *239*, 239–240
Hindbrain, 251
Hippocampal formation, 183
  connections of, 201, *203*, 204
  function of, 204, *205*
Homonymous anopsia, 159, *160*
Horizontal cells, *154*, 155
Horner syndrome, 162, 275, *277*
Huntington disease, 92, *92*
Hydrocephalus, 253, 256–257
Hyperacusis, 167
Hypercarbia, 235–236
Hyperkinesia, in basal ganglia disorders, 94, *94*,
    95
Hyperthermia, hypothalamic lesions and, 213
Hypertonia, in upper motor neuron syndrome, 66, *68*
Hypoglossal hemiplegia syndrome, alternating, 70
Hypoglossal nerve (XII), *26*, *28*, 53, *54*
  lesions of, 53, *54*, 262–263, 294, 294*t*, 297*t*
Hypoglossal nucleus, *48*, 53, *54*
Hypoglossal palsy, 263
Hypokinesia, in basal ganglia disorders, 94–96, *95*
Hypophysial arteries, superior, 238, *239*
Hypophysial portal system, *211*, 212
Hypothalamic sulcus, *42*
Hypothalamic syndrome, 212
Hypothalamus, *37*, *38*, 209–214
  connections of, *206*, 209, 211–214, *211*
  functions of, 212–214, 213*t*
  humoral input to, 211
  humoral output of, 212

  input to, 209, 211, *211*
  lesions of, 212–214, 279, *281*
  nuclei of, 209, *210*, *211*, 213*t*
  output from, *211*, 212
  subdivisions of, 209, *210*
  zones of, 209, *210*, *211*
Hypoxia, 235

I
Ia afferent fibers, 57, *57*
Ib afferent fibers, 58, *58*
Incus, 167, *168*
Inferior alternating hemiplegia, 70
Infranuclear lesion, 66. *See also* Lower motor neu-
    ron syndrome
Intention tremor, 107–108, *107*, 265
Internal capsule, 40, *41*, 188, *189*, 190
  lesions of, *266*, 271, *272*
  vascular accident in, 66–70, *68*, *69*, *70*
Internal ear, 167, *168*
Internuclear ophthalmoplegia, 122
Interpeduncular cistern, 254, *254*, *255*
Interpeduncular fossa, 25
Interposed nucleus, *101*, *103*, 106
Intervertebral disc, *16*
Intervertebral foramen, *15*
Intracranial pressure, 257
Intrafusal muscle fibers, 58–59, *58*
Intraventricular foramen of Monro, 252
Iodopsin, 155
Iris, innervation of, 221*t*
Ischemia, cerebral, 66–70, *68*, *69*, *70*, 237

J
Juxtarestiform body, 74, *75*, *329*

K
Kernicterus, 236
Kinocilium, 117
Klüver-Bucy syndrome, *205*, 207
Korsakoff syndrome, 204, *205*

L
Labyrinth, 73, *74*, 167–168, *168*
Lamina terminalis cistern, 254, *254*, *255*
Laminae, of spinal cord, *18*, *19*
Language
  cortical representation of, *192*, 197–199, *198*
  hemispheric lateralization of, 195–197
  pathway of, 199
Lateral lemniscus, 169
  nuclei of, 170, *170*, *171*, *172*
Lateral ventricles, *41*, *42*, 251–252, *252*
Lateralization, hemispheric, 195–197
Lead-pipe rigidity, 275

in basal ganglia disease, 90
Lemniscus
    lateral, 169, 170, *170, 171, 172*
    medial, 132, *133, 134, 135*
Lentiform nucleus, 83, *85, 86*
Light reflex, 159–160, *161*
Light touch, 127
Limbic system, 149, 201–207
    amygdaloid nucleus of, 205–207
        connections of, 205, *206*
        functions of, 205, 207
    hippocampal formation of, 201–204, *202, 203*
        connections of, 201, *203, 204*
        function of, 204, *205*
    lesions of, 204, *205*, 207
    limbic lobe of, 201, *202*
    septal region of, 207
Lobotomy, prefrontal, 193
Lobule
    inferior parietal, *191*, 194
    paracentral, *40*, 61, *62, 63*, 134, *134*, 138, *138*,
        190, 194, *196*
    superior parietal, *191*, 194
Longitudinal fasciculus (MLF)
    medial, 75, *75, 112*, 113, *119, 120, 121*, 122, *123,
        124*
    superior, *185*, 186, 199
γ-Loop, 58–59, *58*
Loop of Meyer, 157, *158*
Lower motor neuron syndrome, 55, *56*, 59, 67t
    upper motor neuron lesions with, 70–71
Lower motor neurons, 45–59, *46*, 78, 79–80
    brainstem, 46–54, *48*. *See also* Cranial nerve(s)
    lesions of, 45, *55, 56*, 59, 67t
    spinal cord, 54, *55, 56*, 57t
        γ-loop of, 58–59, *58*
        reflex activity of, 57–59, *57*, 57t, *58*
Lumbar puncture, *16*, 17, 255–256
Lung carcinoma, cerebellar metastases from, 271, *274*

M
Macula, of utricle, 73, *74*
Macula lutea, 155
Malleus, 167, *168*
Mamillary bodies, *37*, 38, *41, 203*, 204, *205*
Mandibular nerve, 50, *51*
Mastication, abnormalities of, cranial nerve lesions
        and, 50, *51*
Mechanoreceptors, 110, 128, 129t
Medial forebrain bundle, 207, 211
Medulla
    anatomy of, 23, *24*
    caudal part of, 29, *30*
    lesions of, 275, 277
    rostral part of, 29, *29, 30*

topography of, 25, *26, 27*
transverse sections of, 29, *29, 30, 327, 328*
Medulloblastoma, 114
Melanin, of substantia nigra, 84
Membranous labyrinth, *74*, 167–168, *168*
Meningeal spaces, 9–10, *10*
Meninges, spinal, 15–17, *15*
Micturition, 230
Midbrain
    anatomy of, *24*, 25
    caudal part of, 31, 33, *33*
    coronal section of, *336*
    lesions of, *266*, 275, *276*
    rostral part of, 33, *33*
    topography of, 25, 27
    transverse sections of, 31, 33, *33, 87, 333, 334, 335*
Middle alternating hemiplegia, 70
Middle cerebral artery, *237, 239*, 241–242, *241*
Middle ear, 167, *168*
Midpons, transverse section of, *331*
Motion sense, 128
α-Motoneurons, 45, 78, 79–80. *See also* Lower mo-
        tor neurons
Motor aphasia, *192*, 198
Motor cortex. *See also* Pyramidal system
    primary, 190, *191–192, 196–197*
    supplementary, 190, *196*
Motor end-plate (myoneural junction), 45, *47*
γ-Motor neurons, 46, 58–59, *58*
Motor system, 45, *46, 47*. *See also specific compo-
        nents*
Motor unit, 45–46, *47*
Müller cells, *154*, 155
Multiple sclerosis, 283, *284*
Muscle(s)
    extraocular, 117, *118*, 118t
    innervation of, 45–46, *47*, 54, 57t
    intrafusal fibers of, 58–59, *58*
    inverse myotatic reflex of, 57–58, *58*
    myotatic reflex of, 57, *57*, 57t
    neuronal control of, 79–80
Muscle spindles, 46
Mydriasis, 49, *49*
Myelin sheath, 5, 7, *7*
Myotatic reflex, 57, *57*, 57t
    inverse, 57–58, *58*
Myotome, 54

N
Neglect syndrome, 194
Neocerebellar syndrome, 107–108, *107*
Neocerebellum, 99, *100*
Neospinothalamic system, 136–140, *137, 138, 139,
        140*
Nerve deafness, 170

Nervous system, 1–2, *2*
Neurinoma, acoustic, 169, 267, *270*
Neurogenic bladder, 230, *231*
Neurolemma, 7, *7*
Neuron(s), 1, 2, *3, 4*
  bipolar, 2, *4*
  multipolar, 2, *4*
  of neocortex, 184–186, *184, 185*
  propriospinal system of, 78–79, *78*
  Purkinje, 102, *102,* 106
  of spinal cord, *18,* 19
  unipolar, 2, *4*
Neurotransmitters, 5
  of basal ganglia, 93–94, *93*
Nissl bodies, 2, *3*
Nociceptors, 128, 129*t. See also* Pain
Node of Ranvier, *3,* 7, *7*
Nonfluent aphasia, *192,* 198
Nonreflex neurogenic bladder, 230, *231*
Nuclear lesion. *See also* Lower motor neuron syn-
    drome
Nucleus (nuclei)
  abducent, *48,* 50–52, *51, 330*
  ambiguus, *48, 53, 53, 328, 329*
  amygdaloid, *85, 86,* 205–207, *206, 337, 338*
  basal, *338*
  brainstem, 46–54, *48*
  caudate, *41, 42,* 83, *84, 85, 336, 337, 338, 339*
  centromedian, *38, 336*
  cerebellar, *101, 103,* 106, *328, 329*
  of Clarke, 110, *325*
  cochlear, 169, *328*
  of corpus striatum, 83–84, *84, 85, 86*
  cuneate, 110, *327*
  Deiters, 74
  dentate, *101, 103,* 106, *328, 329*
  facial, *48,* 52, *53, 330*
  fastigial, *101, 103,* 106, *328, 329*
  geniculate, 37, 38, *335*
    lateral, *156,* 157, *157,* 158, 202
    medial, 169, 170, 171, 172
  gracile, *327*
  gustatory, 175, *176, 177, 178*
  hypoglossal, *48,* 53, *54*
  hypothalamic, 209, *210, 211,* 213*t*
  intermediolateral, *325*
  interpeduncular, *336*
  interposed, *101, 103,* 106
  of lateral lemniscus, 170, *170, 171, 172*
  lentiform, 83, *85, 86*
  motor, 73–76, *74, 75, 324, 325, 326*
  oculomotor, 46, *48,* 49, *49, 334, 335*
  olivary, 170, *170, 171, 172*
    inferior, *327, 328, 329*
    superior, *330*

  Onuf, 54
  phrenic, 54
  pontine, *330, 331, 332*
  red, 75–76, *76, 334, 336*
  reticular, *38,* 75, *336*
  salivatory, 218
  sensory, *325, 326*
  solitary, 222, 224, *224, 328*
  spinal, *18,* 19, 54, *326, 327, 328, 329, 330*
  subthalamic, 84, *86,* 92–94, *94, 95, 337*
  thalamic, 37, *38, 41, 42,* 89, 90, *336, 338*
  trigeminal, *48,* 50, *51, 331, 332*
  trochlear, *48,* 49, *50, 333*
  vagal, dorsal, *328*
  vestibular, 73–75, *74, 75,* 118–122, *120, 121, 328,
      329, 330*
Nucleus ambiguus, *48,* 53, *53, 328, 329*
Nystagmus, 119
  optokinetic, 125

O
Obstructive hydrocephalus, 257
Occipital eye field, *124,* 125
Occipital horn, of lateral ventricle, 252, *252*
Occipital lobe, 193*t,* 195, *196–197*
  lesions of, 193*t, 197*
Occipitofrontal fasciculus, 188
Ocular motor system, 66, 117–125
  brainstem gaze centers of, 122, *123*
  conjugate movements of, 122
  cortical gaze centers of, 122–125, *124*
  nuclei of, 117, 118, *118,* 118*t,* 119, *120*
  occipital eye field of, *124,* 125
  superior colliculus of, 125
  vergence movements of, 122
  vestibulo-ocular reflex of, 117–122, *119, 120, 121*
  voluntary movements of, 122
Oculocephalic reflex, 118
Oculomotor hemiplegia, alternating, 70
Oculomotor nerve (III), 26, 46, 49, *49*
  lesions of, 285, *286,* 289, 289*t,* 295*t*
Oculomotor nucleus, 46, *48,* 49, *49, 334, 335*
Oculomotor palsy, 49, *263*
Olfactory bulb, 179, *180*
Olfactory hallucinations, 180
Olfactory nerve (I), *288,* 288*t,* 295*t*
Olfactory receptors, 177, 179, *179*
Olfactory system, 177, 179–180, *179, 180*
  lesions of, 179, 180
  pathways of, 179–180, *179, 180*
  receptors of, 177, 179, *179*
Olfactory trigone, 180, *180*
Oligodendrocytes, *6,* 7
Olivary complex, lesions of, 113
Olivary nucleus, 170, *170, 171, 172*

Olivocerebellar degeneration, 114
Onuf nucleus, 54
Operculum, parietal, 176
Ophthalmic artery, 238, *238*
Ophthalmoplegia, 49, *49*
Optic chiasm, 156, *156*
  lesions of, 159, *160*
Optic disc, 155
Optic nerve (II), lesions of, 160, 161, *288, 288t,*
  295t
Optic tract, *156*, 157
Optokinetic nystagmus, 125
Otoconia, 73
Otolith, 73
Otolithic membrane, 73, *74*
Oval window, 168, *168*
Oxytocin, 212

P
Pain, 128
  cranial pathways of, 145–147, *146*
    first order neurons of, 145, *146*
    lesions of, 147–148, *147*
    second order neurons of, 145
    third order neurons of, 147
  endogenous modulation of, 151
  exogenous modulation of, 151
  fast, 128, *149t*
  modulation of, 150–151, *150*
  referred, 225–226, *225, 226*
  slow, 128, *149t*
    modulation of, 150–151, *150*
    pathways of, 148–150, *148, 149t*
  spinal pathways of, 136–140, *137, 138*
    first order neurons of, 136, *138, 139*
    lesions of, 140–141, *141,* 147–148, *147*
    second order neurons of, 136, *140*
    third order neurons of, 136, 138
  visceral, 224
Paleocerebellum, 99, *100*
Paleospinothalamic system, 136
Pallidum, 83–85, *87,* 89–90, *89*
Palsy
  Bell, 52
  oculomotor, 49
Papez circuit, 201, *203,* 204
Papilledema, 155
Parahippocampal gyrus, 201, *202*
Paralysis
  flaccid, 70
  of tongue, 53
  in upper motor neuron syndrome, 66
  of vocal muscles, 53
Paralysis agitans, 91–92, *91*
Paramedian arteries, *244*

Paramedian pontine reticular formation, 122, *123*
Paraplegia, post-traumatic, 71
Parastriate cortex, 195
Parasympathetic autonomic system, 217–219, *218,*
  218t, 219, 221t
Parietal association area, *191–192,* 194, *196*
Parietal lobe, *191–192,* 193t, 194, *196–197*
  lesions of, *192,* 193t, 283, *285*
Parietal operculum, 176
Parieto-occipital sulcus, 39, *40*
Parkinson disease, 91–92, *91,* 94–96, *95,* 275, *276*
Parotid gland, innervation of, 221t
Patellar reflex, in upper motor neuron syndrome,
  67, *69*
Peduncles
  cerebellar, 99, *101,* 102, 283, *284, 329*
  cerebral, *41*
Perforating arteries, 246–247, *247*
Pericallosal trunk artery, 240, *240*
Peripheral nervous system, 1–2
Photopic vision, 153
Photoreceptors, 153, *154,* 155
Phrenic nucleus, 54
Pia mater, *8, 9,* 15, *15,* 17
Pituitary gland, hypothalamic regulation of, 212
Plantar response, in upper motor neuron syndrome,
  67, 70
Poikilothermy, hypothalamic lesions and, 213
Poliomyelitis, spinal cord lesions in, 267, *268*
Pons
  anatomy of, 23, *24, 25*
  caudal part of, 31, *31*
  lesions of, 267, *269*
  middle part of, 31, *32*
  rostral part of, 31, *32*
    lesions of, *265*
  topography of, 25
  transverse sections of, 31, *31, 32, 330, 331, 332*
Pontomedullary cistern, 253, *254*
Pontomedullary junction, transverse section of, *329*
Position sense, 128
Posterior cerebral artery, 244, 245, *245*
Posterior choroidal artery, *244*
Posterior communicating artery, 237, 238, *238*
Posterior lobe syndrome, 107–108, *107*
Posterior median sulcus, of spinal cord, 18, *18*
Prefrontal cortex, 191–194, *191, 196*
  lesions of, 193–194
Prefrontal lobotomy, 193
Premedullary cistern, *255*
Prepontine cistern, *255*
Pressure sense, 127–128
Projection fibers, 188
Propriospinal neurons, 78–79, *78*
Ptosis, 49, *49*

Pupillary dilation reflex, 161–162, *162*
Pupillary light reflex, 159–160, *161*
Purkinje neurons, 102, *102*, 106
Putamen, *41, 42*
Pyramidal system, 61–71
    corticobulbar (corticonuclear) tract of, *62, 63,*
        65–66, *65*
    lesions of, 61, 66–71, 67*t. See also* Upper motor
        neuron syndrome
    pyramidal (corticospinal) tract of, 61–65, *62, 63,*
        64
Pyramidal tract, 61–65, *62, 63, 64*
    postcapsular lesion recovery of, 78–80, *78*

Q
Quadrigeminal artery, *244*
Quadrigeminal cistern, 253–254, *254, 255*

R
Rage attacks, 214
Receptive aphasia, *192*, 198–199
Receptors
    auditory, 168–169, *171*
    gustatory, 175, *176*
    olfactory, 177, 179, *179*
    somatosensory, 128, 129*t*
    visual, 153, *154*, 155
Recurrent artery of Heubner, 239–240, *239*
Red nucleus, 75–76, *76, 334, 336*
Referred pain, 225–226, *225, 226*
Reflex(es)
    accommodation, 163–164, *163*
    corneal, 145
    light, 159–160, *161*
    myotatic, 57, *57,* 57*t*
        inverse, 57–58, *58*
    oculocephalic, 118
    patellar, 67, *69*
    pupillary, 161–162, *162*
    spinal, 57–59, *57,* 57*t, 58*
    vestibulo-ocular, 117, 118–119, *121*
Reflex circuit, 1, *2*
Reflex neurogenic bladder, 230, *231*
Reissner membrane, 168
Relay circuit, 1, *2*
Reproductive system
    hypothalamic regulation of, 213
    innervation of, 221*t*, 230–232
Restiform body, *329*
Reticular formation, of brainstem, 27, *28*, 75
Retina, 153–156, *154*
    embryology of, 156
    visual pathway of, 156–158, *156, 157, 158*
Rhinencephalon, 176
Rhodopsin, 155

Rigidity, in basal ganglia disease, 90
Rinne tuning fork test, 173
Rods, 153, *154*, 155
Romberg sign, 128
Round window, 168, *168*

S
Saccade, 122
Saccule, 73, *74*
Sacral sparing, in spinal cord trauma, 71
Salivatory nucleus, 218
Schwann cells, 7, *7, 9*
Scotopic vision, 153
Senile dementia, 204
Sensory aphasia, *192*, 198–199
Septal region, of limbic system, *202*, 207
Septum pellucidum, *42*
Sheath of Schwann, 7, *7*
Sleep, hypothalamic regulation of, 213
Small vessel disease, 271, *272*
Solitary nucleus, 222, 224, *224*
Somatosensory cortex, *191–192*, 194, *196–197*
Somatosensory receptors, 128, 129*t*
Somatosensory system, 127–151
    cranial pain pathways of, 145–147
        first order neurons of, 145, *146*
        second order neurons of, 145
        third order neurons of, 147
    cranial tactile pathways of, 142–145, *142, 143*
        first order neurons of, 143–144, *144–145*
        second order neurons of, 144
        third order neurons of, 145
    dermatomes of, 129, *130–131*
    lesions of, 147–148, *147*
    motion sense of, 128
    pain sense of, 128
    peripheral components of, 128–129, 129*t*
    position sense of, 128
    pressure sense of, 127–128
    slow pain pathways of, 148–151, *148*, 149*t, 150*
    somatosensory nerve fibers of, 129, 129*t*
    somatosensory receptors of, 128, 129*t*
    spinal pain pathways of, 136–140, *137, 138*, 141*t*
        first order neurons of, 136, *138, 139*
        lesions of, 140–141, *141*, 147–148, *147*
        paleospinothalamic neurons of, 148–150, *148*
        second order neurons of, 136, *140*
        spinoreticulothalamic neurons of, 148–150,
            148
        third order neurons of, 136, 138
    spinal tactile pathways of, 132–134, *133, 134,*
        135, 141*t*
        clinical significance of, 140, *140*, 141*t*
        lesions of, 140–141, *141*, 147–148, *147*
        second order neurons of, 132, *133, 134, 135*

Somatosensory system—*continued*
    third order neurons of, 132, 134, *134, 135*
    tactile sense of, 127
    temperature sense of, 128
    trigeminal sensory nuclei of, 141–142, *142*
    vibration sense of, 128
Spastic paresis, *263*
Spasticity, in upper motor neuron syndrome, 66, *68*
Speech
    cortical representation of, *192,* 197–199, *198*
    hemispheric lateralization of, 195–197
    pathway of, 199
    in posterior lobe syndrome, 108
Spinal artery (arteries)
    anterior, *238, 239,* 243, 248, *248*
    posterior, 248, *248*
Spinal cord, 13–21, *14*
    anterior horns of, *18,* 19
    anterior median fissure of, 17–18, *18*
    anterolateral cordotomy of, 136, 149
    arachnoid of, 15, *15,* 17
    cervical, *21, 326*
    cortical motor path of, *78,* 79, 80
    dura mater of, *9, 15,* 17
    dural sac of, *16,* 17
    gray matter of, 18–19, *18*
    gross anatomy of, 13–15, *14*
    hemisection of, *147, 261*
    intermediate zones of, *18,* 19
    laminae of, *18,* 19
    lateral horn of, *18,* 19
    lateral motor path of, *78,* 79, 80
    lesions of
        localization of, 259, *260, 261*
        in poliomyelitis, 267, *268*
        pyramidal tract, 70, 71
    lumbar, *20, 325*
    meninges of, 15–17, *15*
    α-motoneurons of, *78,* 79–80
    neurons of, *18,* 19
    nuclei of, *18,* 19, 54, *326, 327, 328, 329, 330*
    pia mater of, *9, 15, 15,* 17
    posterior horns of, *18,* 19
    posterior median sulcus of, 18, *18*
    propriospinal neurons of, 78–79, *78*
    pyramidal tracts of, lesions of, 70, 71
    regional differences of, 19–21, *20, 21*
    sacral, *20, 324*
    segments of, *14,* 15
    somatotopic organization of, 79–80
    supraspinal path of, *78,* 79
    thoracic, *21, 325*
    topography of, 17–18, *18*
    transection of, 71, *260*
    trauma to, 71

    vasculature of, 248, *248*
    veins of, 249
    ventromedial motor path of, *78,* 79, 80
    visceral afferent fibers to, 224
    white matter of, 18, *18*
Spinal nerves, *14, 15,* 17, *18*
Spinal shock, 71
Spinal veins, 249
Spinocerebellar tract, *109,* 110
Spinothalamic tract, 136, *137,* 138, 140, *140*
    lesion of, *265*
Spiral organ, 168–169, *171*
Splenium, *187,* 188
Split brain, 188
Stapedius muscle, 167, *168*
Stapes, 167, *168*
Stereocilia, 73, *74*
Stereognosis, 127
Stomach, innervation of, 221*t*
Stria medullaris, *41*
Striate arteries
    lateral, *238,* 247, *247*
    medial, 246–247, *247*
Stroke, 190, 241, 243
    capsular, 66–70, *68, 69, 70*
Subarachnoid cisterns, 253–255, *254*
Subarachnoid space, 9, *10, 15*
Subdural space, 9, *10*
Subiculum, 201, *202*
Substantia innominata, 204
Substantia nigra, *41,* 84, *87, 333, 337*
    lesions of, 275, *276*
Subthalamic nucleus, 84, *86, 337*
    in hyperkinetic disorders, 94, *94, 95*
    lesions of, 92–94
Subthalamus, 38
Superior alternating hemiplegia, 70
Superior colliculus, 125
Supplementary motor area, 190, *196*
Supranuclear lesion, 66. *See also* Upper motor neuron syndrome
Sylvian cistern, 254–255
Sylvius, cerebral aqueduct of, *24, 25,* 253
Sympathetic autonomic system, *218,* 218*t,* 219–221, *219, 220,* 221*t*
Sympathic shock syndrome, 231, 232
Synapse, 5
Syringomyelia, 136

T
Tabes dorsalis, 140, 164
Tachycardia, 228
Tardive dyskinesia, 93
Taste buds, 175, *176*
Taste sense, 175–176, *176, 177, 178*

Tegmentum, lesions of, *265*
Temperature, body, hypothalamic regulation of, 213
Temperature sense, 128, 136–140, *137, 138, 139, 140*
Temporal horn, of lateral ventricle, 252, *252*
Temporal lobe, *191–192,* 193t, *194–195*
    lesions of, 193t, 195
Temporal lobe epilepsy, 279, *280*
Tensor tympani muscle, 167, *168*
Tentorium cerebelli, *8,* 9
Thalamogeniculate arteries, 247
Thalamoperforate arteries, *238, 244,* 247, *247*
Thalamus, 36–37, *37*
    coronal section of, *336*
    nuclei of, 37, *38, 41, 42,* 176, *336, 337, 338*
Thermoreceptors, 128, 129t
Tic douloureux, 145
Tics, in basal ganglia disease, 91
Tongue, paralysis of, 53
Touch sense, 127, 132–135, *133, 134, 135*
Tract(s)
    corticobulbar (-nuclear), 62, *63,* 65, 65–66, 67t,
        189, 190
    corticospinal (see pyramidal)
        anterior (ventral), *62, 63,* 65
        lateral, *64,* 65, 78, 79, *140*
    central tegmental, 176
    cuneate, 132, *133, 134, 135, 140,* 141t
    dorsal spinocerebellar, *108, 109,* 110
    frontopontine, *104, 105*
    gracile, 132, *133, 134, 135, 140,* 141t, *229*
    habenulointerpeduncular, 207
        of Lissauer, 136, *138, 139,* 140
    mamillotegmental, *211,* 212
    mamillothalamic, *203, 204, 211,* 212
    mesencephalic of trigeminal, 141
    nigro-striatal, *88*
    olfactory, 179, *180,* 180
    optic, *156,* 157, *157, 158,* 159, *160, 161*
    parietotemporo-occipitopontine, *104, 105*
    pyramidal, 61–65, *62, 63, 64,* 67t, 70, 71, 80,
        93–95, 188, *189,* 190
        postcapsular lesion recovery of, 78–80, *78*
    reticulospinal
        lateral, 75, 79, 80
        medial, 75, 79, 80
    rubrobulbar, 76
    rubrospinal, 76
    solitary, 175, *176, 177, 178*
    spinal trigeminal, *142, 143,* 145, *146, 147,* 148
    spinothalamic, 136, *137, 138, 139,* 140, *140,* 141t,
        147, 148, 228, *229*
    striato-nigral, *88*
    trigeminothalamic, *142, 143, 144,* 145, *146, 147,*
        147
    tuberoinfundibular, 212

vestibulospinal
    lateral, *74,* 75, 79, 80
    medial, *74,* 75, 79, 80
Transcutaneous electrical nerve stimulation, 129
Tremor, intention, 107–108, *107,* 265
Trigeminal nerve (V), 26, *28,* 50, *51,* 141–142, *142,*
        143, 144–145
    lesions of, 50, *51, 290,* 290t, 295t
Trigeminal neuralgia, 145
Trigeminal nucleus
    mesencephalic, 141
    motor, *48,* 50, *51, 331*
    principal, 141, *142, 143, 144, 147, 331*
    spinal, 141, *142, 143,* 145, *146, 147, 327, 328,*
        329, 330
Trigeminothalamic tract, 145
Trigone, of lateral ventricle, 251–252, *252*
Trochlear nerve (IV), 26, *27,* 49, *50,* 50–52, *51*
    lesions of, *289,* 289t, 295t
Trochlear nucleus, *48,* 49, *50*
Truncal ataxia, 113–114, *113*
Tuber cinereum, *42*
Two-point sense, 127

U
Uncinate fasciculus, *185, 186,* 188
Uncinate fits, 180
Uncus, 176
    lesions of, 180
Uninhibited reflex bladder, 230, *231*
Upper motor neuron syndrome, 66–71, 67t
    capsular stroke in, 66–69, *68, 69, 70*
    lower motor neuron lesions with, 70–71
    spinal trauma in, 71
Utricle, 73, *74*

V
Vagus nerve (X), 26, *28,* 53, *53*
    lesions of, *264,* 293, 293t, 297t
Venous sinus, *8*
Ventral amygdaloid path, 205, *206,* 211, 214
Ventral anterior nucleus, *89,* 90
Ventricle(s)
    fourth, 26–27, 253
    lateral, *41, 42,* 251–252, *252*
    third, *24, 41,* 253
Vertebral arteries, 242–243, *242, 243*
Vertebral column, 13, *14*
Vestibular membrane, 168
Vestibular nuclei, 73–75, *74, 75,* 118–122, *120, 121,*
        328, 329, 330
Vestibulocerebellum, 99, *100*
Vestibulocochlear nerve (VIII), 26, *28,* 73–74, *74,*
        75
    lesions of, *288,* 288t, 296t

Vestibulo-ocular reflex, 117, 118–119, *121*
    receptors for, 117–118, *119*
Vibration sense, 128
Virchow-Robin space, 236
Viscera
    autonomic afferents of, *221t*, 222–224, *223*, *224*
    sensations of, 224
Visual cortex, 195, *196–197*
Visual fields, 158–159, *158*
    defects of, 159, *160*
Visual system, 153–164
    accommodation reflexes of, 163–164, *163*
    lesions of, 153, 158–164, *160*
    light reflex of, 159–160, *161*
    pupillary dilation reflex of, 161–162, *162*
    retina of, 153–156, *154*
    visual fields of, 158–159, *158*, *159*

    visual pathway of, 156–158, *156*, *157*, *158*
Vocal muscles, paralysis of, 53

W
Wallenberg syndrome, 275, *277*
Weber syndrome, 70
Weber tuning fork test, 173
Wernicke area, 197–199, *198*
Wernicke zone, 157, *157*

Z
Zona incerta, 84
Zone(s)
    dorsal root entry, 136
    of hypothalamus, 209
    of Wernicke, 157
    perforation for penetrating arteries, *239*